WHO REPORT 2005

Global Tuberculosis Control

Surveillance, Planning, Financing

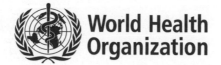

**World Health
Organization**

WHO Library Cataloguing-in-Publication Data

World Health Organization.
Global tuberculosis control : surveillance, planning, financing : WHO report 2005.

1.Tuberculosis, Pulmonary – prevention and control 2.Tuberculosis, Multidrug-resistant – drug therapy
4.Directly observed therapy 5.Treatment outcome 6.National health programs – organization and
administration 7.Financing, Health 7.Statistics I.Title.

ISBN 92 4 156291 9   (NLM classification: WF 300)   WHO/HTM/TB/2005.349

Suggested citation

Global tuberculosis control: surveillance, planning, financing. WHO report 2005. Geneva, World Health Organization
(WHO/HTM/TB/2005.349).

Designed by minimum graphics
Printed in Switzerland

Contents

Acknowledgements

The WHO Global TB Surveillance, Planning and Financing Project is coordinated by Christopher Dye, Léopold Blanc and Katherine Floyd. This year's report was written by Léopold Blanc, Daniel Bleed, Christopher Dye, Katherine Floyd, Giuliano Gargioni, Mehran Hosseini, Knut Lönnroth, Lindsay Martinez, Eva Nathanson, Andrea Pantoja, Amy Piatek, Alasdair Reid, Holger Sawert, Lisa Véron, Catherine Watt, Brian Williams and Abigail Wright.

The following WHO staff assisted in compiling, analysing and editing information:

WHO HQ Geneva: Mohamed Aziz, Karin Bergström, Bernadette Bourdin, Karen Ciceri, José Figueroa-Muñoz, Haileyesus Getahun, Malgosia Grzemska, Anne Guilloux, Ernesto Jaramillo, Fabienne Jouberton, Adalbert Laszlo, Pierre-Yves Norval, Paul Nunn, Salah Ottmani, Mario Raviglione, Krystina Ryszewska, Joanne Sheppard, Mukund Uplekar, Lana Velebit.

WHO African Region: Ayodele Awe (Nigeria), Oumou Bah-Sow (AFRO), Doulourou Coulibaly (AFRO), Jan van den Hombergh (Ethiopia), Joseph Imoko (Uganda), Bah Keita (AFRO, West Africa), Daniel Kibuga (AFRO), Robert Makombe (AFRO), Giampaolo Mezzabotta (Uganda), Vainess Mfungwe (AFRO), Wilfred Nkhoma (AFRO), Lisa Véron (AFRO), Henriette Wembanyama (DR Congo).

WHO Region of the Americas: Ademir Albuquerque (Brazil), Raimond Armengol (El Salvador), Marlene Francis (CAREC), Mirtha del Granado (AMRO), Juan Carlos Millan (Peru), Pilar Ramon-Pardo (AMRO), Rodolfo Rodriguez-Cruz (Brazil).

WHO Eastern Mediterranean Region: Aaiyad Al Dulaymi Munim (Somalia), Samiha Baghdadi (EMRO), Laura Gillini (Pakistan), Sevil Husseinova (Afghanistan), Keiko Inaba (Afghanistan), John Jabbour (EMRO), Akihiro Seita (EMRO), Emanuele Tacconi (Afghanistan).

WHO European Region: Irina Danilova (Russian Federation), Lucica Ditiu (TB Office Balkans), Wieslaw Jakubowiak (Russian Federation), Konstantin Malakhov (Russian Federation), Kestutis Miskinis (TB Office Ukraine), Andrey Mosneaga (Caucasus), Jerod Scholten (EURO), Gombogaram Tsogt (TB Office Central Asia), Richard Zaleskis (EURO).

WHO South-East Asia Region: Marijke Becx-Bleumink (Bangladesh), Erwin Cooreman (SEARO), Christian Gunneberg (Nepal), Asheena Khalakdina (SEARO), Hans Kluge (Myanmar), Franky Loprang (Indonesia), Davide Manissero (Indonesia), Firdosi Mehta (Indonesia), Nani Nair (SEARO), Myo Paing (Myanmar), Emanuele Pontali (SEARO), Suvanand Sahu (India), Fraser Wares (India).

WHO Western Pacific Region: Dongil Ahn (WPRO), Maarten Bosman (Viet Nam), Daniel Chin (China), Philippe Glaziou (WPRO), Pratap Jayavanth (Cambodia), Wang Lixia (China), Pieter van Maaren (WPRO), Michael Voniatis (Philippines).

The primary aim of this report is to share information from national TB control programmes. The data presented here are supplied largely by programme managers, who have been instrumental in driving much of the work on surveillance, planning and financing. We thank all of them, and their staff, for their contributions. The WHO TB Surveillance Project is carried out with the financial backing of USAID. The WHO DOTS Expansion Project is supported by funding from the governments of Australia, Belgium, Canada, Germany, Ireland, the Netherlands, Norway, Switzerland, the United Kingdom and USA. Data for the European Region were collected and validated jointly with EuroTB, a dedicated European TB surveillance network funded by the European Commission; we thank Andrea Infuso and Dennis Falzon of EuroTB for their collaboration. We also thank Pam Baillie, Kreena Govender, Sue Hobbs and Keith Wynn for doing everything necessary to get this report published earlier than ever before, and well in advance of 24 March, World TB Day.

Copies of *Global tuberculosis control* are available from the World Health Organization, 20 Avenue Appia, CH-1211 Geneva 27, Switzerland, and at www.who.int/tb.

Dedication
As this report went to press, we learnt of the tragic death of our colleague Lisa Véron. During her short period in Africa, Lisa contributed enormously to TB control in the region, and especially to the development of the financial monitoring project. We miss her greatly.

Abbreviations

ADB	Asian Development Bank
AFB	Acid fast bacilli
AFR	WHO African Region
AFRO	WHO Regional Office for Africa
AIDS	Acquired immunodeficiency syndrome
AMR	WHO Region of the Americas
AMRO	WHO Regional Office for the Americas
ART	Antiretroviral therapy
BPHS	Basic package of health-care services
BRAC	Bangladesh Rural Advancement Committee
CAREC	Caribbean Epidemiology Centre
CARE International	International relief and development organization
CB DOTS	Community-based DOTS
CCM	Country Coordinating Mechanism (Global Fund)
CDC	Centers for Disease Control and Prevention, Atlanta, GA, USA
CENAT	Centre National Anti-Tuberculeux
CI	Confidence interval
CIDA	Canadian International Development Agency
COOPI	Cooperazione Internazionale (Italian NGO)
COMBI	Communication for behavioural impact
DANIDA	Danish International Development Agency
DCPP	Disease Control Priorities Project
DDC	Department of Disease Control
DEWG	DOTS Expansion Working Group of the Stop TB Partnership
DFB	Damien Foundation Belgium
DFID	UK Department for International Development
DHT	District health team
DoH	Department of Health
DOT	Directly observed treatment
DOTS	The internationally recommended strategy for TB control
DRS	Drug Resistance Surveillance
DST	Drug susceptibility testing
DTC	District TB coordinator
DRS	Drug resistance surveillance
EMR	WHO Eastern Mediterranean Region
EMRO	WHO Regional Office for the Eastern Mediterranean
EQA	External quality assurance
EU	European Union
EUR	WHO European Region
EURO	WHO Regional Office for Europe
FCT	Federal Capital Territory
FDC	Fixed-dose combination (or FDC anti-TB drug)
FIDELIS	Fund for Innovative DOTS Expansion, managed by IUATLD
GDF	Global TB Drug Facility
GFATM	Global Fund to Fight AIDS, Tuberculosis and Malaria
GLC	Green Light Committee
GLRA	German Leprosy and TB Relief Association
GMS	German Medical Service
GNI	Gross national income
GTZ	Deutsche Gesellschaft für Technische Zusammenarbeit (German development agency)
HBC	High-burden country of which there are 22 that account for approximately 80% of all new TB cases arising each year
HIV	Human immunodeficiency virus
HR	Human resource
HRD	Human resource development
HRDP	Human resource development plan
HSD	Health subdistrict
HSSP	Health Sector Strategic Plan
IEC	Information, education, communication
IFRC	International Federation of Red Cross and Red Crescent Societies
IRR	Incidence rate ratio
ISAC	Intensified support and action in countries, an emergency initiative to reach targets for DOTS implementation by 2005
IUATLD	International Union Against Tuberculosis and Lung Disease
JICA	Japan International Cooperation Agency
KIT	Royal Tropical Institute (Netherlands)
KNCV	Royal Netherlands Tuberculosis Association
LEPCO	Tuberculosis and Leprosy Control (German NGO)
LGA	Local government area
MDG	Millennium Development Goal
MDR	Multidrug resistance
MDR-TB	Multidrug-resistant tuberculosis
MEDAIR	An international humanitarian aid organization
MoH	Ministry of Health
MoPH	Ministry of Public Health
MSF	Médecins Sans Frontières
MSH	Management Sciences for Health
NGO	Nongovernmental organization
NHLS	National Health Laboratory Services
NICC	National interagency coordinating committee
NLR	Netherlands Leprosy Relief
NPO	National programme officer (WHO-appointed)
NRL	National reference laboratory
NTI	National TB institute
NTP	National tuberculosis control programme

PAHO	Pan-American Health Organization	TB	Tuberculosis
PAL	Practical Approach to Lung Health	TBCTA	Tuberculosis Coalition for Technical Assistance
PATH	International health NGO that focuses on advancing technologies, strengthening systems and encouraging healthy behaviour	UNAIDS	Joint United Nations Programme on HIV/AIDS
		UNDP	United Nations Development Programme
PHC	Primary health care	USAID	United States Agency for International Development
PHilCAT	Philippines Coalition against TB		
PLWHA	People living with HIV/AIDS	USTP	Uganda Stop TB Partnership
PPM	Public–private or public–public mix	VCT	Voluntary counselling and testing for HIV infection
PPP	Purchasing power parity		
RIT	Research Institute of Tuberculosis, Japan Anti-Tuberculosis Association	WHO	World Health Organization
		WHO-CHOICE	Choosing interventions that are cost-effective, a WHO project
SARS	Severe acute respiratory syndrome		
SEAR	WHO South-East Asia Region	WPR	WHO Western Pacific Region
SEARO	WHO Regional Office for South-East Asia	WPRO	WHO Regional Office for the Western Pacific
STD	Sexually transmitted disease		
STI	Sexually transmitted infection	ZTLS	Zonal TB and leprosy supervisor
SVS	Secretary of health surveillance		

Summary

Background and methods

1. The 9th World Health Organization (WHO) annual report on surveillance, planning and financing for TB control includes data on case notifications and treatment outcomes from all national TB control programmes (NTPs) that have reported to WHO, together with an analysis of plans, budgets, expenditures and progress in DOTS expansion for 22 high-burden countries (HBCs).

2. Ten consecutive years of data (1994–2003) are now available to assess progress towards the Millennium Development Goals (MDGs) for TB control. The five MDG targets directly relevant to TB control are: by 2005, to detect 70% of new smear-positive cases and successfully treat 85% of these cases; by 2015, to have halted and begun to reverse incidence; between 1990 and 2015, to halve TB prevalence and deaths rates.

Improving case detection and treatment

3. A total of 199 countries reported to WHO on their strategies for TB control, and on TB case notifications and/or treatment outcomes.

4. Using surveillance and survey data to update estimates of incidence, we calculate that there were 8.8 million new cases of TB in 2003 (140/100 000 population), of which 3.9 million (62/100 000) were smear-positive and 674 000 (11/100 000) were infected with human immunodeficiency virus (HIV). There were 15.4 million prevalent cases (245/100 000), of which 6.9 million were smear-positive (109/100 000). An estimated 1.7 million people (28/100 000) died from TB in 2003, including those coinfected with HIV (229 000).

5. A total of 182 countries were implementing the DOTS strategy during 2003, two more countries than in 2002. By the end of 2003, 77% of the world's population lived in coun-

tries, or parts of countries, covered by DOTS. DOTS programmes notified 3.7 million new and relapse TB cases, of which 1.8 million were new smear-positive. In total, 17.1 million TB patients, and 8.6 million smear-positive patients, were treated in DOTS programmes between 1995 and 2003.

6. The 1.8 million smear-positive cases notified by DOTS programmes in 2003 represent a case detection rate of 45%. The increment in smear-positive cases notified under DOTS between 2002 and 2003 (324 000) was greater than ever before (the average annual increment from 1995–2000 was 134 000). The acceleration in notifications was more pronounced for all TB cases, which increased by 693 000 between 2002 and 2003, compared with the average annual increment of 270 000 in the interval 1995–2000.

7. While the number of TB cases reported by DOTS programmes appears to have been accelerating since 2000, the total number of TB cases reported to WHO (all forms from all sources) increased very little over the period 1995–2003 (average detection rate 42%). The number of smear-positive cases reported from all sources has been increasing (50% detection rate in 2003), but much more slowly than the increases reported under DOTS.

8. Of the additional smear-positive cases reported under DOTS in 2003, 63% were in just two countries: India and China. Among those individuals who are thought to have developed smear-positive TB in 2003, but were not detected by DOTS programmes, 67% were living in just eight countries: Bangladesh, China, Ethiopia, India, Indonesia, Nigeria, Pakistan and the Russian Federation.

9. As DOTS programmes have expanded geographically, the new smear-positive case detection rate within DOTS areas has remained roughly constant since 1995 (average 52%),

although there are signs of a slow increase in the HBCs, especially in Bangladesh, India, Myanmar and the Philippines.

10. The rate of treatment success in the 2002 DOTS cohort was 82% on average, unchanged since 2000. As in previous years, the treatment success rate was substantially below average in the WHO African Region (73%) and the WHO European Region (76%). Low treatment success rates in these two regions can be attributed, in part, to the complications of TB/HIV coinfection and drug resistance, respectively. Equally important, though, is the failure of DOTS programmes in these two regions to monitor the outcome of treatment for all patients.

11. Based on case reports and WHO-estimates, 22 countries had reached the targets for case detection and treatment success by the end of 2003. Viet Nam was still the only member of the current group of HBCs[1] among them, although Cambodia, Myanmar and the Philippines are within reach.

Epidemiological trends and DOTS impact

12. In 2003, the TB incidence rate was falling or stable in five out of six WHO regions, but growing at 1.0% per year globally. The exception is the African Region, where incidence has been rising more quickly in countries with higher HIV prevalence rates. In Eastern Europe the incidence rate increased during the 1990s, but peaked around 2001, and has since fallen. The rise in global incidence is slowing because HIV epidemics are slowing in Africa, but it is unclear when the global incidence rate will begin to decline.

13. We calculate that, as a consequence of DOTS expansion between 1990 and 2003, the global TB preva-

---

[1] Peru was excluded from the original group of high-burden countries, having met the targets and successfully reduced incidence.

lence rate fell from 309 to 245 per 100 000 (including HIV-positive TB patients), and by 5% between 2002 and 2003, even though incidence continued to rise. The global mortality rate peaked during the 1990s, and fell at 2.5% (including HIV-positive TB patients) or 3.5% per year (excluding HIV-positive TB patient) between 2002 and 2003. But for the strongly adverse trends in Africa, prevalence and death rates would be falling more quickly worldwide.

Planning and DOTS implementation

14. All HBCs have a strategic plan for DOTS expansion and, during 2005, many will begin a new planning cycle, ideally working towards the MDG target year of 2015. Although the health systems of many countries are still undergoing reform and restructuring, all HBCs except the Russian Federation and Thailand reported that TB control functions are fully integrated with essential national health services.

15. Among the obstacles to DOTS expansion, five are of overriding importance: shortages of trained staff; lack of political commitment; weak laboratory services; and inadequate management of multidrug-resistant TB (MDR-TB), and of TB in people infected with HIV. Concerning drug resistance, few countries have national policies for the diagnosis and treatment of MDR-TB; even in those that do, treatment commonly fails to meet acceptable standards. Concerning TB/HIV, NTPs reported that few TB patients are tested for HIV (3% of notified cases), still fewer are assessed for antiretroviral therapy (ART) and a very small fraction begin ART (1349 patients reported in 2003). The report discusses a wide range of remedial actions to overcome these constraints.

16. Intensified support and action in countries (ISAC) is a new initiative designed to catalyse and accelerate DOTS expansion towards 2005 targets. The goal of ISAC is to improve technical capacity so as to facilitate the spending of large grants from the Global Fund to Fight AIDS, Tuberculosis and Malaria (GFATM) and other

major donors. Participants in 2004 included China, India, Indonesia, Kenya, Pakistan, Romania, the Russian Federation and Uganda.

17. The increasing contributions of nongovernmental organizations (NGOs) and community groups are clear expressions of the growing commitment of civil society to TB control. The work of these groups puts patients at the centre of the DOTS strategy, and improves access to TB services in remote areas and among disadvantaged and marginalized populations.

18. Public–private and public–public mix (PPM) projects are showing a measurable impact on case detection in several Asian countries, and may prove to be a mechanism for expanding TB control services in African cities.

Financing DOTS expansion

19. Financial data were received from 134 out of 211 (64%) countries, up from 123 in 2003. Complete budget and expenditure data were provided by 70 and 69 countries, respectively. Data were received from all 22 HBCs, except South Africa.

20. There has been a big increase in NTP budgets and a big improvement in the funding available for TB control in the HBCs since 2002, with particularly large increases between 2003 and 2004. The NTP budgets reported for 2005 total US$ 741 million. The total estimated costs of TB control are projected to be US$ 1.3 billion in 2005, and available funding is US$ 1.2 billion. The large increase in available funding is almost entirely due to additional government funding in China, Indonesia and the Russian Federation, and to GFATM grants.

21. The countries with the largest NTP budgets in 2005 are China, India, Indonesia and the Russian Federation. When costs beyond those included in NTP budgets are also considered, China, India, the Russian Federation and South Africa account for US$ 946 million (73%) of the US$ 1.3 billion total. Eight HBCs have total costs of US$ 20–50 million in 2005; the rest are US$ 18 million or less.

22. Per patient treated, there is considerable variation in budgets for first-line drugs, in total NTP budgets and in total costs for each year 2002–2005. Among HBCs, the NTP budget per patient is lowest in India (US$ 34). Most countries have budgets in the range US$ 100–200 per patient, and costs in the region of US$ 150–300. The Russian Federation and South Africa are notable exceptions, with costs per patient treated above US$ 1000. Budgets per patient treated are generally stable or increasing, and as a consequence costs per patient treated are also generally stable or increasing.

23. In 2005, HBC governments are providing 62% of NTP budgets (including loans), the GFATM 15%, and grants from other sources 7%, leaving a gap equivalent to 16% of the reported budgets. HBC governments contribute more (79%) to total costs than to NTP budgets because they finance the general health services staff and infrastructure used for TB control. High average contributions to the financing of TB control by HBC governments conceal the fact that many HBCs rely extensively on grant funding.

24. Despite progress in securing additional funding, HBCs reported a funding gap of US$ 119 million in 2005. This is higher than the gaps reported for 2003 and 2004. The largest funding gaps are those reported by China, India, Pakistan, the Russian Federation and Zimbabwe (US$ 93 million, or 78% of the total gap). Proportional to budgets, the largest gaps are in Kenya, Nigeria, Pakistan, Uganda and Zimbabwe.

25. Planned activities are not in line with meeting the case detection target in 2005 in 12 countries. In addition, the budgets for collaborative TB/HIV activities and for second-line drugs to treat MDR-TB are currently small. This means that the gaps currently reported by NTPs could be regarded as underestimates, and that the total resources required for TB will be higher than US$ 1.3 billion in future.

26. Absorption capacity is a major issue for HBCs that have secured substantial amounts of additional funding. Expenditures were lower than available funding in 2003; it remains to be seen whether NTPs can effectively spend the extra money available in 2004 and 2005.

27. In financing terms, the HBCs fall into four categories: (a) four countries (India, Myanmar, the Philippines and Viet Nam) that have budgets consistent with reaching the 2005 targets, and which are likely to have minimal or no funding shortfall; (b) four countries that have adequate budgets, but which need to make up funding shortfalls (Cambodia, China), or where it is unclear how many more cases will be detected and successfully treated as a result of the substantial additional funds now available (Bangladesh, Indonesia); (c) five countries whose plans are not in line with meeting the 2005 targets, but which report minimal or no funding gaps; (d) nine countries that report large funding gaps and whose plans are less than required to meet the targets for case detection (eight countries) and/or it is not clear if they are sufficient to meet the target for treatment success. These nine countries merit particular attention from donors and other support agencies.

Progress towards the Millennium Development Goals

28. If the improvement in case-finding between 2002 and 2003 can be maintained, the case detection rate will be 60% in 2005. To reach the 70% target, DOTS programmes must recruit TB patients from non-participating clinics and hospitals, especially in the private sector in Asia, and from beyond the present limits of public health systems in Africa. To reach the target of 85% treatment success, a special effort must be made to improve cure rates in Africa and Eastern Europe.

29. Our analysis of epidemiological trends suggests that the TB incidence rate is still slowly rising globally, but prevalence and death rates are falling. Whether the burden of TB can be reduced sufficiently to reach the MDGs by 2015 depends on how rapidly DOTS programmes can be implemented by a diversity of health-care providers, and how effectively they can be adapted to meet the challenges presented by HIV coinfection (especially in Africa) and drug resistance (especially in eastern Europe).

30. Financing for global TB control has improved since 2002, dramatically in some countries. Some HBCs now have sufficient funds to meet targets, but must show that they can spend them effectively; some have no apparent shortfall, but should verify that their budgets are sufficient; some have an obvious funding gap, and must focus on raising the money needed to improve programme performance.

Key epidemiological and financial indicators

EPIDEMIOLOGICAL INDICATORS (WORLD)	MDG TARGET	TARGET YEAR	ESTIMATE 2003	CHANGE, REFERENCE YEAR TO 2003 (%)	REFERENCE YEAR
DOTS case detection (%)	70	2005	45	+7.5	2002
DOTS treatment success (%)	85	2005	82 (2002 cohort)	0.0	2001 cohort
Incidence rate (per 100 000 per year exc HIV)	falling	2015	129	+0.6	2002
Incidence rate (per 100 000 per year inc HIV)*			140	+1.0	2002
Prevalence rate (per 100 000 exc HIV)	half 1990 level	2015	240	−22	1990
Prevalence rate (per 100 000 inc HIV)			245	−21	1990
Mortality rate (per 100 000 per year exc HIV)	half 1990 level	2015	24	−12	1990
Mortality rate (per 100 000 per year inc HIV)			28	−1.6	1990

FINANCIAL INDICATORS (HIGH-BURDEN COUNTRIES)	ESTIMATE 2005	CHANGE, 2002–2005 (%)	REFERENCE YEAR
Total costs of TB control (US$ millions)	1321	+49	2002
NTP budgets for TB control (US$ millions)	741	+79	2002
Total funding available for TB control (US$ millions):	1202	+36	2002
Government (excl. loans)	982	+26	2002
Loans	56	+102	2002
Grants (excl. GFATM)	55	+29	2002
GFATM	109	NA	2002
Funding gap as reported by NTPs (US$ millions)	119	+34	2002
Costs per patient (US$) (median values)			
Total cost	213	+22	2002
NTP budget	133	+45	2002
First-line drugs budget	28	−12	2002

* inc HIV: including HIV+ TB patients; MDG indicators for TB exclude HIV+ patients, but these statistics are also useful in TB control.
NA: not applicable; funds first distributed in 2003.

Résumé

Contexte et méthodes

1. Le neuvième rapport annuel de l'Organisation Mondiale de la Santé (OMS) sur la surveillance, la planification et le financement de la lutte antituberculeuse contient des informations sur le nombre de cas notifiés et les résultats du traitement en provenance de tous les programmes nationaux de lutte antituberculeuse (PNT) qui ont envoyé des rapports à l'OMS, ainsi qu'une analyse des plans, budgets, dépenses et progrès concernant l'extension de la stratégie DOTS dans les 22 pays les plus touchés par la tuberculose.

2. On dispose désormais de données s'étendant sur dix années consécutives (1994-2003) pour évaluer les progrès accomplis en vue d'atteindre les objectifs du Millénaire pour le développement (OMD) qui concernent la lutte antituberculeuse. Les cinq objectifs des OMD concernant directement la lutte contre la tuberculose sont: d'ici 2005, dépister 70 % des nouveaux cas à frottis positif et traiter avec succès 85 % d'entre eux ; d'ici 2015, arrêter l'augmentation de l'incidence et commencer à inverser la tendance ; entre 1990 et 2015, diminuer de moitié le taux de prévalence de la tuberculose et le taux de mortalité.

Améliorer le dépistage et le traitement

3. Au total, 199 pays ont présenté à l'OMS un rapport sur leur stratégie pour lutter contre la tuberculose, sur le nombre de cas de tuberculose notifiés et/ou les résultats du traitement.

4. Nous avons calculé, en utilisant les données de surveillance et d'enquête pour établir de nouvelles estimations de l'incidence, qu'il y a eu 8,8 millions de nouveaux cas de tuberculose en 2003 (140 pour 100 000 habitants), dont 3,9 millions (62 pour 100 000) avaient un frottis positif et 674 000 (11 pour 100 000) étaient porteurs du virus de l'immunodéficience humaine (VIH). Le nombre total de cas était de 15,4 millions (245 pour 100 000), sur lesquels 6,9 millions avaient un frottis positif (109 pour 100 000). Le nombre de décès dus à la tuberculose en 2003 est estimé à 1,7 millions (28/100 000); ce chiffre englobe les cas de co-infection tuberculose-VIH (229 000).

5. En 2003, 182 pays au total appliquaient la stratégie DOTS, soit 2 de plus qu'en 2002. A la fin de 2003, 77 % de la population mondiale vivaient dans des pays, ou des régions de pays, où la stratégie était appliquée. Les programmes ont rapporté 3,7 millions de cas nouveaux et de rechutes, parmi lesquels on recense 1,8 millions de cas nouveaux à frottis positif. Au total, 17,1 millions de tuberculeux et 8,6 millions de sujets à frottis positif ont suivi un traitement dans le cadre des programmes DOTS entre 1995 et 2003.

6. Les 1,8 million de cas à frottis positif signalés par les programmes DOTS en 2003 représentent un taux de détection de 45 %. L'augmentation du nombre de cas à frottis positif notifiés dans le cadre de la stratégie DOTS n'a jamais été aussi forte qu'entre 2002 et 2003 (324 000) (l'augmentation annuelle moyenne entre 1995 et 2000 était de 134 000). L'augmentation des cas notifiés a été plus marquée encore pour tous les cas de tuberculose confondus : elle a été de 693 000 entre 2002 et 2003, alors que l'augmentation annuelle moyenne était de 270 000 pendant la période 1995-2000.

7. Alors que l'augmentation du nombre de cas de tuberculose notifiés par les programmes DOTS semble s'accélérer depuis 2000 le nombre total de cas notifiés à l'OMS (toutes formes et toutes sources confondues) n'a que très peu augmenté entre 1995 et 2003 (taux moyen de notification de 42 %). Le nombre de cas à frottis positif raporté par toutes les sources a augmenté (taux de notification de 50 % en 2003), mais bien plus lentement que la hausse dont il est fait état dans le cadre de la stratégie DOTS.

8. Deux pays, l'Inde et la Chine, concentraient à eux seuls 63 % de tous les cas supplémentaires à frottis positif signalés dans le cadre de la stratégie DOTS en 2003. Parmi les personnes qui ont développé une tuberculose à crachat positif en 2003 (nombre estimé) mais qui n'ont pas été détectées par les programmes DOTS, 67% habitaient dans seulement 8 pays: le Bangladesh, la Chine, l'Ethiopie, la Fédération de Russie, l'Inde, l'Indonésie, le Nigéria et le Pakistan.

9. Alors que les programmes DOTS se sont étendus géographiquement, le taux de détection des cas nouveaux à frottis positif dans les zones couvertes par la stratégie DOTS est resté relativement constant depuis 1995 (52 % en moyenne), encore qu'on observe une légère hausse dans les pays les plus touchés, en particulier au Bangladesh, en Inde, au Myanmar et aux Philippines.

10. Le taux de succès thérapeutique dans la cohorte DOTS de 2002 était de 82 % en moyenne, inchangé depuis 2000. Comme pour les années précédentes, il était nettement inférieur à la moyenne dans la Région africaine (73 %) et dans la Région européenne (76 %). Cela s'explique en partie par les complications de la co-infection tuberculose-VIH dans la Région africaine et par la pharmacorésistance dans la Région européenne. Un autre facteur tout aussi important dans ces deux régions est l'ncapacité des programmes DOTS à documenter les résultats du traitement pour tous les patients.

11. D'après les cas déclarés et les estimations de l'OMS, 22 pays avaient atteint à la fin de 2003 les objectifs en matière de détection et de succès thérapeutique. Le Viet Nam est cependant le seul pays du groupe des pays les plus touchés[1] parmi eux, mais le Cambodge, le Myanmar et les Philippines ne sont pas loin d'atteindre les objectifs.

Tendances épidémiologiques et impact de la stratégie DOTS

12. En 2003, le taux d'incidence de la tuberculose fléchissait ou se stabilisait dans cinq des six Régions de l'OMS, mais augmentait de 1,0 % à l'échelle mondiale. La région qui fait exception est la Région africaine, où l'incidence a augmenté plus rapidement dans les pays à plus haut taux de prévalence VIH. En Europe de l'Est, les taux d'incidence ont augmenté pendant les années 90 pour atteindre un pic vers 2001 et ont baissé depuis. La hausse de l'incidence mondiale ralentit parce que les épidémies d'infection au VIH ralentissent en Afrique, mais on ignore encore quand l'incidence mondiale de la tuberculose commencera à décroître.

13. Nous calculons que, suite à l'extension de la stratégie DOTS entre 1990 et 2003, le taux de prévalence mondial est passé de 309 à 245 pour 100 000 (cas de co-infection tuberculose-VIH compris), et a diminué de 5 % entre 2002 et 2003 alors que l'incidence continuait d'augmenter. Le taux de mortalité mondial a atteint un record dans les années 90, puis a diminué à 2,5 % (cas de co-infection tuberculose-VIH compris) ou 3,5 % par an (cas de co-infection tuberculose-VIH non compris) entre 2002 et 2003. Si les tendances n'étaient pas si contraires en Afrique, les taux de prévalence et de mortalité baisseraient beaucoup plus rapidement à l'échelle mondiale.

Planification et mise en oeuvre de la stratégie DOTS

14. Tous les pays les plus touchés ont un plan stratégique d'extension de la stratégie DOTS et beaucoup d'entre

eux commenceront en 2005 un nouveau cycle de planification, de préférence axé sur l'année cible des OMD, 2015. Bien que les systèmes de santé de nombreux pays subissent encore des réformes et des restructurations, tous les pays les plus touchés, sauf la Fédération de Russie et la Thaïlande, indiquent que les fonctions de lutte antituberculeuse sont entièrement intégrées aux services de santé nationaux généraux.

15. L'extension de la stratégie DOTS se heurte à cinq obstacles d'une importance capitale : pénurie de personnel qualifié, absence d'engagement politique, insuffisance des services de laboratoire, prise en charge inadéquate de la tuberculose multirésistante et de la tuberculose associée au VIH. En ce qui concerne la pharmacorésistance, les pays sont peu nombreux à avoir une politique nationale en matière de diagnostic et de traitement de la tuberculose résistante, et même dans ceux qui en ont une, le traitement n'est souvent pas conforme aux normes acceptables. En ce qui concerne la co-infection tuberculose-VIH, les programmes nationaux de lutte antituberculeuse indiquent que peu de tuberculeux ont un test de dépistage du VIH (3 % des cas notifiés), qu'ils sont moins nombreux encore à être examinés en vue de bénéficier d'un traitement antirétroviral et qu'une très faible proportion commence un traitement de ce type (1347 patients recensés en 2003). Le rapport discute une série de mesures pour remédier à cette situation.

16. L'intensification du soutien et de l'action dans les pays (ISAC) est une nouvelle initiative destinée à catalyser et à accélérer l'extension de la stratégie DOTS en vue d'atteindre les objectifs de 2005. L'initiative a pour but d'améliorer les capacités techniques afin de faciliter l'utilisation des subventions importantes provenant du Fonds Mondial de lutte contre le SIDA, la Tuberculose et le Paludisme (FMSTP) et autres bailleurs de fonds importants. En 2004, ont participé à l'initiative la Chine, la Fédération de Russie, l'Inde, l'Indonésie, le Kenya, l'Ouganda, le Pakistan et la Roumanie.

17. Les contributions croissantes des organisations non gouvernementales (ONG) et de groupes communautaires manifestent clairement l'engagement de plus en plus important de la société civile en faveur de la lutte antituberculeuse. L'action de ces groupes place les patients au centre de la stratégie DOTS et améliore l'accès aux services antituberculeux dans les zones éloignées et au sein des populations défavorisées et marginalisées.

18. Les projets public-privé et public-public ont des effets mesurables sur le dépistage des cas dans plusieurs pays d'Asie, et pourraient être un moyen d'élargir les services de lutte antituberculeuse dans les villes africaines.

Financement de l'extension des programmes DOTS

19. Des données financières ont été reçues de 134 pays sur 211 (64 %), contre 123 en 2003 ; 70 et 69 pays ont fourni des données complètes concernant respectivement le budget et les dépenses. Les 22 pays les plus touchés ont tous fourni des données sauf l'Afrique du Sud.

20. On a observé une forte augmentation des budgets des PNT ainsi qu'un net accroissement des fonds disponibles pour la lutte antituberculeuse dans les pays les plus touchés depuis 2002, avec des augmentations particulièrement importantes entre 2003 et 2004. Les budgets PNT prévus pour 2005 atteignent au total US $741 millions. La projection des coûts totaux estimés de la lutte antituberculeuse s'élève à US $1,3 milliard en 2005 et les fonds disponibles à US $1,2 milliard. La forte augmentation des crédits disponibles est pratiquement entièrement due à des fonds publics supplémentaires aloués par la Chine, la Fédération de Russie et l'Indonésie et à des subventions du fond mondial (FMSTP).

21. Les pays dont le budget du PNT pour 2005 est le plus important sont la Chine, la Fédération de Russie, l'Inde et l'Indonésie. Si l'on prend également en considération des coûts non inclus dans les budgets PNT, l'Afrique du Sud, la Chine, la Fédération

---

[1] Le Pérou a été exclu du groupe initial des pays les plus touchés car ce pays a atteint les objectifs de détection et de succès thérapeutique et a réussi à réduire l'incidence de la tuberculose.

de Russie et l'Inde représentent à elles seules US $946 millions (73 %) du montant total de US $1,3 milliard. Huit pays parmi les plus touchés prévoient des coûts totaux de US $20–50 millions en 2005 ; le reste représente US $18 millions ou moins.

22. On observe des variations considérables, par patient traité, dans les budgets pour les médicaments de première ligne, dans les budgets PNT totaux et dans les coûts totaux pour chaque année entre 2002 et 2005. Parmi les pays les plus touchés, le budget PNT par patient est le plus faible en Inde (US $34). Dans la plupart des pays, les budgets se situent entre US $100 et 200 par patient et les coûts entre US $150 et 300. L'Afrique du Sud et la Fédération de Russie sont des exceptions notables, avec des coûts par patient traité supérieurs à US $1000. Les budgets par patient traité sont généralement stables ou en augmentation et, par conséquent, les coûts par patient traité le sont aussi.

23. En 2005, les gouvernements des pays les plus touchés financent 62 % des budgets des PNT (y compris par des prêts), le FMSTP 15 % et 7 % proviennent d'autres sources, ce qui correspond à un déficit équivalent à 16 % des budgets prévus. Les gouvernements des pays les plus touchés contribuent davantage (79 %) aux coûts totaux qu'aux budgets PNT parce qu'ils financent le personnel des services de santé généraux et les infrastructures utilisées pour la lutte antituberculeuse. Les contributions moyennes au financement de la lutte antituberculeuse des gouvernements des pays les plus touchés sont élevées et masquent le fait que nombre de ces pays sont largement dépendants de subventions.

24. Malgré des progrès dans la mobilisation de crédits supplémentaires, les pays les plus touchés ont signalé un déficit de financement de US $119 millions en 2005. Ce chiffre est plus élevé que ceux qui avaient été enregistrés en 2003 et 2004. Les plus importants déficits de financement sont signalés par la Chine, la Fédération de Russie, l'Inde, le Pakistan et le Zimbabwe (US $93 millions, soit 78 % du déficit total). Proportionnellement aux budgets, les déficits les plus importants sont ceux du Kenya, du Nigéria, de l'Ouganda, du Pakistan et du Zimbabwe.

25. Les activités planifiées ne sont pas en mesure d'atteindre les objectifs fixés pour le dépistage des cas en 2005 dans 12 pays. En outre, les budgets pour les activités concertées contre la tuberculose et le VIH et pour les médicaments de deuxième ligne pour traiter la tuberculose multirésistante sont actuellement peu élevés. Cela veut dire que l'on peut considérer que les déficits actuellement rapportés par les PNT sont sous-estimés et que les ressources nécessaires pour la tuberculose seront dans le futur plus élevées que US $1,3 milliard.

26. La capacité d'absorption est l'un des grands problèmes pour les pays les plus touchés qui sont parvenus à mobiliser un important financement supplémentaire. En 2003, les dépenses ont été inférieures au financement disponible ; reste à évaluer si les PNT peuvent effectivement dépenser les crédits supplémentaires disponibles en 2004 et 2005.

27. En termes financiers, les pays les plus touchés entrent dans quatre catégories : a) quatre pays (l'Inde, le Myanmar, les Philippines et le Viet Nam) dont les budgets devraient permettre d'atteindre les objectifs de 2005, et qui auront sans doute un déficit de financement minime, voire nul; b) quatre pays dont les budgets sont suffisants, mais qui devront combler des déficits de financement (Cambodge, Chine), ou qui ne savent pas très bien combien de cas supplémentaires seront détectés et traités avec succès grâce aux fonds supplémentaires importants désormais disponibles (Bangladesh, Indonésie) ; c) cinq pays dont les plans ne sont pas de nature à leur permettre d'atteindre les objectifs de 2005, mais qui signalent des déficits de financement minimes ou nuls ; d) neuf pays qui signalent d'importants déficits de financement et dont les plans sont loin d'être de nature à leur permettre d'atteindre les objectifs de détection des cas (huit pays) et/ou dont on ne sait pas s'ils seront suffisants pour atteindre l'objectif de succès thérapeutique. Ces neuf pays méritent une attention particulière de la part des donateurs et d'autres organismes d'aide.

Progrès vers la réalisation des objectifs du Millénaire pour le développement

28. Si l'amélioration de la détection des cas observée entre 2002 et 2003 peut être maintenue, le taux de détection des cas sera de 60 % en 2005. Pour atteindre l'objectif de 70 %, les programmes DOTS doivent recruter des patients tuberculeux dans les centres de santé et les hôpitaux qui ne participent pas encore aux programmes, notamment dans le secteur privé en Asie, et au-delà des limites actuelles des systèmes de santé publique en Afrique. Pour atteindre l'objectif de 85 % de succès thérapeutique, un effort particulier doit être fait afin d'améliorer les taux de guérison en Afrique et en Europe de l'Est.

29. Notre analyse des tendances épidémiologiques laisse supposer que le taux d'incidence de la tuberculose est encore en légère augmentation dans le monde, mais que les taux de prévalence et de mortalité sont en diminution. Quant à savoir si la diminution du poids de la tuberculose sera suffisante pour atteindre les OMD d'ici 2015, dépendra de la rapidité avec laquelle les programmes DOTS seront mis en œuvre par les divers prestataires de soins, et de l'efficacité avec laquelle les programmes seront adaptés pour répondre aux problèmes que présentent la co-infection tuberculose-VIH (notamment en Afrique) et la pharmacorésistance (notamment en Europe de l'Est).

30. Le financement de l'effort mondial de lutte antituberculeuse s'est amélioré depuis 2002, de façon spectaculaire dans certains pays. Certains des pays les plus touchés disposent désormais de fonds suffisants pour atteindre les objectifs, mais doivent encore montrer qu'ils sont capables de les utiliser efficacement ; certains n'ont pas de déficit apparent, mais

Principaux indicateurs epidemiologiques et financiers

INDICATEURS ÉPIDÉMIOLOGIQUES (MONDE)	CIBLE OMD	ANNÉE CIBLE	ESTIMATION 2003	EVOLUTION PAR RAPPORT À 2003 (%)	ANNÉE DE RÉFÉRENCE
DOTS détection des cas (%)	70	2005	45	+7,5	2002
DOTS succès thérapeutique (%)	85	2005	82 (cohorte 2002)	0,0	cohorte 2001
Taux d'incidence (pour 100 000 par an, VIH exclus)	En diminution	2015	129	+0,6	2002
Taux d'incidence (pour 100 000 par an, VIH inclus*)			140	+1,0	2002
Taux de prévalence (pour 100 000, VIH exclus)	moitié du niveau de 1990	2015	240	-22	1990
Taux de prévalence (pour 100 000, VIH inclus)			245	-21	1990
Taux de mortalité (pour 100 000 par an, VIH exclus)	moitié du niveau 1990	2015	24	-12	1990
Taux de mortalité (pour 100 000 par an, VIH inclus)			28	-1,6	1990

INDICATEURS FINANCIERS (PAYS LES PLUS TOUCHÉS)	ESTIMATION 2005	EVOLUTION 2002–2005 (%)	ANNÉE DE RÉFÉRENCE
Dépenses totales pour la lutte antituberculeuse (US $ millions)	1321	+49	2002
Budget PNT pour la lutte antituberculeuse (US $ millions)	741	+79	2002
Total des fonds disponibles pour la lutte contre la tuberculose (US $ millions)	1202	+36	2002
Etat (à l'exclusion des prêts)	982	+26	2002
Prêts	56	+102	2002
Subventions (à l'exclusion du FMSTP)	55	+29	2002
FMSTP	109	NA	2002
Déficit de financement tel que raporté par les PNT (US$ millions)	119	+34	2002
Coûts par patient (US $) (valeurs médianes)			
Coût total	213	+22	2002
Budget PNT	133	+45	2002
Budget pour les médicaments de première ligne	28	-12	2002

* VIH inclus: y compris les patients souffrant à la fois de tuberculose et d'une infection à VIH ; les indicateurs OMD pour la tuberculose excluent les patients également atteints d'infection à VIH cependant ces statistiques sont également utiles dans la lutte antituberculeuse.

NA: non applicable car les fonds ont été distribués pour la première fois en 2003

devraient vérifier que leurs budgets sont suffisants ; certains ont un déficit de financement évident et doivent se concentrer sur la mobilisation des fonds nécessaires pour améliorer la performance du programme.

Resumen

Antecedentes y métodos

1. El noveno informe anual de la Organización Mundial de la Salud (OMS) sobre vigilancia, planificación y financiación de la lucha contra la tuberculosis (TB) incluye datos sobre las notificaciones de casos y los resultados del tratamiento procedentes de todos los programas nacionales de lucha contra la TB (PNT) que han informado a la OMS, así como un análisis de los planes, presupuestos y gastos, y de los progresos de la expansión de la estrategia DOTS en 22 países con alta carga de TB (PACT).

2. En la actualidad se dispone de datos reunidos durante diez años consecutivos (1994–2003), que permiten evaluar los progresos realizados para alcanzar los Objetivos de Desarrollo del Milenio (ODM) relativos a la lucha contra la TB. Las cinco metas de los ODM que guardan relación directa con la lucha antituberculosa son: para 2005, detectar el 70% de los nuevos casos bacilíferos y tratar con éxito el 85% de esos casos; para 2015, haber detenido y comenzado a reducir la incidencia; entre 1990 y 2015, reducir a la mitad las tasas de prevalencia y de mortalidad de la TB.

Mejorar la detección y el tratamiento de los casos

3. Un total de 199 países han informado a la OMS de sus estrategias de lucha contra la TB, así como de las notificaciones de casos y/o de los resultados del tratamiento.

4. Tras actualizar las estimaciones de la incidencia tomando como base los datos de la vigilancia y de las encuestas, hemos calculado que en 2003 hubo 8,8 millones de nuevos casos de TB (140/100 000 habitantes), de los cuales 3,9 millones (62/100 000) eran bacilíferos y 674 000 (11/100 000) estaban infectados por el virus de la inmunodeficiencia humana (VIH). Hubo 15,4 millones de casos prevalentes (245/100 000), de los cuales 6,9 millones eran bacilíferos (109/100 000). Se estima que 1,7 millones de personas (28/100 000) murieron de TB en 2003, incluidos los casos de coinfección por el VIH (229 000).

5. Ciento ochenta y dos países aplicaron la estrategia DOTS en 2003, dos más que en 2002. A finales de 2003, el 77% de la población mundial vivía en países (o regiones de países) que disponían de cobertura de DOTS. Los programas DOTS notificaron 3,7 millones de casos de TB nuevos y recidivantes, de los cuales 1,8 millones eran nuevos bacilíferos. Entre 1995 y 2003, 17,1 millones de pacientes con TB y 8,6 millones de pacientes bacilíferos recibieron tratamiento en los programas DOTS.

6. Los 1,8 millones de casos bacilíferos notificados por los programas DOTS en 2003 representan una tasa de detección del 45%. El aumento de los casos bacilíferos notificados en el ámbito de los programas DOTS entre 2002 y 2003 (324 000) fue mayor que nunca (el incremento medio anual entre 1995 y 2000 había sido de 134 000). El aumento de las notificaciones fue todavía mayor si se consideran todos los casos de TB: 693 000 entre 2002 y 2003, en comparación con un incremento medio anual de 270 000 en el periodo 1995–2000.

7. Mientras que el número de casos de TB notificados por los programas DOTS parece haber crecido de forma acelerada desde 2000, el número total de casos de TB notificados a la OMS (todas las formas, de todas las fuentes) aumentó muy poco entre 1995 y 2003 (tasa media de detección del 42%). El número de casos bacilíferos notificados por la totalidad de las fuentes ha ido en aumento (tasa de detección del 50% en 2003), pero mucho más lentamente que los notificados en el marco del DOTS.

8. El 63% de los casos bacilíferos adicionales notificados a través de DOTS en 2003 provenían de tan sólo dos países: China e India. Dos tercios (67%) de los nuevos casos estimados para 2003 que no fueron detectados por medio de los programas DOTS procedían de ocho países: Bangladesh, China, Etiopía, la Federación de Rusia, la India, Indonesia, Nigeria y Pakistán.

9. A medida que los programas DOTS se han extendido geográficamente, la tasa de detección de nuevos casos bacilíferos en las zonas donde se aplica la estrategia DOTS ha permanecido prácticamente constante desde 1995 (media del 52%), aunque hay signos de un lento aumento en los PACT, sobre todo en Bangladesh, Filipinas, la India y Myanmar.

10. La tasa media de éxito del tratamiento en la cohorte de DOTS de 2002 fue del 82%, la misma que se viene observando desde 2000. Como en años anteriores, dicha tasa fue considerablemente inferior a la media en las regiones de África (73%) y Europa (76%). Las bajas tasas de éxito del tratamiento en esas dos regiones pueden atribuirse en parte a la coinfección por el VIH y a la farmacorresistencia, respectivamente. Sin embargo, igualmente importante es el fracaso de los programas DOTS en la vigilancia de los resultados del tratamiento en todos los pacientes en esas dos regiones.

11. Con base en los casos notificados y las estimaciones de la OMS, 22 países habían alcanzado a finales de 2003 las metas fijadas en materia de detección de casos y éxito del tratamiento. Viet Nam era aún el único miembro del actual grupo de PACT[1] entre ellos, aunque Camboya, Filipinas y Myanmar están a punto de lograrlo.

---

[1] Perú ha sido excluido del grupo original de PACT, ya que ha alcanzado la metas y la incidencia ha disminuido.

Tendencias epidemiológicas e impacto de la estrategia DOTS

12. En 2003, la tasa de incidencia de TB estaba disminuyendo o era estable en cinco de las seis regiones de la OMS, pero aumentando en todo el mundo a razón de 1,0% al año. La excepción fue la región de África, donde la incidencia ha aumentado con mayor rapidez en los países con mayores tasas de prevalencia de infección por VIH. En Europa Oriental, las tasas de incidencia aumentaron en la década de los noventa, pero alcanzaron su valor máximo en 2001, y desde entonces han disminuido. El aumento de la incidencia mundial se está haciendo más lento debido a la desaceleración de la epidemia de VIH en África, pero aún no está claro cuándo comenzará a disminuir la tasa de incidencia mundial.

13. Hemos calculado que, debido a la expansión de la estrategia DOTS entre 1990 y 2003, la tasa mundial de prevalencia de TB disminuyó de 309 a 245 por 100 000 (incluidos los pacientes tuberculosos con VIH), y en un 5% entre 2002 y 2003, aun cuando la incidencia siguió aumentando. La tasa mundial de mortalidad alcanzó su valor máximo en la década de los noventa y disminuyó al 2,5% (incluidos los pacientes VIH-positivos con TB) o al 3,5% anual (excluidos los pacientes VIH-positivos) entre 2002 y 2003. De no ser por las tendencias extremadamente adversas que se observan en África, las tasas de prevalencia y de mortalidad estarían disminuyendo más rápidamente en todo el mundo.

Planificación y aplicación de la estrategia DOTS

14. Todos los PACT disponen de un plan estratégico de expansión de la estrategia DOTS; en 2005, muchos comenzarán un nuevo ciclo de planificación con miras a alcanzar la meta de 2015 fijada por los ODM. Si bien los sistemas de salud de numerosos países todavía son objeto de reformas y de reestructuración, todos los PACT, salvo la Federación de Rusia y Tailandia, informaron que las funciones relacionadas con la lucha anti-tuberculosa están completamente integradas en los servicios de salud esenciales de la nación.

15. Entre los obstáculos con que se enfrenta la expansión de la estrategia DOTS, hay cinco de importancia capital: la escasez de personal capacitado, la falta de compromiso político, la debilidad de los servicios de laboratorio y la gestión inadecuada de la tuberculosis multirresistente (MDR-TB) y de la TB asociada al VIH. Con respecto a la farmacorresistencia, pocos países cuentan con políticas nacionales para el diagnóstico y el tratamiento de la MDR-TB, e incluso en aquellos que disponen de ellas, el tratamiento no suele estar a la altura del nivel exigido. Por lo que se refiere a TB-VIH, los PNT informaron que son pocos los pacientes con TB sometidos a pruebas de detección del VIH (el 3% de los casos notificados), aún menos los evaluados con vistas a la administración de tratamiento antir-retrovírico y que sólo una fracción pequeña inicia dicho tratamiento (1347 pacientes en 2003). Este informe examina un amplio abanico de medidas correctivas para superar dichos obstáculos.

16. ISAC (actuaciones y apoyo intensificados en los países) es una nueva iniciativa destinada a catalizar y acelerar la expansión de DOTS con miras a las metas de 2005. Su objetivo consiste en mejorar la capacidad técnica para facilitar el gasto de grandes subsidios del Fondo Mundial de Lucha contra el SIDA, la Tuberculosis y la Malaria (FMSTM) y de otros donantes importantes. En 2004, los participantes fueron China, la Federación de Rusia, la India, Indonesia, Kenya, Pakistán, Rumania y Uganda.

17. Las contribuciones cada vez más importantes de las organizaciones no gubernamentales y de los grupos comunitarios constituyen una clara manifestación del compromiso creciente de la sociedad civil en la lucha contra la TB. El trabajo de esos grupos sitúa a los pacientes en el centro de la estrategia DOTS y mejora el acceso a los servicios relacionados con la TB en zonas remotas y entre las poblaciones desfavorecidas y marginadas.

18. Los proyectos mixtos de carácter publicoprivado y público-público están ejerciendo un impacto perceptible en la detección de casos en varios países asiáticos y podrían llegar a constituir un mecanismo de expansión de los servicios de lucha contra la TB en las ciudades africanas.

Financiación de la expansión de la estrategia DOTS

19. Se ha recibido información financiera de 134 países sobre un total de 211 (64%), en comparación con 123 en 2003. Han presentado datos completos en materia de presupuesto y gasto 70 y 69 países, respectivamente. Se recibieron datos de los 22 PACT, con excepción de Sudáfrica.

20. Desde 2002 ha habido un gran aumento de los presupuestos de los PNT y de la financiación disponible para la lucha antituberculosa en los PACT, en particular entre 2003 y 2004. Los presupuestos de los PNT previstos para 2005 ascienden a US$ 741 millones. Se calcula que los costos totales de la lucha contra la TB en 2005 serán de US$ 1,3 mil millones, y los fondos disponibles son de US$ 1,2 mil millones. El gran aumento de fondos disponibles se debe casi por completo a nuevos recursos proporcionados por los gobiernos de China, la Federación de Rusia e Indonesia, así como a subsidios del FMSTM.

21. Los países que disponen de mayores presupuestos para sus PNT en 2005 son China, la Federación de Rusia, la India e Indonesia. Si también se toman en consideración los costos que no figuran en los presupuestos de los PNT, los costos de China, la Federación de Rusia, la India y Sudáfrica reflejan el 73% del costo total (US$ 946 millones de US$ 1,3 mil millones). En otros ocho PACT, los costos totales oscilan entre US$ 20 y US$ 50 millones, y en el resto de los PACT ascienden a US$ 18 millones, o menos.

22. Por paciente tratado, hay variaciones considerables en los presupuestos destinados a medicamentos de primera línea, en los presupuestos de los PNT y en los costos totales en cada uno de los años del período 2002–2005. Entre los PACT, la India es el país con menor presupuesto de PNT por paciente (US$ 34). La mayoría de los países tienen presupuestos que van de US$ 100 a US$ 200 por paciente, y costos que varían entre US$ 150 y US$ 300. La Federación de Rusia y Sudáfrica constituyen excepciones notables, con costos por paciente tratado que superan los US$ 1000. En general, los presupuestos por paciente tratado son estables o tienden a aumentar, de modo que los costos por paciente tratado también son generalmente estables o tienden al alza.

23. En 2005, el 62% de los presupuestos de los PNT (incluidos los préstamos) será proporcionado por los gobiernos de los PACT, el 15% por el FMSTM, el 7% por subsidios de otras fuentes, con lo que queda un déficit del 16% con respecto a los presupuestos notificados. Los gobiernos de los PACT contribuyen más a los costos totales (79%) que a los presupuestos de los PNT, pues financian el personal y las infraestructuras de los servicios de salud generales utilizados en la lucha contra la tuberculosis. La elevada contribución media de los gobiernos de los PACT a la financiación de la lucha antituberculosa oculta el hecho de que muchos de esos países dependen en gran medida de la financiación bajo la forma de subsidios.

24. A pesar de los progresos realizados en la obtención de fondos adicionales, los PACT acusan un déficit financiero de US$ 119 millones en 2005, cifra que es superior a las registradas en 2003 y 2004. Los mayores déficit corresponden a China, la Federación de Rusia, la India, Pakistán y Zimbabwe (US$ 93 millones, es decir, el 78% del déficit total). Proporcionalmente a los presupuestos, los mayores déficit corresponden a Kenya, Nigeria, Pakistán, Uganda y Zimbabwe.

25. En 12 países las actividades planificadas no son compatibles con el logro de la meta de detección de casos para 2005. Además, los presupuestos actuales para las actividades de colaboración TB-VIH y para los medicamentos de segunda línea para el tratamiento MDR-TB son pequeños. Esto significa que los déficit notificados por los PNT pueden estar subestimados, y que el total de recursos necesarios para el control de TB será superior a US$ 1,3 mil millones en el futuro.

26. Una cuestión fundamental para los PACT que han conseguido cuantiosos fondos adicionales es su capacidad de absorberlos. En 2003, los gastos fueron inferiores a los fondos disponibles, y queda por ver si los PNT pueden gastar eficazmente el dinero extra disponible en 2004 y 2005.

27. En materia de financiación, los PACT pueden clasificarse en cuatro categorías: a) cuatro países cuyos presupuestos son compatibles con el logro de las metas para 2005 y que probablemente no tendrán déficit de fondos o, en el caso de que los tengan, serán mínimos (Filipinas, la India, Myanmar, y Viet Nam); b) cuatro países cuyos presupuestos son suficientes, pero que tendrán que encontrar la forma de completar los fondos que les faltan (Camboya y China) o en los que no está claro cuántos casos adicionales se detectarán y tratarán con éxito como resultado de los considerables fondos adicionales de que disponen actualmente (Bangladesh e Indonesia); c) cinco países cuyos planes no se ajustan al logro de las metas para 2005, pero que tienen un pequeño o nulo déficit de fondos, y d) nueve países con un gran déficit de fondos y cuyos planes están por debajo de lo necesario para alcanzar las metas de detección de casos (ocho países) y/o en los que no está claro si los fondos son suficientes para alcanzar el objetivo del éxito del tratamiento. Estos nueve países merecen especial atención por parte de los organismos donantes y de otros organismos de apoyo.

Progresos en la consecución de los Objetivos de Desarrollo del Milenio

28. Si se mantiene la mejora en la detección de casos que se produjo entre 2002 y 2003, la tasa de detección de casos será del 60% en 2005. Para alcanzar la meta del 70%, los programas DOTS deben reclutar pacientes con TB de clínicas y hospitales que no participan en esos programas, especialmente los del sector privado en Asia, y los que están fuera de los límites actuales de los sistemas de salud pública en África. Para lograr la meta del 85% de éxito del tratamiento habrá que hacer un esfuerzo especial por mejorar las tasas de curación en África y Europa Oriental.

29. Nuestro análisis de las tendencias epidemiológicas indica que la tasa de incidencia de la TB sigue aumentando lentamente en todo el mundo, pero que las tasas de prevalencia y de mortalidad están descendiendo. Que la carga de TB pueda disminuir lo suficiente como para alcanzar los ODM en 2015 dependerá de la rapidez con que los diversos prestadores de atención de salud puedan poner en marcha los programas DOTS, y de cuán eficazmente se puedan adaptar esos programas para hacer frente a los retos que suponen la coinfección por VIH (especialmente en África) y a la farmacorresistencia (especialmente en Europa Oriental).

30. La financiación de la lucha mundial contra la TB ha mejorado desde 2002, y en algunos países lo ha hecho de forma espectacular. Algunos PACT disponen ahora de fondos suficientes para alcanzar las metas, pero deben demostrar que son capaces de utilizarlos de forma eficaz, otros no tienen déficit aparente, pero deben comprobar que disponen de suficiente presupuesto, y otros presentan un déficit financiero evidente y deben centrarse en conseguir el dinero necesario para mejorar el rendimiento del programa.

Principales indicadores epidemiológicos y financieros

INDICADORES EPIDEMIOLÓGICOS (NIVEL MUNDIAL)	META DE LOS ODM	AÑO DE CONSECUCIÓN PREVISTO	ESTIMACIÓN 2003	CAMBIO, DEL AÑO DE REFERENCIA A 2003 (%)	AÑO DE REFERENCIA
Detección de casos bajo DOTS (%)	70	2005	45	+7,5	2002
Éxito del tratamiento bajo DOTS (%)	85	2005	82 (cohorte de 2002)	0,0	2001
Tasa de incidencia (por 100 000 por año, excluido VIH)	En descenso	2015	129	+0,6	2002
Tasa de incidencia (por 100 000 por año, incluido VIH)*			140	+1,0	2002
Tasa de prevalencia (por 100 000, excluido VIH)	Mitad del nivel de 1990	2015	240	-22	1990
Tasa de prevalencia (por 100 000, incluido VIH)			245	-21	1990
Tasa de mortalidad (por 100 000 por año, excluido VIH)	Mitad del nivel de 1990	2015	24	-12	1990
Tasa de mortalidad (por 100 000 por año, incluido VIH)			28	-1,6	1990

INDICADORES FINANCIEROS (PACT)	ESTIMACIÓN 2005	CAMBIO, DE 2002 A 2005 (%)	AÑO DE REFERENCIA
Costos totales del control de la TB (en millones de US$)	1321	+49	2002
Presupuestos de los PNT para el control de la TB (en millones de US$)	741	+79	2002
Fondos disponibles totales para el control de la TB (en millones de US$)	1202	+36	2002
Gobierno (excluidos préstamos)	982	+26	2002
Préstamos	56	+102	2002
Subsidios (excluidos los del FMSTM)	55	+29	2002
FMSTM	109	NA	2002
Déficit financiero según los PNT (en millones de US$)	119	+34	2002
Costos por paciente (US$) (valores medianos)			
Costo total	213	+22	2002
Presupuesto de los PNT	133	+45	2002
Presupuesto para medicamentos de primera línea	28	-12	2002

* Incluido VIH: incluidos los pacientes con TB VIH-positivos; los indicadores de los ODM para la TB excluyen a los pacientes VIH-positivos, pero estas estadísticas también son útiles en el control de la TB.

NA: no aplicable, puesto que los recursos fueron distribuidos por primera vez en 2003.

Introduction

The goal of this series of annual reports is to chart progress in global TB control and, in particular, to evaluate progress in implementing the DOTS strategy.[1,2] The first targets set for global TB control were ratified in 1991 by WHO's World Health Assembly.[3] They are to detect 70% of new smear-positive TB cases, and to successfully treat 85% of these cases. Since these targets were not reached by the end of year 2000 as originally planned, the target year was deferred to 2005.[4]

In 2000, the United Nations created a new framework for monitoring progress in human development, the MDGs. Among 18 MDG targets, the eighth is to "have halted by 2015 and begun to reverse the incidence of malaria and other major diseases". Although the objective is expressed in terms of incidence, the MDGs also specify that progress should be measured in terms of the reduction in TB prevalence and deaths. The target for these two indicators, based on a resolution passed at the 2000 Okinawa (Japan) summit of G8 industrialized nations, and now adopted by the Stop TB Partnership, is to halve TB prevalence and death rates (all forms of TB) between 1990 and 2015. All three measures of impact (incidence, prevalence and death rates) have been added to the two traditional measures of DOTS implementation (case detection and treatment success), so that the MDG framework includes five principal indicators of progress in TB control. All five MDG indicators will, from now on, be evaluated by WHO's Global TB Surveillance, Planning and Financing Project. The focus is on the performance of NTPs in 22 HBCs, and in priority countries in WHO's six regions.

Some other MDGs are indirectly relevant to TB control. For example, Goal 1 is to eradicate extreme poverty and hunger, and Goal 3 is to promote gender equality and empower women. Goal 8 is to develop a global partnership for development, in which the Stop TB Partnership will have a role. A discussion of these goals is beyond the scope of this report, but further details can be found at web site: unstats.un.org/unsd.

While the MDGs set out the main objectives for global TB control, numerous specific activities must be carried out to meet these larger goals. This technical report, the ninth in the series, describes many of the details. It presents plans and budgets for DOTS expansion, and costs, expenditures and sources of funding. It also summarizes the progress made on special initiatives such as collaborative TB/HIV activities, improvements in the laboratory network and DOTS-Plus projects for the management of drug-resistant TB.

Since 1980, 81 million TB patients have been reported through WHO's surveillance system, including 17 million notified by DOTS programmes since 1995. The financial monitoring system has accounted for US$ 4.3 billion spent on TB control in the HBCs since its inception in 2002. Thus, the Global TB Surveillance, Planning and Financing Project has become a formidable instrument for monitoring and evaluating progress in TB control.

---

[1] *Framework for effective tuberculosis control*. Geneva, World Health Organization (WHO/TB/94.179).

[2] *An expanded DOTS framework for effective tuberculosis control*. Geneva, World Health Organization (WHO/CDS/TB/2002.297).

[3] Resolution WHA44.8. Tuberculosis control programme. In: *Handbook of resolutions and decisions of the World Health Assembly and the Executive Board*. Volume III, 3rd edition (1985–1992). Geneva, World Health Organization, 1993 (WHA44/1991/REC/1).

[4] *Stop Tuberculosis Initiative. Report by the Director-General*. Fifty-third World Health Assembly. Geneva, 15–20 May 2000 (A53/5, 5 May 2000); available at http://www.who.int/gb/ebwha/pdf_files/WHA53/ea5.pdf, accessed 11 January 2005).

Methods

Monitoring progress towards the Millennium Development Goals

MDGs for tuberculosis control

The MDG framework consists of a hierarchy of indicators that measure progress towards "targets", which are the specific achievements needed to satisfy higher "goals". Those most directly relevant to TB control are Goal 6 (to combat HIV/AIDS, malaria and other diseases) and Target 8 (to have halted by 2015 and begun to reverse the incidence of malaria and other major diseases, including TB). Among the indicators for Target 8 are two groups that can be used to evaluate the implementation and impact of TB control:

> **Indicator 23**: between 1990 and 2015, to halve the prevalence and death rates associated with tuberculosis; and
>
> **Indicator 24**: by 2005, to detect 70% of new smear-positive TB cases arising annually, and to successfully treat 85% of these cases.

The MDG indicators exclude HIV-positive TB patients, mainly to avoid double-counting in death statistics (deaths of HIV-positive people are recorded as AIDS deaths by WHO). However, we routinely calculate all TB indicators with and without HIV-positive TB patient, because TB control programmes need to know both.

This report focuses on the five principal indicators: incidence, prevalence, deaths, case detection and treatment success. The objective of reducing incidence is made explicit by Target 8; the targets for case detection and treatment success have been set by WHO's World Health Assembly;[3] the targets for prevalence and deaths are based on a resolution of the year 2000 meeting of the Group of Eight (G8) industrialized countries, held in Okinawa, Japan.

Data collection and verification

Every year, WHO requests information from TB control programmes (or relevant public health authorities) in 211 countries or territories via a standard data collection form. The latest form was distributed in mid 2004. The section dealing with monitoring and surveillance asked for the following data: TB control strategies implemented up to the end of 2003; TB case notifications in 2003; and treatment outcomes for TB patients registered during 2002, following definitions given in Table 1. The most recent form can be downloaded from www.who.int/tb.

The data collection form is a tool for collecting aggregated national data. The process of national and international reporting is quite distinct from WHO's recommendations about procedures for recording and reporting data within NTPs. The information gathered from the form includes a core set of data (questions remain more or less the same each year), plus new or timely information (questions may change from year to year). In the latest form, there are new questions about TB/HIV collaboration, about financing (the second year of collection but somewhat expanded), and about the outcomes of re-treatment, for patients who have received two or more courses of anti-TB drugs.

Completed forms are collected and reviewed at all levels of WHO – in WHO country offices, regional offices and at headquarters – and an acknowledgement form that tabulates all data submitted and shows WHO's calculations of principal indicators, is sent back to the national correspondent in order to complete any missing responses and to resolve any inconsistencies.

In the WHO European Region only, data collection and verification are performed jointly by the regional office and a WHO collaborating centre, EuroTB (Paris), using a different format. EuroTB subsequently publishes an annual report with additional analyses, using more detailed data for the European Region (see: www.eurotb.org).

High-burden countries and WHO regions

Much of the data submitted to WHO is shown, country by country, in the annexes of this report. The analysis and interpretation that precedes these annexes focuses on 22 HBCs and the six WHO regions. The 22 HBCs account for approximately 80% of the estimated number of new TB cases (all forms) arising worldwide each year. These countries are the focus of intensified efforts in DOTS expansion (Annex 1). The HBCs are not necessarily those with the highest incidence

---

TABLE 1

Technical elements of the WHO TB control strategy (DOTS)[a]

MICROSCOPY Case detection among symptomatic patients self-reporting to health services, using sputum smear microscopy.[b]

SCC/DOT Standardized short-course chemotherapy using regimens of 6–8 months for at least all confirmed smear-positive cases. Good case management includes directly observed treatment (DOT) during the intensive phase for all new smear-positive cases, during the continuation phase of regimens containing rifampicin, and during the entirety of a re-treatment regimen.[c]

DRUG SUPPLY Establishment and maintenance of a system to supply all essential anti-tuberculosis drugs, and to ensure no interruption in their availability.

RECORDING AND REPORTING Establishment and maintenance of a standardized recording and reporting system, allowing assessment of treatment results (see Table 2).

[a] The DOTS strategy comprises five elements in all, including political commitment.

[b] Sputum culture is also used for diagnosis, but direct sputum smear microscopy should still be performed for all suspected cases.

[c] In countries that have consistently documented high treatment success rates, direct observation of treatment may be reserved for a subset of patients, as long as cohort analysis of treatment results is provided to document the outcome of all cases.

TABLE 2

Definitions of tuberculosis cases and treatment outcomes

A. DEFINITIONS OF TUBERCULOSIS CASES

CASE OF TUBERCULOSIS A case of TB which has been bacteriologically confirmed, or has been diagnosed by a clinician.

DEFINITE CASE Patient with positive culture for the *Mycobacterium tuberculosis* complex. In countries where culture is not routinely available a patient with two sputum smears positive for acid-fast bacilli (AFB+) is also considered a definite case.

PULMONARY CASE A case of TB disease involving the lung parenchyma.

SMEAR-POSITIVE PULMONARY CASE At least two initial sputum smear examinations (direct smear microscopy) AFB+; or one sputum examination AFB+ and radiographic abnormalities consistent with active pulmonary tuberculosis as determined by a clinician; or one sputum specimen AFB+ and culture positive for *M. tuberculosis*.

SMEAR-NEGATIVE PULMONARY CASE Pulmonary tuberculosis not meeting the above criteria for smear-positive disease. Diagnostic criteria should include: at least three sputum smear examinations negative for AFB; and radiographic abnormalities consistent with active pulmonary TB; and no response to a course of broad-spectrum antibiotics; and decision by a clinician to treat with a full course of anti-tuberculosis therapy; or positive culture but negative AFB sputum examinations.

EXTRAPULMONARY CASE Patient with tuberculosis of organs other than the lungs e.g. pleura, lymph nodes, abdomen, genitourinary tract, skin, joints and bones, meninges. Diagnosis should be based on one culture-positive specimen, or histological or strong clinical evidence consistent with active extrapulmonary disease, followed by a decision by a clinician to treat with a full course of anti-tuberculosis chemotherapy. Note: a patient diagnosed with both pulmonary and extrapulmonary tuberculosis should be classified as a case of pulmonary tuberculosis.

NEW CASE Patient who has never had treatment for tuberculosis, or who has taken anti-tuberculosis drugs for less than one month.[a]

RELAPSE CASE Patient previously declared cured but with a new episode of bacteriologically positive (sputum smear or culture) tuberculosis.[b]

RE-TREATMENT CASE Patient previously treated for tuberculosis, undergoing treatment for a new episode of bacteriologically positive tuberculosis.[b]

B. DEFINITIONS OF TREATMENT OUTCOMES

(expressed as a percentage of the number registered in the cohort)

CURED Initially smear-positive patient who was smear-negative in the last month of treatment, and on at least one previous occasion.[b]

COMPLETED TREATMENT Patient who completed treatment but did not meet the criteria for cure or failure.

DIED Patient who died for any reason during treatment.

FAILED Smear-positive patient who remained smear-positive at five months or later during treatment.

DEFAULTED Patient whose treatment was interrupted for two consecutive months or more.

TRANSFERRED OUT Patient who transferred to another reporting unit and for whom the treatment outcome is not known.

SUCCESSFULLY TREATED Patients who were cured *and* those that completed treatment.

COHORT A group of TB cases diagnosed (and in principal notified and started on treatment) during a specified time period, e.g., the cohort of new smear-positive cases for the calendar year 2003. This group forms the denominator for calculating treatment outcomes. The sum of the above treatment outcomes, plus any cases for which no outcome is recorded (e.g. still on treatment) should equal the number registered. Some countries monitor outcomes among cohorts defined by smear and/or culture, and define cure and failure according to the best laboratory evidence available for each patient.

[a] Cases reported as "history unknown" in the European Region are included as new cases in this report.

[b] In the EuroTB database, bacteriologically positive re-treatment cases for some countries could not be distinguished from other re-treatment cases. For the purposes of this report, where this occurred, all relapse cases were included in the category "relapse", and the remainder of re-treatment cases (after default and after failure) were included as "re-treatment excluding relapse" (applies to countries in the European Region only).

rates per capita; many of the latter are medium-sized African countries with high rates of TB/HIV coinfection.

The WHO regions are the African Region, the Region of the Americas, the Eastern Mediterranean Region, the European Region, the South-East Asia Region and the Western Pacific Region. All essential statistics are summarized for each of these regions and globally. However, to make clear the differences in epidemiological trends within regions, we divide the African Region into countries that have low and high rates of HIV infection (boundary at an estimated infection rate of 4% in adults aged 15–49 years), and include those countries in the Eastern Mediterranean Region which are actually on the African continent (Djibouti, Somalia and Sudan) in the low-HIV Africa group. Furthermore, we distinguish central from eastern Europe (countries of the former Soviet Union plus Bulgaria and Romania), and combine western European countries with the other established market economies. The countries within each of the resulting nine regions are listed in the legend to Figure 6.

DOTS classification

DOTS is the internationally recommended approach to TB control. It is not simply a clinical approach to patient management, but rather a strategy for TB control primarily within public health systems. Countries reporting to WHO classify themselves as DOTS or non-DOTS, referring to the elements listed in Table 2. DOTS countries must have officially accepted and adopted the strategy, and must have implemented the essential components of DOTS in at least part of the country (Annex 2). Based on NTP responses to standard questions about policy, and usually on further discussion with the NTP, WHO accepts or revises each country's own determination of its DOTS status.

DOTS coverage

Coverage in any country is defined as the percentage of the national population living in areas where health services have adopted DOTS. "Areas" are the lowest administrative or management units in the country –

townships, districts, counties, etc. If an area (with its one or more health facilities) is considered by the NTP to be a DOTS area in 2003, then all the cases registered and reported by the NTP in that area are considered DOTS cases, and the population living within the boundaries of that area counts towards the national DOTS coverage. In some cases, treatment providers who are not following DOTS guidelines (for example private practitioners, or public health services outside the NTP such as those within prisons) notify cases to the NTP. These cases are considered non-DOTS cases, even if they are notified from within DOTS areas. However, when certain groups of patients treated by DOTS services receive special regimens or management (for example nomads placed on long-course treatment), these are considered as DOTS cases. Where possible, additional information about these special groups of patients is provided in the country notes in Annex 2.

Coverage is a crude indicator, which is easy to calculate, and which is most useful during the early stages of DOTS expansion. As a measure of patient access to diagnosis and treatment under DOTS, coverage is an approximation, and usually an overestimate. Where countries are able to provide more precise information about access to DOTS services this information is reported in the country notes of Annex 2. The case detection rate (defined below) is more precise, but also more demanding of data.

Estimating TB incidence, prevalence and death rates
Estimates of incidence, prevalence and deaths are based on a consultative and analytical process; they are revised annually to reflect new information gathered through surveillance and from special studies, such as prevalence surveys. The details of estimation are described elsewhere.[5,6] In brief, estimates of incidence (number of new cases per year) for each country are derived by one or more of four approaches, depending on the available data:

$$(1) \quad \text{incidence} = \frac{\text{case notifications}}{\text{proportion of cases detected}}$$

$$(2) \quad \text{incidence} = \frac{\text{prevalence}}{\text{duration of condition}}$$

$$(3) \quad \text{incidence} = \text{annual risk of infection} \times \text{Stýblo coefficient}$$

$$(4) \quad \text{incidence} = \frac{\text{deaths}}{\text{proportion of incident cases that die}}$$

The "Stýblo coefficient" in equation (3) is taken to be a constant, with an empirically derived value in the range 40–60, relating risk of infection (%) to the incidence of smear-positive cases (per 100 000 per year). Given two of the quantities in any of these equations, we can calculate the third, and any of these formulae can be rearranged to estimate incidence, prevalence and death rates. The available data differ from country to country but include case notifications and death records (from routine surveillance and vital registration), and measures of the prevalence of infection and disease (from population-based surveys).

For each country, estimates of incidence for each year in the period 1995–2003 are made as follows. We first select a reference year for which we have a best estimate of incidence; this may be the year in which a survey was carried out, or the year in which incidence was first estimated. We then use the series of case notifications (all forms of TB) to determine how incidence changed before and after that reference year. The time series of estimated incidence rates is constructed from the notification series in two ways: if the rate of change of incidence is roughly constant through time, we fit exponential trends to the notifications; if the rate of change varies (eastern Europe, central Europe and high-HIV Africa), we use a three-year moving average of the notification rates. If the notifications for any country are considered to be an unreliable guide to trend (e.g. because reporting effort is known to have changed), we apply the aggregated trend for all other countries with reliable data from the same epidemiological region. For China, exceptionally, we have used an assessment of the trend in incidence

based on risk of infection derived from tuberculin surveys. For those countries that have no reliable data from which to assess trends in incidence (e.g. for countries such as Iraq, for which data are hard to interpret, and which are atypical within their own regions), we assume incidence is stable. Further details are available at www.who.int/tb.

For countries that have not yet measured HIV infection rates in TB patients directly, an indirect estimate can be obtained from the incidence rate ratio (IRR, the TB incidence rate in HIV-infected people divided by the incidence rate in HIV-uninfected people), as described elsewhere.[6] The prevalence of MDR-TB among previously untreated TB patients has also been estimated in a separate exercise,[7] supplemented with data from more recent surveys.[8]

Estimates of incidence form the denominator of the case detection rate. Trends in incidence are determined by underlying epidemiological processes, modified by control programmes. The impact of control on prevalence is determined by the trend in incidence, and by the estimated

---

[5] Dye C et al. Global burden of tuberculosis: estimated incidence, prevalence and mortality by country. *Journal of the American Medical Association*, 1999, 282: 677–686.

[6] Corbett EL et al. The growing burden of tuberculosis: global trends and interactions with the HIV epidemic. *Archives of Internal Medicine*, 2003, 163:1009–1021.

[7] Dye C et al. Worldwide incidence of multidrug-resistant tuberculosis. *Journal of Infectious Diseases*, 2002, 185:1197–1202.

[8] *Anti-tuberculosis drug resistance in the world. Report No.3.* WHO/IUATLD Global Project on Anti-Tuberculosis Drug Resistance Surveillance. Geneva, World Health Organization, 2004 (WHO/HTM/TB/2004.343).

reduction in the duration of the condition, e.g. smear-positive disease. The impact of control on deaths is determined by the trend in incidence, and by the estimated reduction in case fatality (proportion of incident cases that ever die from TB).[5,6]

Where population sizes are needed to calculate TB indicators, we use the latest revision of estimates provided by the United Nations Population Division,[9] even though these estimates sometimes differ from those made by the countries themselves (some of which are based on more recent census data). The estimates of some TB indicators, such as the case detection rate, are derived from data and calculations that use only rates per capita, and discrepancies in population sizes do not affect these indicators. Where rates per capita are used as a basis for calculating numbers of TB cases, these discrepancies sometimes do make a difference. Some examples of important differences are given in the country notes in Annex 2.

Case detection rate
Smear-positive cases are the focus of DOTS programmes because they are the principal sources of infection to others, because sputum smear microscopy is a highly-specific (if somewhat insensitive) method of diagnosis, and because patients with smear-positive disease typically suffer higher rates of morbidity and mortality than smear-negative patients. As a measure of the quality of diagnosis, we calculate the proportion of new sputum smear-positive cases out of all new pulmonary cases, which has an expected value of 65–80% in areas with negligible HIV prevalence.[10] However, this report presents the numbers of all TB cases notified, smear-positive and smear-negative pulmonary cases, in addition to those in whom extra-pulmonary disease is diagnosed.

The term "case detection", as used here, means that TB is diagnosed (correctly or incorrectly) in a patient, and is reported within the national surveillance system, and then to WHO. The case detection rate is calculated as the ratio of the number of notified smear-positive cases to the number of new smear-positive cases esti-

mated for that year. Detection is presented in two ways – as the case detection rate (countrywide) and as the DOTS case detection rate (by DOTS programmes):

$$
\text{(5)} \quad \text{case detection rate} = \frac{\text{annual new smear-positive notifications (country)}}{\text{estimated annual new smear-positive incidence (country)}}
$$

$$
\text{(6)} \quad \text{DOTS case detection rate} = \frac{\text{annual new smear-positive notifications (DOTS)}}{\text{estimated annual new smear-positive incidence (country)}}
$$

The case detection rate and the DOTS case detection rate are identical when a country reports only from DOTS areas. This generally happens when DOTS coverage is 100% but, in some countries where DOTS is implemented in only part of the country, no TB notifications are received from the non-DOTS areas. Furthermore, in some countries where DOTS coverage is 100%, patients may choose to seek treatment from non-DOTS providers, who in some cases notify TB cases to the national authorities.

Both of the above definitions of the case detection rate refer to smear-positive cases, although we also present the detection rate for all forms of TB. The detection rate of all forms is similarly presented in two ways: detection by DOTS programmes, and detection countrywide.

Although these indices are termed "rates", they are actually ratios. The number of cases notified is usually smaller than estimated incidence because of incomplete coverage by health services, under-diagnosis, or deficient recording and reporting. However, the calculated detection rate can exceed 100% if case-finding has been intense in an area that has a backlog of chronic cases, if there has been over-reporting (e.g. double-counting) or over-diagnosis, or if estimates of incidence are too low. If the expected number of cases per year is very low (especially if it is less than one), the case detection rate can vary markedly from year to year due to chance. Whenever this index comes close to or exceeds 100%, we attempt to investigate, as part of the joint planning and evaluation process with NTPs, which of these explanations is correct.

The ratio of the DOTS case detec-

tion rate to coverage estimates the case detection rate within DOTS areas (as distinct from the case detection rate nationwide), assuming that the TB incidence rate is homogeneous across counties, districts, provinces, or other administrative units. Ideally, this ratio would have a value of 70% or more as DOTS coverage increases within any country. Where the value of this indicator is much lower, it is clear that the DOTS programme has been poorly implemented, at least in some parts of the designated DOTS area. Changes in the value of this ratio through time are a measure of changes in the quality of TB control, after the DOTS programme has been established.

Treatment success
Treatment success in DOTS programmes is the percentage of new smear-positive patients that are cured (negative on sputum smear examination), plus the percentage that complete a course of treatment, without bacteriological confirmation of cure (Table 2).[11] Cure and completion are among the six mutually exclusive outcomes.[12] The sum of cases assigned to these outcomes, plus any additional cases registered but not assigned to

[9] *World population prospects – the 2002 revision.* New York, United Nations Population Division, 2003.

[10] *Tuberculosis handbook.* Geneva, World Health Organization, 1998 (WHO/TB/ 98.253).

[11] TB control programmes should ensure high treatment success before expanding case detection. The reason is that a proportion of patients given less than a fully-curative course of treatment remain chronically infectious, and continue to spread TB. Thus DOTS programmes must be shown to achieve high cure rates in pilot projects before attempting countrywide coverage.

[12] *Treatment of tuberculosis: Guidelines for national programmes.* Third edition. Geneva, World Health Organization, 2003 (WHO/CDS/TB/2003.313).

an outcome, adds up to 100% of cases registered (i.e. the treatment cohort).

We also compare the number of new smear-positive cases registered for treatment (for this report, in 2002) with the number of cases notified as smear-positive (also in 2002). All notified cases should be registered for treatment, and the numbers notified and registered should therefore be the same (discrepancies arise e.g. when subnational reports are not received at national level). If the number registered for treatment is not provided we take, as the denominator for treatment outcomes, the number notified for that cohort year. If the sum of the six outcome categories is greater than the number registered (or the number notified), we use this sum as the denominator.

Because the number of patients presenting for a second or subsequent course of treatment, and the outcome of further treatment, are indicative of NTP performance and levels of drug resistance, we have begun to compile these data in this report. We present the numbers of patients registered for re-treatment, and the outcomes of re-treatment, for each of three registration types: re-treatment after relapse, failure or default. However, some countries do not yet compile data on cases registered for re-treatment after failure and default separately at national level. Furthermore, some countries do not have outcome data for each of these re-treament case types.

The assessment of outcomes for a given calendar year always lags notifications by one year to ensure that all patients registered during that calendar year have completed treatment. A DOTS country must report treatment outcomes, unless it is newly-classified as DOTS, in which case it would take an additional year to report outcomes from the first cohort of patients treated.

Overview of data in annexes

Annex 1 presents data on epidemiology and surveillance, and planning and financing for each of the 22 HBCs. Data on policy and strategy are collected for both DOTS and non-DOTS areas separately.

Annex 2 contains the estimates needed to evaluate MDG Target 8 and indicators 23 and 24. These data include case detection and treatment success rates to monitor DOTS implementation, and incidence, prevalence and death rates to monitor the impact of TB control.

These data are presented, for each of the six WHO regions, as follows:

- TB control policies for each country, stating which technical components of the DOTS strategy have been implemented;

- incidence, prevalence and death rates for 1990 (MDG reference year) and 2003;

- case notifications, detection rates, and DOTS coverage: nationally, and separately for DOTS and non-DOTS programmes. Notifications include new pulmonary cases (smear-positive, smear-negative and laboratory-confirmed), new extrapulmonary and re-treatment cases;

- treatment outcomes for 2002 cohorts: both the new smear-positive and the re-treatment cohorts from DOTS programmes (relapse, re-treatment after default and re-treatment after failure are presented separately where possible, as well as all re-treatment cases combined), and the new smear-positive treatment outcomes (where available) from non-DOTS programmes;

- new smear-positive notification rates by age and sex for the whole country;

- new smear-positive notifications (numbers) by age and sex, from DOTS and non-DOTS programmes;

- notification rates and numbers since 1980, for all forms of TB;

- notification rates and numbers since 1995, for new smear-positive cases;

- country notes: remarks that may help to explain data reported by selected countries (e.g. additional breakdown of cases of interest, late-reported data, reasons for incomplete data, discrepancies in estimated population sizes).

The data in Annex 2 are available as Excel spreadsheets from www.who.int/tb.

Planning and DOTS implementation

The information on strategic planning analysed and presented in this report reflects activities from July 2003 to June 2004. Country plans and activities are monitored through several mechanisms, including direct discussion with NTP managers, analysis of a questionnaire on planning and implementation sent by WHO to all HBCs during 2004 (available from www.who.int/tb), collaboration with international technical agencies, monitoring missions, comprehensive programme reviews, GFATM applications, regional NTP managers' meetings, and the annual meeting of the DOTS Expansion Working Group (DEWG) of the Stop TB Partnership. In writing this report, WHO staff worked with NTP managers of the 22 HBCs to:

- assess national TB control activities planned and carried out during 2004, focusing on activities to improve political commitment, expand access to DOTS, strengthen diagnosis, improve treatment outcomes, ensure adequate staffing, and improve programme monitoring and supervision;

- update the country profiles to summarize progress made by the end of 2004 in implementing, or scaling up, national plans for DOTS expansion;

- analyse constraints to reaching the targets for detection and treatment success;

- review and revise the list of partners operating in, or on behalf of, each country;

- assess levels of drug resistance and activities planned to address MDR-TB, including mechanisms of drug-resistance surveillance, MDR-TB diagnosis and treatment policies, and the availability of second-line drugs;

- determine the status of collaborative TB/HIV activities;

- determine the status of additional strategies to expand DOTS, and to involve community and health-care providers not currently participating in the provision of DOTS.

Planning activities carried out in 2003
In preparation for the 5th DEWG meeting (Paris, France, 27–28 October 2004), NTP managers for the 22 HBCs were asked to summarize what activities had been planned for implementation during 2003, which of those activities were implemented, which were not and why, and what corrective actions were taken so that these activities could be implemented in 2004. The information from these DEWG summary tables, supplemented with additional information provided by NTP managers and by WHO staff, is incorporated into the country profiles (Annex 1).

Update of country profiles
Country profiles (Annex 1) were updated by incorporating information from the following sources: summary tables prepared for the 5th DEWG; country posters presented by the 22 HBCs at the DEWG meeting; questionnaires submitted by the 22 HBCs; and consultations with, and reviews of, the country profiles by NTP staff and collaborating technical agencies.

Constraints and remedial actions
Following the previous analysis of constraints to DOTS expansion and remedial actions proposed,[13] this year's report provides an update. Constraints and remedial actions were assessed with information provided at the DEWG meeting, and through personal communications with NTP managers and staff. Special attention was devoted to constraints related to laboratory services and human resources.

Partnerships and coordination
The list of donors and collaborating organizations was updated in consultation with NTP managers, WHO regional and country offices and partners. Major technical agencies, along with financial partners, are listed in each country profile. The coordination of these numerous agencies is vital for the efficient use of limited resources within countries, and is facilitated through a formal coordination mechanism, such as the national interagency coordinating committee (NICC).

Management of drug resistance
Data on the prevalence of drug resistance are collected through the WHO/IUATLD Global Project on Anti-tuberculosis Drug Resistance Surveillance (DRS), which began in 1994, and which published its third report in 2004.[8] Profiles of the 22 HBCs contain estimates of the national prevalence of MDR-TB among previously untreated TB patients based on survey data for those countries participating in the WHO/IUATLD project. For those countries that have not carried out surveys, figures given in the country profiles are estimates.

WHO develops global policy on the management of MDR-TB and facilitates access to second-line drugs through the Green Light Committee (GLC).[14] As part of this process, and under the continuous monitoring of the GLC, several DOTS-Plus pilot projects are evaluating the feasibility and cost-effectiveness of using second-line drugs for managing MDR-TB in countries with limited resources. Projects approved by the GLC have access to quality-assured, second-line drugs at reduced prices and benefit from technical support and external monitoring. This report summarizes the number and status of GLC-approved DOTS-Plus projects that had been established by 2004.

Collaborative TB/HIV activities
WHO has published an interim policy on collaborative TB/HIV activities[15] that outlines the methods and benefits of collaboration between HIV and TB programmes. Three main areas of collaboration are recommended. First, organizational structures should be set up to plan and manage collaborative TB/HIV activities. Second, people infected with HIV should be screened for TB, treated if they have active disease, and offered isoniazid preventive therapy as needed. Third, TB patients should be offered voluntary counselling and testing for HIV infection (VCT); if positive, they should be offered co-trimoxazole preventive therapy and, wherever possible, ART. WHO has also developed a guide for monitoring and evaluating collaborative TB/HIV activities that defines indicators for each of the key activities recommended in the interim policy.[16]

To investigate progress in implementing the recommended collaborative TB/HIV activities, countries were asked, via the standard WHO data collection form, to report on the extent to which TB patients were tested for HIV, assessed for ART and provided with ART during 2003. A supplementary questionnaire (available at www.who.int/tb) was sent to the 41 countries that have the highest incidence rates of TB with HIV coinfection. This questionnaire asked specifically about policy developments between 2002 and 2003. The data obtained from both forms were reviewed at WHO regional offices and headquarters, and any inconsistencies or missing data were discussed with the national correspondent before being included in the analysis.

Additional strategies for DOTS expansion
This report covers three areas:

- PPM initiatives that aim to bring a greater diversity of health-care providers into DOTS programmes, promoting the essential package of patient care and improving reporting and monitoring procedures;

- community participation that improves access to care and fosters a patient-centered approach to the management of TB. While the type and scope of community involve-

---

[13] *Global tuberculosis control: surveillance, planning, financing. WHO report 2004.* Geneva, World Health Organization (WHO/HTM/TB/2004.331).

[14] Gupta R et al. Increasing transparency in partnerships for health – introducing the Green Light Committee. *Tropical Medicine and International Health*, 2002, 7:970–976.

[15] *Interim policy on collaborative TB/HIV activities.* Geneva, World Health Organization, 2004 (WHO/HTM/TB/2004.330; WHO/HTM/HIV/2004.1).

[16] *A guide to monitoring and evaluation for collaborative TB/HIV activities.* Geneva, World Health Organization, 2004 (WHO/HTM/TB/2004.342; WHO/HIV/2004.09).

ment depends upon location and context, many HBCs regard civil society as an essential partner in providing support to patients and their families;

- the feasibility of implementing the Practical Approach to Lung Health (PAL), which several countries are examining, and assessing its potential impact on TB case detection and on the rationalization of drug prescriptions.

In addition to the findings presented in this report, further details of PPM, TB/HIV, PAL and other projects can be found at www.who.int/tb.

Financing DOTS expansion

The financial analysis in this series of annual reports on global TB control has evolved and improved since being introduced in 2002.[17] The main developments in this year's report are: (a) to place greater emphasis on the presentation and analysis of trends, with each HBC profile including budget and cost data for four years; and (b) to provide a more complete analysis of data for countries other than the HBCs. The report has eight objectives:

- for each HBC, and for all HBCs combined, to present trends in total NTP budgets and expenditures for the period 2002–2005, with breakdowns by funding source and line item;

- for each HBC and for all HBCs combined, to present trends in total TB control costs[18] for the period 2002–2005, with breakdowns by funding source and line item;

- for each HBC and for all HBCs combined, to assess trends in NTP budgets and total TB control costs, giving particular attention to where progress has been made and where major funding gaps persist;

- for each HBC, to estimate and compare per patient costs, budgets and available funding for the period 2002–2005 and per patient expenditures for 2002 and 2003;

- for HBCs, to assess the relationship between gross national income (GNI) per capita and (a) per

patient costs and (b) the fraction of funds contributed by the government;

- for HBCs, to assess whether projected budgets and available funding will be sufficient to achieve the global targets for case detection and treatment success;

- to assess the contribution of the GFATM to funding for TB control;

- for countries other than the HBCs, to quantify NTP budgets and funding gaps in 2004 and 2005.

Data collection

We collected data from five main sources: NTPs, the WHO-CHOICE web site,[19] costing guidelines developed for the "Disease Control Priorities in Developing Countries" project (DCPP),[20] GFATM proposals and databases, and previous WHO reports in this series. In 2004, data were collected directly from countries by means of a two-page questionnaire included in the standard WHO data collection form. NTP managers were asked to complete three tables. The first two tables required a summary of the NTP budget for fiscal years 2004 and 2005 in US$, broken down by line item and funding source (including a column for funding gaps). The third table requested NTP expenditure data for 2003, broken down by line item and source of funding. The form also requested information about dedicated TB control infrastructure and the way in which general health infrastructure is used for TB control – for example, the number of dedicated TB beds that exist, the number of outpatient visits that patients need to make to a health facility during treatment and the average number of days for which patients are hospitalized. We also asked for an estimate of the number of patients that would be treated in 2004 and 2005. We used the WHO-CHOICE web site to identify the average costs, in international dollars (I$), of a hospital bed-day and an outpatient clinic visit in every country. The costing guidelines for the DCPP and the WHO-CHOICE web site were used to identify the purchasing power parity (PPP) exchange rates re-

quired for conversion of I$ costs to costs in US$ (for consistency with budget and expenditure data reported on the data collection form).

Data entry and analysis

High-burden countries. Data entry and analysis focused on the 22 HBCs. We created a standardized spreadsheet, with one worksheet for each country. Additional worksheets were included for summary analyses and for the data required as inputs to the analyses in each country worksheet (e.g. notification data, unit costs for bed-days and outpatient clinic visits, and the typical number of outpatient clinic visits and days in hospital for different types of patient during treatment). For each country worksheet, seven tables were created. These were:

- NTP budget by source of funding for each year 2002–2005, with the funding sources defined according to the 2004 data collection form i.e. government (excluding loans), loans, grants (excluding GFATM), GFATM and budget gap;

- NTP budget by line item for each year 2002–2005, with the line items defined according to the 2004 data collection form i.e. first-line drugs, second-line drugs, dedicated NTP staff, initiatives to increase case detection and cure rates, collaborative TB/HIV activities, buildings/equipment and other;

- NTP expenditures by source of funding for 2002 and 2003, with funding sources as defined for NTP budgets;

- NTP expenditures by line item for 2002 and 2003, with line items defined as for NTP budgets;

[17] *Global tuberculosis control: surveillance, planning, financing. WHO report 2002.* Geneva, World Health Organization, 2002 (WHO/CDS/TB/2002.295).

[18] i.e. including costs not reflected in NTP budget data.

[19] www3.who.int/whosis/cea/prices/unit.

[20] *DCPP guidelines for authors*, pp. 74–77, (available at www.fic.nih.gov/dcpp/authorguide.pdf, accessed 11 January 2005).

- total TB control costs by funding source for each year 2002–2005, with funding sources defined as for NTP budgets;

- total TB control costs by line item for each year 2002–2005, with the line items defined as NTP budget items, hospitalization and clinic visits;

- per patient costs, NTP budget, available funding, expenditures and budget for first-line drugs.

Budget data for 2004 and 2005 were taken from the 2004 data collection form. Budget data for 2002 and 2003 were taken from the 2002 and 2004 annual reports, respectively. Expenditure data for 2002 and 2003 were based on the 2003 and 2004 data collection forms, respectively. Total TB control costs were estimated by adding costs for hospitalization and outpatient clinic visits to either NTP expenditures (for 2002 and 2003) or NTP budgets (for 2004 and 2005).[21] Expenditures were used in preference to budgets for 2002 and 2003 because they reflect actual costs, whereas budgets can be higher than actual expenditures (for example, when large budgetary funding gaps exist or the NTP does not spend all the available funding). When expenditures are known for 2004 and 2005, they will be used instead of budget data to calculate, retrospectively, the total cost of TB control in these years. For some HBCs, expenditures were not available for 2002 and 2003. When this was the case, we estimated expenditures based on available funding, which was calculated as the total budget minus the funding gap.

The cost of outpatient clinic visits was estimated in three steps. First, we converted I$ prices for clinic visits reported on the WHO-CHOICE web site into US$ prices using the DCPP exchange rates. Second, we multiplied the average number of visits required per patient (estimated on the WHO data collection form) by the average cost (in US$) per clinic visit, to give the cost per patient treated. Third, we multiplied the cost per patient treated by the number of patients notified (for 2002 or 2003) or the number of pa-

tients that the NTP projects will be treated (for 2004 and 2005). The cost of hospitalization was generally calculated in the same way, replacing the unit cost of a clinic visit with the unit cost of a bed-day. The procedure differed for eight countries that have dedicated TB beds, and where the total cost of these beds is higher than implied by multiplying bed-days per patient by the number of patients treated (this applied to Brazil, Cambodia, India, Nigeria, the Russian Federation, the United Republic of Tanzania, Viet Nam and Zimbabwe). We assumed that all clinic visits and hospitalization are funded by the government.

Per patient costs, budgets, available funding and expenditures were calculated by dividing the relevant total by the number of cases notified (for 2002 and 2003) and the number of patients that the NTP projects will be treated (for 2004 and 2005). Since the total costs of TB control for 2002 and 2003 were based on expenditure data, it is possible for the total TB control cost per patient treated to be less than the NTP budget per patient treated when the funding gap is large or there is an important budgetary under-spend. In addition, for 2002 and 2003, the expenditure per patient was sometimes higher than the available funding per patient. This can occur when some of the NTP budget funding gap is closed following the reporting of budget data to WHO.

All data are reported in nominal prices (i.e. they have not been adjusted for inflation) rather than constant prices (i.e. all data are adjusted to a common year of prices) for two reasons. First, this avoids adjustment of values reported in the 2002–2004 reports in this series, which makes it easier for country staff to review the data for previous years. Second, the adjustment will make only a limited difference to the numbers reported (about 5% to 2002 values and less for other years). However, as data are collected for an increasing number of years, presentation of data in constant prices will be necessary.

Following data entry, text on data sources and assumptions were added. Where there were questions

about the data, these were discussed with NTP staff and the appropriate WHO regional and country office. These discussions were used to produce a final set of charts. Four of these charts appear in the profiles for each country at Annex 1: NTP budget by funding source, NTP budget by line item, total TB control costs by line item, and per patient costs, budgets, available funding, expenditures and budget for first-line drugs. These charts were selected because they illustrate the most important trends in financing, while other data are referred to in the text. A full set of charts and data is available upon request. In some instances, the review process led to revisions to data included in previous annual reports. For this reason, figures sometimes differ from those reported in the 2002, 2003 and 2004 reports.

Finally, we compared the total costs of TB control with total government health expenditures to estimate the percentage of total government health expenditures used for TB control. Total government health expenditures were estimated by multiplying the government health expenditure per capita in US$ (as estimated in the WHO national health accounts database)[22] by population size. We also explored the association between GNI per capita in 2003 and (a) government contributions to total NTP budgets and TB control costs, and (b) the cost per patient treated. Data on GNI per capita were taken from *World development indicators 2004*.[23]

Other countries. The data provided by countries other than the HBCs were less complete, and as a consequence our analyses to date are more superficial. We used the data provided on the 2004 data collection form to assess NTP budgets by region, and com-

---

[21] The exception was South Africa, because no data on hospitalization and clinic visits, or on NTP budgets, were provided in the data collection form. Costs were therefore estimated based on recent costing studies, as described in previous WHO reports in this series.

[22] www.who.int/nha/country/en/.

[23] www.worldbank.org/data/wdi2004/.

pared these with the budgets reported by the HBCs. Only countries that submitted complete data of sufficient quality (e.g. subtotals and totals were consistent by both line item and funding source) were used.

GFATM contribution to TB control
We assessed GFATM funding for both HBCs and other countries, as announced after the first four rounds of funding. We assessed total approved funding at the end of 2004, how the amounts in signed grant agreements compared with those in the original proposals, disbursements to the end of 2004, the time taken between approval of a proposal and the signature of grant agreements, and the time taken between the signing of the grant agreement and the first disbursement of funds.

Results

Progress towards the Millennium Development Goals

Countries reporting to WHO

By the end of 2004, 199 (94%) of 211 countries and territories reported case notifications for 2003 and/or treatment outcomes for patients registered in 2002. These countries include 99% of the world's population. WHO received reports from all 22 HBCs.

Case notifications and incidence

The 199 countries reporting to WHO in 2003 notified 4.4 million new and relapse cases, of which 1.9 million (44%) were new sputum smear-positive (Table 3; Figure 1). Among these notifications, 3.7 million were from DOTS areas, including 1.8 million smear-positives. A total of 17.1 million cases, and 8.6 million smear-positives, were notified by DOTS programmes between 1995 and 2003. Based on surveillance and survey data, we estimate that there were 8.8 million new cases of TB in 2003 (140 per 100 000), including 3.9 million (62 per 100 000) smear-positive cases (Table 4; Figure 2).

The African Region (24%), South-East Asia Region (35%), and Western Pacific Region (22%) together ac-counted for 82% of all notified cases and similar proportions of new smear-positive cases. Because DOTS emphasizes diagnosis by sputum smear microscopy, 47% of all new and relapse cases were smear-positive (45–60% expected) in DOTS areas, compared with 29% elsewhere. Similarly, 58% of new pulmonary cases were smear-positive under DOTS (55–70% expected), compared with 35% elsewhere (Table 3).

The ranking of countries by number of incident TB cases has drawn attention to the 22 HBCs, but the magnitude of the TB burden in individual

TABLE 3
Case notifications, 2003

	ALL NEW AND RELAPSE CASES		NEW SMEAR-POSITIVE		NEW SMEAR-NEGATIVE OR SMEAR UNKNOWN		NEW EXTRAPULMONARY		RE-TREATMENT CASES EXCLUDING RELAPSE		OTHER[a]		% OF NEW PULMONARY CASES SMEAR POSITIVE[b]	
	DOTS	NON-DOTS	DOTS	NON-DOTS	DOTS	NON-DOTS	DOTS	NON-DOTS	DOTS	NON-DOTS	DOTS	NON-DOTS	DOTS	NON-DOTS
1 India	836 768	236 297	372 088	61 183	305 921	153 503	112 064	20 189	102 542	13 247	–	–	55	29
2 China	553 677	62 191	257 287	10 127	206 493	42 312	27 804	2 964	64 887	2 822	–	–	55	19
3 Indonesia	178 260	–	92 566	–	77 561	–	4 047	–	–	–	–	–	54	–
4 Nigeria	44 184	–	28 173	–	13 276	–	1 525	–	2 151	–	261	–	68	–
5 Bangladesh	88 156	–	53 618	–	24 913	–	7 120	–	–	–	–	–	68	–
6 Pakistan	73 100	–	20 962	–	34 447	–	12 874	–	3 184	–	–	–	38	–
7 Ethiopia	117 600	–	39 698	–	35 141	–	40 883	–	676	–	–	–	53	–
8 South Africa	227 278	42	116 331	33	56 535	5	37 682	4	28 094	8	–	–	67	87
9 Philippines	134 375	–	72 670	–	55 942	–	1 693	–	–	–	–	–	57	–
10 Kenya	91 522	–	38 158	–	37 135	–	13 403	–	1 127	–	2 661	–	51	–
11 DR Congo	84 687	–	53 578	–	9 352	–	18 357	–	1 641	–	387	–	85	–
12 Russian Federation	21 064	102 977	6 322	22 546	12 780	72 252	1 016	3 648	–	22 512	851	4 840	33	24
13 Viet Nam	92 741	–	55 937	–	16 791	–	14 564	–	680	–	–	–	77	–
14 UR Tanzania	61 579	–	24 899	–	21 911	–	12 959	–	378	–	2 708	–	53	–
15 Brazil	16 560	63 554	9 061	30 877	4 795	18 727	1 503	9 081	799	3 663	1 256	2 690	65	62
16 Uganda	41 805	–	20 320	–	16 612	–	3 249	–	–	–	1 096	–	55	–
17 Thailand	54 504	–	28 459	–	17 596	–	6 756	–	–	–	–	–	62	–
18 Mozambique	28 602	–	16 138	–	7 847	–	3 441	–	505	–	–	–	67	–
19 Zimbabwe	53 183	–	14 488	–	28 246	–	8 916	–	–	–	3 934	–	34	–
20 Myanmar	75 744	–	27 448	–	26 006	–	17 796	–	2 451	–	–	–	51	–
21 Afghanistan	13 808	–	6 510	–	3 440	–	3 254	–	141	–	–	–	65	–
22 Cambodia	28 216	–	18 923	–	4 307	–	4 232	–	79	–	91	–	81	–
High-burden countries	**2 917 413**	**465 061**	**1 373 634**	**124 766**	**1 017 047**	**286 799**	**355 138**	**35 886**	**209 335**	**42 252**	**13 245**	**7 530**	**57**	**30**
AFR	1 061 882	10 789	503 217	6 947	319 715	2 513	193 812	1 013	39 548	403	19 902	–	61	73
AMR	142 409	85 142	82 479	43 324	31 761	24 210	19 936	11 835	4 208	4 259	5 909	3 154	72	64
EMR	206 160	3 781	80 822	191	63 703	2 099	51 417	1 488	4 015	–	178	–	56	8
EUR	142 760	195 883	44 673	50 839	64 716	96 592	16 547	12 085	7 334	25 316	22 292	54 198	41	34
SEAR	1 314 983	240 402	610 079	62 799	481 487	155 219	160 093	20 772	107 746	13 408	9 845	583	56	29
WPR	879 827	108 100	431 396	23 336	313 113	63 566	59 422	11 084	66 352	3 563	3 262	3 746	58	27
Global	**3 748 021**	**644 097**	**1 752 666**	**187 436**	**1 274 495**	**344 199**	**501 227**	**58 277**	**229 203**	**46 949**	**61 388**	**61 681**	**58**	**35**

– Indicates not applicable or not available.

[a] Cases not included elsewhere in table.

[b] Expected percentage of new pulmonary cases that are smear-positive is 65–80%.

FIGURE 1
Tuberculosis notification rates, 2003

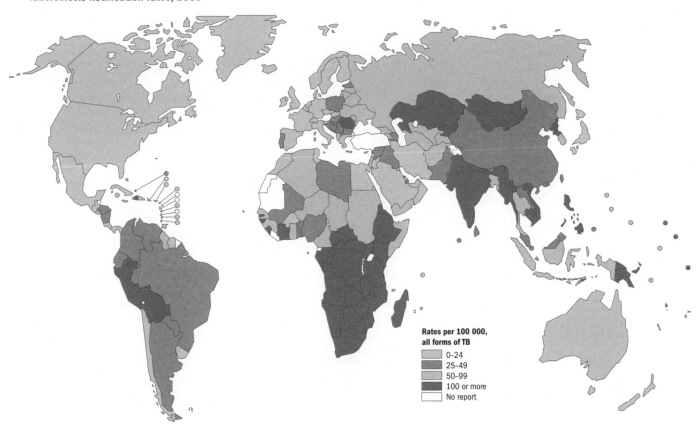

Rates per 100 000,
all forms of TB
- 0–24
- 25–49
- 50–99
- 100 or more
- No report

FIGURE 2
Estimated TB incidence rates, 2003

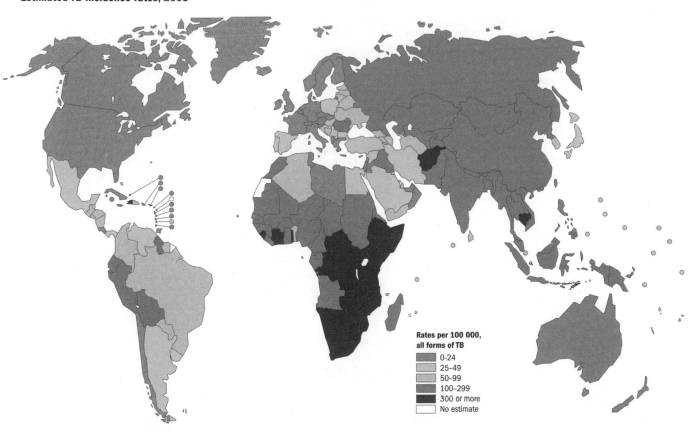

Rates per 100 000,
all forms of TB
- 0–24
- 25–49
- 50–99
- 100–299
- 300 or more
- No estimate

TABLE 4
Estimated TB burden, 2003

| | | INCIDENCE | | | | PREVALENCE | | MORTALITY | |
| | | ALL CASES | | SMEAR-POSITIVE CASES | | ALL FORMS OF TB, INCLUDING IN HIV-INFECTED PEOPLE | | | |
	POPULATION 1000s	NUMBER 1000s	RATE PER 100 000 POP.	NUMBER 1000s	RATE PER 100 000 POP.	NUMBER 1000s	RATE PER 100 000 POP.	NUMBER 1000s	RATE PER 100 000 POP.
1 India	1 065 462	1 788	168	798	75	3 086	290	352	33
2 China	1 304 196	1 334	102	600	46	3 203	246	236	18
3 Indonesia	219 883	627	285	282	128	1 484	675	143	65
4 Nigeria	124 009	363	293	156	126	677	546	105	85
5 Bangladesh	146 736	361	246	162	111	719	490	84	57
6 Pakistan	153 578	278	181	125	82	551	359	67	43
7 Ethiopia	70 678	252	356	109	155	377	533	56	79
8 South Africa	45 026	242	536	98	218	206	458	33	73
9 Philippines	79 999	237	296	107	133	366	458	39	49
10 Kenya	31 987	195	610	84	262	283	884	43	133
11 DR Congo	52 771	195	369	85	160	298	564	43	81
12 Russian Federation	143 246	161	112	72	50	229	160	29	20
13 Viet Nam	81 377	145	178	65	80	195	240	19	23
14 UR Tanzania	36 977	137	371	58	157	194	524	32	86
15 Brazil	178 470	110	62	49	28	164	92	15	8
16 Uganda	25 827	106	411	46	179	168	652	25	96
17 Thailand	62 833	89	142	40	63	130	208	12	19
18 Mozambique	18 863	86	457	36	190	120	636	24	129
19 Zimbabwe	12 891	85	659	34	265	85	660	20	153
20 Myanmar	49 485	85	171	38	76	92	187	12	25
21 Afghanistan	23 897	80	333	36	150	160	671	22	93
22 Cambodia	14 144	72	508	32	225	108	762	13	95
High-burden countries	**3 942 338**	**7 027**	**178**	**3 112**	**79**	**12 896**	**327**	**1 423**	**36**
AFR	687 405	2 372	345	1 013	147	3 487	507	538	78
AMR	867 768	370	43	165	19	503	58	54	6
EMR	518 063	634	122	285	55	1 120	216	144	28
EUR	878 902	439	50	196	22	577	66	67	8
SEAR	1 614 648	3 062	190	1 370	85	5 662	351	617	38
WPR	1 732 104	1 933	112	868	50	4 081	236	327	19
Global	**6 298 890**	**8 810**	**140**	**3 897**	**62**	**15 430**	**245**	**1 747**	**28**

FIGURE 3

Fifteen countries with the highest estimated TB incidence rates per capita (all ages, all forms; grey bars) and corresponding incidence rates of HIV-infected TB (among adults aged 15–49 years; blue bars), 2003

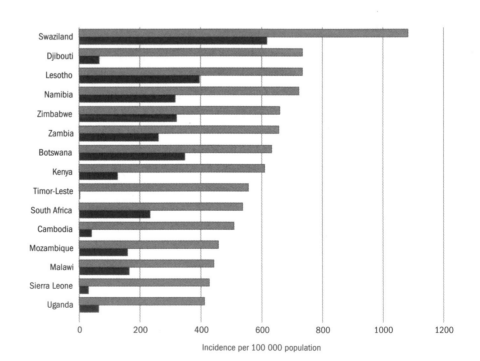

Incidence per 100 000 population

countries is better expressed as the incidence rate per capita. Among the 15 countries with the highest estimated TB incidence rates per capita, 12 are in Africa (Figure 3).

Case notifications from African countries show other patterns that are likely to be associated with HIV infection. First, women aged 15–24 years make up a higher proportion of TB cases in countries with higher rates of HIV infection (Figure 4a). This is consistent with the observation that HIV prevalence tends to be higher in women than men in this age range, and the difference between the sexes is bigger where HIV infection rates are higher. Second, the average age of smear-positive TB cases is typically lower where HIV infection rates are higher, especially for women (Figure 4b). This is another sign that younger rather than older women are more likely to be infected with HIV. Third, the proportion of smear-negative cases among all pulmonary TB cases tends to be higher in African countries with higher rates of HIV infection (data not shown). However, this last association is weak ($R^2 = 0.16$, $P = 0.02$) and could be confounded by the quality of diagnosis if, for example, smear microscopy has become less reliable where the number of HIV-infected TB patients has increased substantially.

Some patterns in the case notification data are striking, but not easy to explain. For example, the number of extrapulmonary TB cases as a proportion of the total reported is consistently different among WHO regions. Between 1995 and 2003, the proportion was lowest in the Western Pacific Region (mostly <5%) and highest in the Eastern Mediterranean Region (20–30%; see Figure 5). We do not know whether these are real epidemiological differences, or due to regional diagnostic biases. Surprisingly, the proportion of cases diagnosed as extrapulmonary disease has not increased in the African Region, despite the growing impact of HIV on the TB epidemic. This raises the question of whether NTPs in Africa are missing extrapulmonary cases.

Using the series of notifications of all TB cases from countries thought to have reliable data, and scaling by

FIGURE 4

(a) The proportion of notified TB patients aged 15–24 years that were women, in relation to HIV prevalence in adults aged 15–49 years ($R^2 = 0.63$, $P<0.0001$). (b) Average age of women with smear-positive TB, in relation to HIV prevalence in adults aged 15–49 years ($R^2 = 0.46$, $P<0.0001$). Data are for countries in Africa.

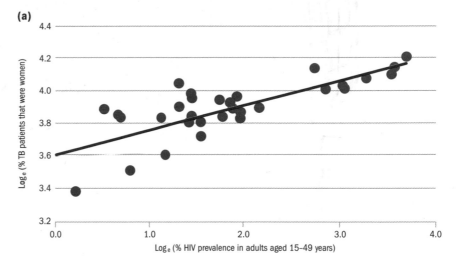

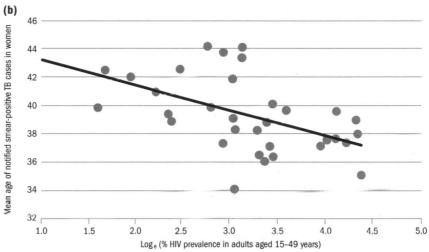

FIGURE 5

The number of extrapulmonary TB cases as a percentage of the total number of cases reported, for each of the six WHO regions

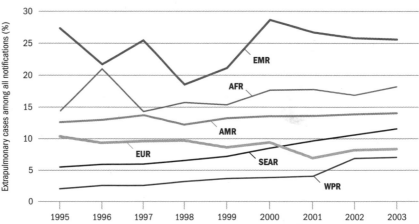

FIGURE 6

Trends in estimated TB incidence rates (all forms; blue lines), and the annual change in incidence rates (black lines), for nine groups of countries, 1990–2003

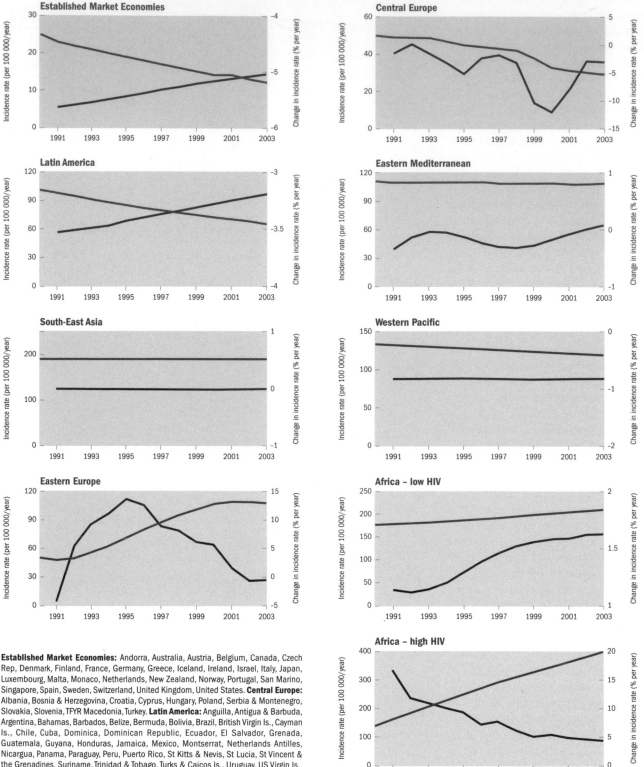

Established Market Economies: Andorra, Australia, Austria, Belgium, Canada, Czech Rep, Denmark, Finland, France, Germany, Greece, Iceland, Ireland, Israel, Italy, Japan, Luxembourg, Malta, Monaco, Netherlands, New Zealand, Norway, Portugal, San Marino, Singapore, Spain, Sweden, Switzerland, United Kingdom, United States. **Central Europe:** Albania, Bosnia & Herzegovina, Croatia, Cyprus, Hungary, Poland, Serbia & Montenegro, Slovakia, Slovenia, TFYR Macedonia, Turkey. **Latin America:** Anguilla, Antigua & Barbuda, Argentina, Bahamas, Barbados, Belize, Bermuda, Bolivia, Brazil, British Virgin Is., Cayman Is., Chile, Cuba, Dominica, Dominican Republic, Ecuador, El Salvador, Grenada, Guatemala, Guyana, Honduras, Jamaica, Mexico, Montserrat, Netherlands Antilles, Nicargua, Panama, Paraguay, Peru, Puerto Rico, St Kitts & Nevis, St Lucia, St Vincent & the Grenadines, Suriname, Trinidad & Tobago, Turks & Caicos Is., Uruguay, US Virgin Is., Venezuela. **Eastern Mediterranean:** Afghanistan, Bahrain, Egypt, Iran, Iraq, Jordan, Kuwait, Lebanon, Libyan Arab Jamahiriya, Morocco, Oman, Pakistan, Qatar, Saudi Arabia, Syrian Arab Rep., Tunisia, United Arab Emirates, West Bank & Gaza Strip, Yemen. **South-East Asia:** Bangladesh, Bhutan, DPR Korea, India, Indonesia, Maldives, Myanmar, Nepal, Sri Lanka, Thailand, Timor-Leste. **Western Pacific:** Amerian Samoa, Brunei Darussalam, Cambodia, China, China Hong Kong SAR, China Macao SAR, Cook Is., Fiji, French Polynesia, Guam, Kiribati, Lao PDR, Malaysia, Marshall Is., Micronesia, Mongolia, Nauru, New Caledonia, Niue, N. Mariana Is., Palau, Papua New Guinea, Philippines, Rep. Korea, Samoa, Solomon Is., Tokelau, Tonga, Vanuatu, Viet Nam, Wallis & Futuan Is. **Eastern Europe:** Armenia, Azerbaijan, Belarus, Bulgaria, Estonia, Georgia, Kazakhstan, Kyrgystan, Latvia, Lithuania, Rep. Moldova, Romania, Russian Federation, Tajikistan, Turkmenistan,

Ukraine, Uzbekistan. **Africa – low HIV:** Algeria, Angola, Benin, Burkina Faso, Cape Verde, Chad, Comoros, Djibouti, Equatorial Guinea, Eritrea, Gambia, Ghana, Guinea, Guinea-Bissau, Liberia, Madagascar, Mali, Mauritania, Mauritius, Niger, Sao Tome & Principe, Senegal, Seychelles, Sierra Leone, Somalia, Sudan, Togo. **Africa – high HIV:** Botswana, Burundi, Cameroon, Central African Rep., Congo, Côte d'Ivoire, DR Congo, Ethiopia, Gabon, Kenya, Lesotho, Malawi, Mozambique, Namibia, Rwanda, South Africa, Swaziland, Uganda, UR Tanzania, Zambia, Zimbabwe.

the estimated rates of case detection, we have estimated the trends in TB incidence rate (all forms) for nine epidemiologically distinct regions of the world (Figure 6). In six of these regions, the trend in the incidence rate has been downward.

Incidence rates have been increasing for most of the period since 1990 in African countries with low and high rates of HIV infection, and in eastern Europe, although the patterns of change in the three regions are quite different. In African countries with high HIV infection, incidence has been pushed upwards by the spread of HIV, but the rate of increase has fallen from a maximum exceeding 15% per year in the early 1990s (Figure 6). In African countries with lower rates of HIV infection, the rate of increase in TB has never been as high (2–3% per year), but neither are there signs that the increase is slowing. In eastern Europe, the rate of increase reached nearly 15% annually by 1995, but the increase now appears to have been halted, and incidence is once again in decline.

The global trend is obtained by summing the estimated numbers of TB cases across all nine regions (Figure 7). Worldwide, the incidence rate of TB was growing at a maximum of around 1.5% per year in 1995, but less than 1% per year by 2003.

TB and HIV
Some countries have carried out surveys of the prevalence of HIV in TB patients, either nationally or locally, and the results have been reported via the data collection form or the supplementary TB/HIV questionnaire. Although the accuracy of the data is not known because, for example, the design of the surveys has not been fully described, a growing number of countries are testing TB patients for HIV infection.

The prevalence of HIV infection in TB patients can be derived from the incidence rate ratio (IRR). IRR is estimated from the relationship between HIV prevalence in adult TB patients and HIV prevalence in the adult population, where both have been measured together (Figure 8). The IRR derived from the national surveys in this set of data is 8.3 (95% CI, 6.1–

FIGURE 7

Trends in the estimated global TB incidence rate (blue line), and the annual change in incidence rate (black line), 1990–2003

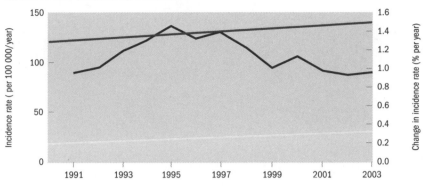

FIGURE 8

The prevalence of HIV in TB patients as measured in national surveys (blue dots) and subnational surveys (data reported to WHO; black dots), plotted against the prevalence of HIV in adults aged 15–49 years (data from UNAIDS). The incidence rate ratio is 8.3 (6.1–10.8; P = 0.0036) for the national survey data and 8.4 (7.9–10.0; P = 0.0029) for the subnational surveys. The countries are: BFA Burkina Faso; BOT Botswana; BUU Burundi; CAE Cameroon; CAF Central African Republic; CAM Cambodia; CNG Congo; COD DR Congo; DJI Djibouti; ETH Ethiopia; GHA Ghana; HAI Haiti; IVC Côte d'Ivoire; KEN Kenya; LES Lesotho; MAL Malawi; MOZ Mozambique; NIE Nigeria; RWA Rwanda; SOA South Africa; TAN UR Tanzania; ZIM Zimbabwe.

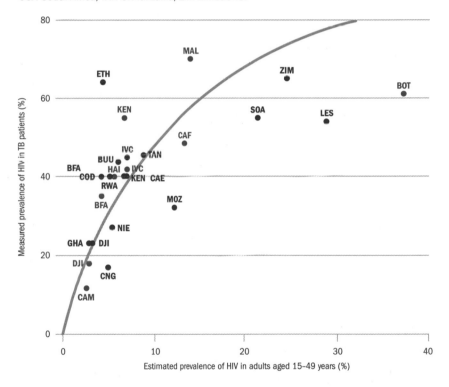

FIGURE 9
Estimated HIV prevalence in TB cases, 2003

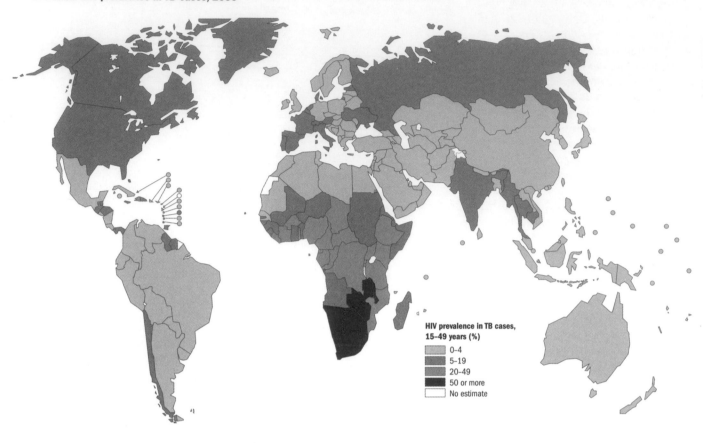

HIV prevalence in TB cases,
15–49 years (%)

- 0–4
- 5–19
- 20–49
- 50 or more
- No estimate

FIGURE 10
Number of countries implementing DOTS (out of a total of 211 countries), 1991–2003

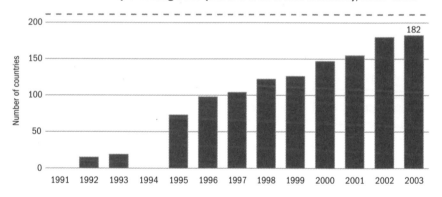

FIGURE 11
DOTS coverage, 1995–2003

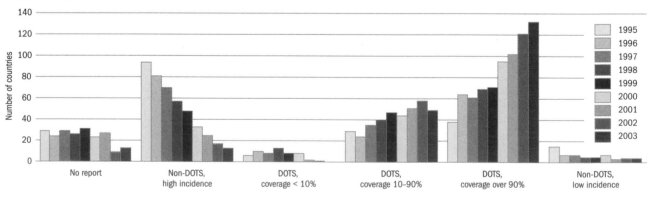

10.8), which is higher than, but not significantly different from, the previously published estimate of 6.0 (3.1–8.0).[24]

Further HIV surveys among TB patients will give, once the data have been validated, better direct measures of the TB/HIV association for the countries surveyed and, through the IRR, better indirect estimates for countries that do not yet test TB patients for HIV infection, thereby improving the distribution map in Figure 9.

DOTS coverage

The total number of countries implementing DOTS increased by two during 2003, bringing the total to 182 out of 211 (Figure 10). All 22 HBCs have had DOTS programmes since 2000; many of these programmes have been established for much longer.

DOTS coverage within countries has steadily increased since 1995 (Figure 11; Table 5). By the end of 2003, 77% of the world's population lived in counties, districts, oblasts and provinces of countries that had adopted DOTS. Coverage was reported to be more than 70% in all regions except Europe (Figure 12).

Case detection

The 4.4 million cases of TB (new and relapse) notified in 2003 represent half (50%) of the 8.8 million estimated new cases; the 1.9 million new smear-positive cases notified also account for half (50%) of the 3.9 million estimated (Table 3, Table 4). In parallel with trends in case notifications, the detection rate of all TB cases, from DOTS and non-DOTS programmes, has remained stable since 1995, while the detection rate of smear-positive cases has slowly increased (Figure 13). Therefore, the proportion of all cases diagnosed as smear-positive has been rising.

DOTS programmes detected an estimated 43% of all new and relapse cases, and 45% of new smear-positive cases, in 2003. The detection rate achieved by DOTS programmes has

[24] Corbett EL et al. The growing burden of tuberculosis: global trends and interactions with the HIV epidemic. *Archives of Internal Medicine*, 2003, 163:1009–1021.

TABLE 5
Progress in DOTS implementation, 1995–2003

	PERCENTAGE OF POPULATION COVERED BY DOTS								
	1995	1996	1997	1998	1999	2000	2001	2002	2003
1 India	1.5	2	2.3	9	13.5	30	45	51.6	67.2
2 China	49	60.4	64.2	63.9	64	68	68	77.6	91
3 Indonesia	6	13.7	28.3	80	90	98	98	98	98
4 Nigeria	47	30	40	45	45	47	55	55	60
5 Bangladesh	40.5	65	80	90	90	92	95	95	99
6 Pakistan	2	8	–	8	8	9	24	45	63
7 Ethiopia	39	39	48	64.4	63	85	70	95	95
8 South Africa	–	0	13	22	66	77	77	98	99.5
9 Philippines	4.3	2	15	16.9	43	89.6	95	98	100
10 Kenya	15	100	100	100	100	100	100	100	100
11 DR Congo	47	51.4	60	60	62	70	70	70	75
12 Russian Federation	–	2.3	2.3	5	5	12	16	25	25
13 Viet Nam	50	95	93	96	98.5	99.8	99.8	99.9	100
14 UR Tanzania	98	100	100	100	100	100	100	100	100
15 Brazil	–	0	0	3	7	7	32	25	33.6
16 Uganda	–	0	100	100	100	100	100	100	100
17 Thailand	–	1.1	4	32	59	70	82	100	100
18 Mozambique	97	100	84	95	–	100	100	100	100
19 Zimbabwe	–	0	0	100	11.6	100	100	100	100
20 Myanmar	–	59	60	60.3	64	77	84	88.3	95
21 Afghanistan	–	–	12	11	13.5	15	12	38	53
22 Cambodia	60	80	88	100	100	99	100	100	100
High-burden countries	**24**	**32**	**36**	**43**	**46**	**55**	**61**	**68**	**79**
AFR	43	47	56	62	56	70	70	81	85
AMR	12	48	50	55	65	68	73	73	78
EMR	23	11	18	33	51	66	72	77	86
EUR	5.4	8.2	17	22	23	26	32	40	41
SEAR	6.7	12	16	30	36	50	61	66	77
WPR	43	55	57	58	57	67	68	77	90
Global	**22**	**32**	**37**	**44**	**47**	**57**	**62**	**69**	**77**

0 Indicates that a report was received, but the country had not implemented DOTS.

– Indicates that no report was received.

FIGURE 12
DOTS population coverage by WHO region, 2003. The shaded portion of each bar shows the DOTS coverage as a percentage of the population. The numbers in each bar show the population (in millions) within (dark portion) or outside (light portion) DOTS areas.

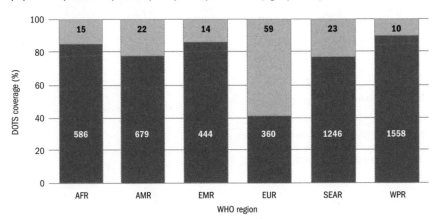

FIGURE 13

Progress towards the 70% case detection target. (a) Open circles mark the number of smear-positive cases notified under DOTS 1995–2003, expressed as a percentage of estimated new cases in each year. The solid line through these points indicates the average annual increment from 1995 to 2000 of about 134 000 new cases, compared with the increment from 2002 to 2003 of 324 000 cases; the steeper line represents a higher annual increment of approximately 488 000 cases per year needed to reach the 70% target by 2005. Closed circles show the total number of smear-positive cases notified (DOTS and non-DOTS) as a percentage of estimated cases. (b) As (a), but for all forms of TB.

(a)

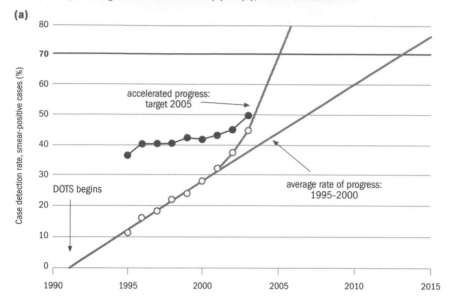

(b)

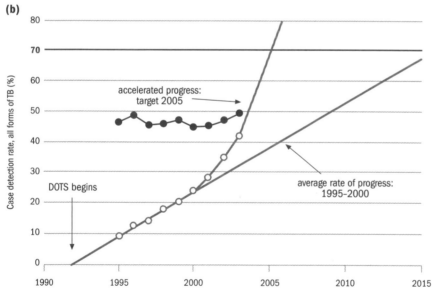

been rising more quickly than the overall case detection rate, and has accelerated since 2000. The 7.5% increase in DOTS case detection between 2002 and 2003, an additional 324 000 smear-positive cases, is the largest annual increase so far reported. If this rate of increase is maintained, the estimated detection rate will be 60% in 2005. To reach the 70% target by 2005, DOTS programmes must find and treat an extra 488 000 cases in each of the two remaining years.

Because case detection under DOTS has increased faster than the overall rate of case detection, the proportion of notified smear-positive cases that were notified by DOTS programmes has also increased, reaching 90% in 2003. DOTS programmes have continued to recruit largely from the pool of patients that would have been detected anyway in the public sector.

Although more cases are recruited to DOTS programmes each year, the case detection rate within DOTS areas (measured by the ratio of case detection to population coverage) has changed little, averaging 52% worldwide between 1996 and 2003 (Figure 14). There are signs of a slow rise in the HBCs, from 35% in 1995 to 56% in 2003, due mostly to improvements in Bangladesh, India, Indonesia, Myanmar and the Philippines.

Smear-positive case detection rates by DOTS programmes in 2003 were lowest in the European Region (23%) and highest in the African Region, Region of the Americas and Western Pacific Region (all 50%; see Figure 15, Table 6). The rate of improvement in case detection by DOTS pro-

FIGURE 14

Smear-positive case detection rate within DOTS areas for high-burden countries (blue) and the world (grey), 1995–2003. DOTS case detection rate divided by DOTS coverage, expressed as percentage.

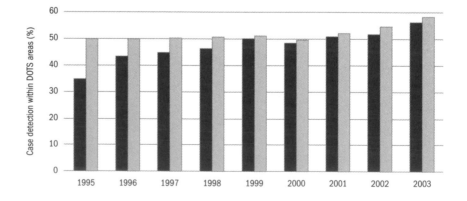

FIGURE 15

Smear-positive case detection rate by DOTS programmes, by WHO region, 1995–2003.
Heavy line shows global DOTS case detection rate.

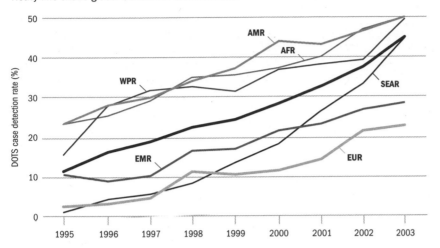

TABLE 6

Case detection rate of new smear-positive cases (%), 1995–2003

	DOTS PROGRAMMES									WHOLE COUNTRY								
	1995	1996	1997	1998	1999	2000	2001	2002	2003	1995	1996	1997	1998	1999	2000	2001	2002	2003
1 India	0.3	0.9	1.1	1.7	7.1	12	24	31	47	38	41	38	38	46	46	50	50	54
2 China	15	28	32	32	29	31	31	30	43	22	34	39	33	33	34	34	32	45
3 Indonesia	1.4	4.6	7.5	12	18	19	20	27	33	13	*	*	*	*	19	*	*	*
4 Nigeria	12	12	12	12	14	14	14	13	18	*	*	*	*	*	*	17	15	*
5 Bangladesh	6.7	14	18	23	23	23	25	29	33	15	21	23	26	25	25	26	29	*
6 Pakistan	1.0	1.8	–	3.8	2.0	2.8	5.2	13	17	2.5	*	–	14	5.5	*	9.2	13	*
7 Ethiopia	16	21	23	25	26	35	35	36	36	*	*	*	*	27	*	*	*	*
8 South Africa	–	–	6.1	22	70	75	81	105	118	41	69	80	91	93	91	95	106	118
9 Philippines	0.4	0.5	3.2	10	20	48	57	62	68	96	87	80	68	71	65	*	*	*
10 Kenya	53	54	50	54	52	44	47	46	46	*	*	*	*	*	48	*	*	*
11 DR Congo	43	49	46	57	56	53	58	57	63	47	*	*	57	*	*	*	*	*
12 Russian Federation	–	0.5	1.0	1.0	1.7	4.6	5.2	6.9	8.8	72	69	64	60	29	35	34	37	40
13 Viet Nam	30	60	79	83	84	83	84	88	86	60	77	*	86	84	*	*	88	*
14 UR Tanzania	55	54	51	52	50	47	46	43	43	*	*	*	*	*	*	*	*	*
15 Brazil	–	–	–	4.1	3.9	7.5	8.0	10	18	79	79	78	80	78	79	75	82	81
16 Uganda	–	–	58	58	58	50	46	46	44	49	54	*	*	*	*	*	*	*
17 Thailand	–	0.3	5.0	21	39	46	73	65	72	55	46	35	*	*	*	*	*	*
18 Mozambique	56	50	48	48	–	45	44	45	45	*	*	*	*	47	*	*	*	*
19 Zimbabwe	–	–	–	51	49	46	46	47	42	50	54	57	*	*	*	*	*	*
20 Myanmar	–	26	26	29	32	48	56	65	73	26	28	28	*	*	*	58	*	*
21 Afghanistan	–	–	2.0	5.9	5.3	9.0	14	19	18	–	–	*	*	*	*	*	*	*
22 Cambodia	40	34	44	47	53	49	47	55	60	*	42	*	*	*	*	*	*	*
High-burden countries	**8.5**	**14**	**17**	**20**	**23**	**27**	**31**	**35**	**44**	**33**	**37**	**37**	**37**	**39**	**39**	**41**	**43**	**48**
AFR	24	26	29	35	36	37	40	47	50	38	43	41	45	45	43	44	47	50
AMR	23	28	30	34	37	44	43	46	50	72	72	77	77	76	74	75	76	76
EMR	11	9.1	10	17	17	22	23	27	28	20	25	24	30	27	23	26	27	28
EUR	2.6	3.4	4.5	11	11	12	14	22	23	63	62	57	57	45	47	43	42	49
SEAR	1.5	4.2	5.6	8.2	14	18	27	33	45	30	30	30	30	37	39	42	45	49
WPR	16	28	32	33	31	37	38	39	50	37	45	48	44	44	43	43	43	52
Global	**11**	**16**	**18**	**22**	**24**	**28**	**32**	**37**	**45**	**37**	**40**	**40**	**40**	**42**	**42**	**43**	**45**	**50**

– Indicates not available.
* No additional data beyond DOTS report, either because country is 100% DOTS, or because no non-DOTS report was received.

FIGURE 16

Proportion of estimated new smear-positive (a) and of all estimated new cases (b) notified under DOTS (grey portion of bars) and non-DOTS (blue portion of bars), 2003.
Figures indicate the number of cases (in thousands) represented by each portion of each bar.

(a) Smear-positive

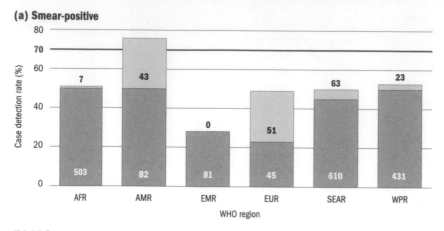

(b) All forms

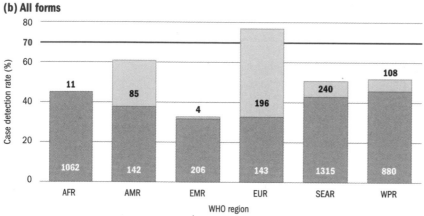

FIGURE 17

Contributions to the global increase in case detection made by high-burden countries, 2002–2003

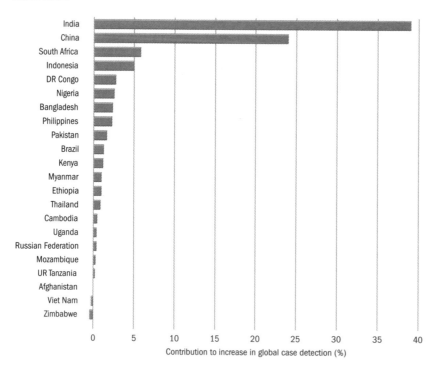

grammes has been roughly the same in all WHO regions except the South-East Asia Region, where the acceleration in case-finding has been visible since 1998, driven mainly by DOTS expansion in India.

In the Region of the Americas, European Region and South-East Asia Region, significant numbers of smear-positive cases were reported, as usual, from outside DOTS programmes (Figure 16a). In the Region of the Americas, the estimated proportion of smear-positive cases detected from all sources exceeded 70%. Thus, the target for case detection would have been reached in this region if all patients in whom TB had been diagnosed had been treated under DOTS. There were similar differences among regions in the detection rates of all TB cases (Figure 16b).

Of the additional smear-positive cases reported by DOTS programmes in 2003 (compared with 2002), 63% were in India (39%) and China (24%; Figure 17). Although China and India have made big improvements in case detection, these two countries still account for an estimated 36% of all undetected smear-positive cases (Figure 18). They are among eight countries that together account for two thirds (67%) of all undetected cases in 2003. In order of importance, these are: India, China, Indonesia, Nigeria, Bangladesh, Pakistan, Ethiopia and the Russian Federation.

Outcomes of treatment
More than 1.4 million new sputum smear-positive cases were registered for treatment in DOTS programmes in 2002, approximately the same number that were notified that year (Table 7, Annex 2). Discrepancies between the numbers of cases notified and registered for treatment were small globally, by region and for most HBCs, the largest differences being in Kenya and the Philippines (where about 10% of notified cases were not registered for treatment) and Afghanistan (where 20% of cases registered for treatment were not notified).

The cure rate among all cases registered under DOTS was 73%, and a further 9% completed treatment (no laboratory confirmation of cure), giv-

FIGURE 18
Smear-positive TB cases undetected by DOTS programmes in six high-burden countries, 2003. Figures indicate the percentage of all cases missed globally which are missed by each country.

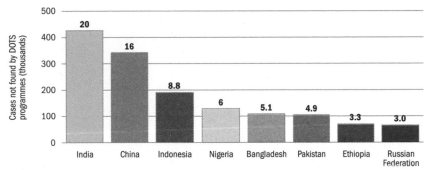

TABLE 7

Treatment outcomes for new smear-positive cases, DOTS strategy, 2002 cohort[a]

	NOTIFIED[c]	REGISTERED[d] NUMBER	%	TREATMENT OUTCOMES (%)[b] CURED	COMPLETED TREATMENT	DIED	FAILED	DEFAULTED	TRANS-FERRED	NOT EVAL[e]	TREATMENT SUCCESS (%)	% ESTIMATED[f] CASES SUCCESSFULLY TREATED UNDER DOTS
1 India	245 135	244 859	100	86	1.0	4.4	2.5	6.1	0.4	0.0	87 †	27
2 China	180 239	180 239	100	90	2.5	1.3	0.9	1.0	1.8	2.6	93 †	28
3 Indonesia	76 230	76 230	100	72	15	2.0	1.3	4.9	2.6	3.0	86 †	24
4 Nigeria	19 596	20 559	105	69	10	1.7	6.7	11	1.5	0.0	79	11
5 Bangladesh	45 741	46 811	102	81	2.9	4.7	0.7	7.0	3.5	0.2	84	25
6 Pakistan	15 331	14 314	93	65	13	3.0	1.2	14	3.8	0.8	77	9.1
7 Ethiopia	36 541	36 541	100	59	17	6.6	0.7	5.0	9.8	1.7	76	27
8 South Africa	97 656	98 090	100	54	14	8.5	1.3	13	9.3	0.0	68	71
9 Philippines	65 148	59 453	91	77	11	2.6	1.1	5.3	2.9	0.5	88 †	49
10 Kenya	34 337	30 966	90	65	14	4.9	0.4	8.9	6.5	0.0	79	33
11 DR Congo	44 518	45 013	101	71	7.8	6.6	1.0	7.8	4.5	1.7	78	45
12 Russian Federation	5 179	5 171	100	64	2.7	13	9.1	7.2	4.1	0.0	67	4.6
13 Viet Nam	56 698	56 590	100	90	1.8	3.4	0.8	1.5	2.0	0.0	92 †	81
14 UR Tanzania	24 136	24 136	100	76	4.3	11	0.3	4.1	4.4	0.1	80	35
15 Brazil	4 835	4 606	95	46	29	6.2	0.3	7.8	11	0.0	75	6.9
16 Uganda	19 088	19 098	100	30	31	6.2	0.4	19	6.6	7.3	60	27
17 Thailand	25 593	26 559	104	69	5.3	11	1.7	9.5	4	0.0	74	50
18 Mozambique	15 236	15 236	100	77	1.4	11	1.3	7.4	2.3	0.3	78	35
19 Zimbabwe	15 941	15 941	100	62	5.6	11	0.1	6.6	15	0.0	67	32
20 Myanmar	24 162	23 922	99	71	10	5.4	1.9	9.2	2.4	0.0	81	52
21 Afghanistan	6 509	7 780	120	60	27	4.0	1.8	4.7	2.6	0.0	87 †	20
22 Cambodia	17 258	17 396	101	89	3.0	3.8	0.3	2.4	1.1	0.0	92 †	51
High-burden countries	**1 075 107**	**1 069 510**	**99**	**76**	**7.0**	**4.6**	**1.5**	**6.2**	**3.3**	**1.0**	**83**	**29**
AFR	442 729	437 873	99	60	13	7.2	1.4	11	6.6	1.4	73	31
AMR	82 312	78 180	95	64	17	4.8	1.0	5.4	3.4	4.3	81	38
EMR	74 450	74 799	100	72	12	3.1	1.4	7.8	2.6	1.5	84	22
EUR	43 112	40 307	93	63	13	6.2	6.2	5.9	2.2	3.1	76	16
SEAR	449 615	451 162	100	81	4.3	4.4	2.1	6.3	1.5	0.5	85 †	28
WPR	340 666	339 754	100	84	6.2	2.4	1.0	2.3	2.3	1.5	91 †	35
Global (DOTS)	**1 432 884**	**1 422 075**	**99**	**73**	**8.7**	**4.8**	**1.6**	**6.7**	**3.4**	**1.4**	**82**	**30**

[a] Cases diagnosed during 2002 and treated/followed-up through 2003.

[b] See Table 2 and accompanying text for definitions of treatment outcomes.

[c] For AMR and EUR, the regional total of notified cases includes the number of laboratory confirmed (as opposed to smear-positive) cases for one country: USA and Israel, respectively.

[d] If the number registered was provided, this (or the sum of the outcomes, if greater) was used as the denominator for calculating treatment outcomes. If the number registered was missing, then the number notified (or the sum of the outcomes, if greater) was used as the denominator. The number used as the denominator is shown in column labelled "Registered".

[e] Eval: evaluated.

[f] Estimated: estimated number of cases for 2002 (as opposed to notified or registered).

† Treatment success ≥85%.

TABLE 8
Treatment outcomes for new smear-positive cases, non-DOTS strategy, 2002 cohort[a]

	NOTIFIED	REGISTERED[a]	REGST'D (%)	TREATMENT OUTCOMES (%)[a]							TREATMENT SUCCESS (%)
				CURED	COMPLETED TREATMENT[a]	DIED	FAILED	DEFAULTED	TRANS-FERRED	NOT EVAL	
1 India	150 698	41 368	27	41	17	1.5	1.4	30	9.3	0.0	58
2 China	14 733	13 681	93	85	7.4	1.1	1.0	2.4	1.2	2.2	92 †
3 Indonesia	–	–	–	–	–	–	–	–	–	–	–
4 Nigeria	2 340	–	–	–	–	–	–	–	–	–	–
5 Bangladesh	1 070	–	–	–	–	–	–	–	–	–	–
6 Pakistan	934	–	–	–	–	–	–	–	–	–	–
7 Ethiopia	–	–	–	–	–	–	–	–	–	–	–
8 South Africa	1 143	1 239	108	59	6.2	5.4	2.4	13	8.2	5.6	65
9 Philippines	–	–	–	–	–	–	–	–	–	–	–
10 Kenya	–	–	–	–	–	–	–	–	–	–	–
11 DR Congo	–	–	–	–	–	–	–	–	–	–	–
12 Russian Federation	22 686	–	–	–	–	–	–	–	–	–	–
13 Viet Nam	–	–	–	–	–	–	–	–	–	–	–
14 UR Tanzania	–	–	–	–	–	–	–	–	–	–	–
15 Brazil	36 536	24 246	66	24	57	5.9	0.3	12	0.6	0.0	81
16 Uganda	–	–	–	–	–	–	–	–	–	–	–
17 Thailand	–	–	–	–	–	–	–	–	–	–	–
18 Mozambique	–	–	–	–	–	–	–	–	–	–	–
19 Zimbabwe	–	–	–	–	–	–	–	–	–	–	–
20 Myanmar	–	–	–	–	–	–	–	–	–	–	–
21 Afghanistan	–	–	–	–	–	–	–	–	–	–	–
22 Cambodia	–	–	–	–	–	–	–	–	–	–	–
High-burden countries	**203 140**	**80 534**	**35**	**44**	**27**	**2.8**	**1.0**	**20**	**5.3**	**0.5**	**71**
AFR	11 714	9 332	80	42	22	10	7.8	10	8.5	0.8	63
AMR	49 603	30 985	62	29	49	5.8	0.5	13	2.0	0.5	78
EMR	1 323	334	25	28	49	1.5	0.6	15	4.8	0.0	78
EUR	40 450	8 622	21	47	21	4.4	4.5	6.6	0.7	15	69
SEAR	157 115	43 784	28	42	17	1.6	1.5	28	9.0	0.1	59
WPR	31 442	18 982	60	64	9.9	1.9	1.4	2.0	12	8.7	74
Global (non-DOTS)	**291 647**	**112 039**	**38**	**43**	**25**	**3.7**	**2.0**	**16**	**6.9**	**2.9**	**68**

– Indicates not available.

[a] See notes for Table 7.

ing a reported, overall treatment success rate of 82%. An estimated 30% of all smear-positive cases arising in 2002 were treated successfully by DOTS programmes. In non-DOTS areas, the quality of reporting was worse: only four HBCs provided data for the 2002 cohort (Table 8).

By WHO region, the documented treatment success rates by DOTS programmes varied from 73% in the African Region to 85% in the South-East Asia Region and 91% in the Western Pacific Region, the latter two regions having met the 85% target (Table 7, Figure 19). Fatal outcomes were most common in the African Region (7%), where a higher fraction of cases are HIV-positive, and in the European Region (6%), where a higher fraction of cases are drug resistant

(eastern Europe), or occur among the elderly (western Europe). Treatment interruption (default) was most frequent in the African Region (11%) and the Eastern Mediterranean Region (8%). Transfer without follow-up was also especially high in the African Region (7%). Treatment failure was conspicuously high in the European Region (6%), mainly because a high proportion of patients in eastern Europe are recorded as failures.

DOTS treatment success exceeded 85% in seven HBCs (Table 7). It was under 70% in the Russian Federation, South Africa, Uganda and Zimbabwe. Treatment results for individual African countries once again point to the effects of HIV: cohort death rates were 9% or more in Mozambique, South Africa, the United Republic of

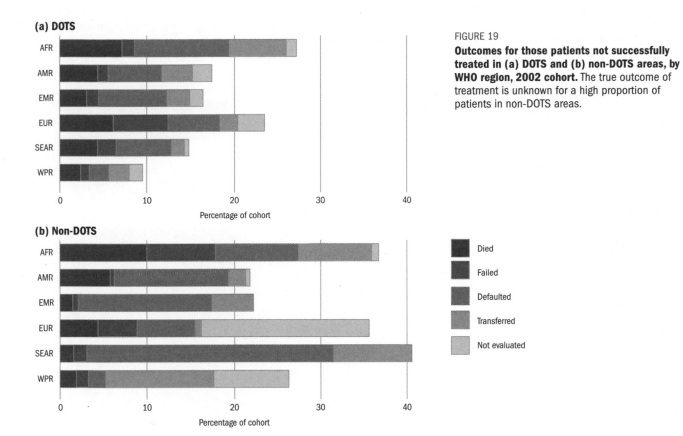

(a) DOTS

(b) Non-DOTS

FIGURE 19

Outcomes for those patients not successfully treated in (a) DOTS and (b) non-DOTS areas, by WHO region, 2002 cohort. The true outcome of treatment is unknown for a high proportion of patients in non-DOTS areas.

Legend:
- Died
- Failed
- Defaulted
- Transferred
- Not evaluated

TABLE 9
Treatment success for new smear-positive cases (%), 1994–2002 cohorts[a]

	DOTS PROGRAMMES									WHOLE COUNTRY								
	1994	1995	1996	1997	1998	1999	2000	2001	2002	1994	1995	1996	1997	1998	1999	2000	2001	2002
1 India	83	79	79	82	84	82	84	85	87	*	25	21	18	27	21	77	54	83
2 China	94	96	96	96	97	96	95	96	93	91	93	94	95	95	95	93	95	92
3 Indonesia	94	91	81	54	58	50	87	86	86	*	*	*	*	*	*	*	*	*
4 Nigeria	65	49	32	73	73	75	79	79	79	*	*	*	*	*	*	*	*	*
5 Bangladesh	73	71	72	78	80	81	83	84	84	*	*	63	73	77	79	81	83	*
6 Pakistan	74	70	–	67	66	70	74	77	77	69	*	–	*	23	*	*	*	*
7 Ethiopia	74	61	73	72	74	76	80	76	76	*	*	71	*	*	74	*	*	*
8 South Africa	–	–	69	73	74	60	66	65	68	78	58	61	68	72	57	63	61	68
9 Philippines	80	–	82	83	84	87	88	88	88	88	60	35	78	71	*	*	*	*
10 Kenya	73	75	77	65	77	78	80	80	79	*	*	*	*	*	79	*	*	*
11 DR Congo	71	80	48	64	70	69	78	77	78	72	74	48	64	*	*	*	*	*
12 Russian Federation	–	65	62	67	68	65	68	67	67	–	*	57	*	*	*	*	*	*
13 Viet Nam	91	91	90	85	93	92	92	93	92	*	89	89	85	92	92	*	*	*
14 UR Tanzania	80	73	76	77	76	78	78	81	80	*	*	*	*	*	*	*	*	*
15 Brazil	–	–	–	–	91	89	73	67	75	70	17	20	27	40	78	71	55	80
16 Uganda	–	–	33	40	62	61	63	56	60	–	44	*	*	*	*	*	*	*
17 Thailand	–	–	78	62	68	77	69	75	74	58	64	*	58	*	*	*	*	*
18 Mozambique	67	39	54	67	–	71	75	77	78	*	*	55	65	–	*	*	*	*
19 Zimbabwe	–	–	–	–	70	73	69	71	67	52	53	32	69	*	*	*	*	*
20 Myanmar	–	66	79	82	82	81	82	81	81	77	67	79	*	*	*	*	*	*
21 Afghanistan	–	–	–	45	33	87	86	84	87	–	–	–	*	*	86	85	*	*
22 Cambodia	84	91	94	91	95	93	91	92	92	*	*	*	*	*	*	*	*	*
High-burden countries	**87**	**83**	**78**	**81**	**83**	**81**	**84**	**84**	**83**	**83**	**53**	**50**	**56**	**62**	**60**	**81**	**72**	**83**
AFR	59	62	57	63	70	69	72	71	73	60	60	56	64	70	68	71	70	72
AMR	77	77	81	81	80	83	81	83	81	65	50	51	58	67	79	77	72	80
EMR	82	87	86	79	76	83	83	83	84	79	79	66	73	56	79	81	83	84
EUR	68	69	72	72	76	77	77	75	76	67	67	58	72	63	75	75	72	75
SEAR	80	74	77	72	72	73	83	84	85	66	33	31	29	40	34	79	63	83
WPR	90	91	93	93	95	94	92	93	91	87	80	72	91	92	91	90	91	90
Global	**77**	**79**	**77**	**79**	**81**	**80**	**82**	**82**	**82**	**75**	**57**	**54**	**60**	**64**	**64**	**80**	**73**	**81**

– Indicates not available.

* No additional data beyond DOTS report, either because country is 100%, or because no non-DOTS report was received.

[a] See notes for Table 7.

Tanzania and Zimbabwe. But programme performance also remains poor in some African countries. For example, more than 15% of patients were lost to follow-up in Ethiopia, Kenya, South Africa, Uganda and Zimbabwe. Large proportions of patients completed treatment without confirming cure (a final, negative sputum smear) in Ethiopia (17%) and Uganda (31%). Uganda reported the lowest proportion of successful treatments among the 22 HBCs (60%). The aggregated treatment results for the European Region are strongly influenced by the performance in the Russian Federation, where 13% of patients died, 9% failed treatment and 11% were lost to follow-up.

A comparison of treatment results for nine consecutive cohorts (1994–2002) shows that the overall success rates have been 80% or more in DOTS areas since 1998 (Table 9). Treatment success rates have been persistently poor outside DOTS programmes in all regions, principally because large fractions of cases are not registered or evaluated.

In DOTS areas, about 250 000 cases were registered for re-treatment in 2002 (Table 10; Annex 2). Some patients remain on treatment (included with those "not evaluated"), but the latest data give an overall treatment success rate of 72%. When the three registration types (re-treatment after relapse, failure and default) are distinguished and compared with new TB patients, three patterns emerge. First, the comparative success of re-treatment was consistent with expectations: lower on average for re-treatment (72%) than for new cases (82%), but higher for relapses (71%), intermediate for defaulters (68%) and lowest for failures (58%). The rank order relapse > default > failed held for six out of eight HBCs that provided data, and for five out of six WHO regions. Second, patients who defaulted from their first course of treatment tended to default when treated again (17% of patients that were re-treated after default failed to complete the subsequent course of treatment, compared with 11% among all re-treated patients and 7% of patients on their first course of treatment). This was true in all six WHO

TABLE 10

Re-treatment outcomes for smear-positive cases, DOTS strategy, 2002 cohort[a]

	REGISTERED[a]	TREATMENT OUTCOMES (%)[a]							TREATMENT SUCCESS (%)
		CURED	COMPLETED TREATMENT[a]	DIED	FAILED	DEFAULTED	TRANS-FERRED	NOT EVAL	
1 India	84 078	68	3.3	7.2	6.1	14	0.7	0.0	72
2 China	46 932	83	5.2	2.6	3.8	2.0	1.0	0.0	88 †
3 Indonesia	3 731	60	17	2.2	3.3	5.4	3.1	8.4	78
4 Nigeria	2 373	63	11	4.7	7.6	11	1.1	2.5	73
5 Bangladesh	4 360	66	2.6	4.3	1.9	10	2.9	12	69
6 Pakistan	2 871	33	43	4.5	1.8	11	5.2	1.9	76
7 Ethiopia	1 716	52	8.6	6.9	2.8	5.3	2.4	22	60
8 South Africa	28 755	43	10	11	2.1	17	10	6.8	53
9 Philippines	–	–	–	–	–	–	–	–	–
10 Kenya	2 476	65	12	10	0.4	6.7	5.8	0.0	77
11 DR Congo	4 618	61	5.8	9.3	3.6	9.8	7.3	3.3	67
12 Russian Federation	962	37	9.4	12	26	8.6	8.1	0.0	46
13 Viet Nam	6 079	79	5.5	4.9	5.4	2.3	2.4	0.0	85 †
14 UR Tanzania	2 081	71	6.4	13	0.7	4.6	3.7	0.5	77
15 Brazil	640	36	24	7.0	1.1	18	13	0.0	60
16 Uganda	2 555	28	27	10	0.9	16	5.3	13	55
17 Thailand	1 990	55	6.4	17	6.7	9.3	5.7	0.0	62
18 Mozambique	1 721	65	1.2	12	2.2	9.4	4.0	5.7	67
19 Zimbabwe	1 371	58	4.7	20	0.9	7.6	8.7	0.0	63
20 Myanmar	8 036	65	10	7.8	3.9	10	3.7	0.2	75
21 Afghanistan	–	–	–	–	–	–	–	–	–
22 Cambodia	875	86	2.9	5.8	1.5	2.7	1.1	0.0	89 †
High-burden countries	**208 220**	**66**	**6.5**	**6.8**	**4.5**	**11**	**2.9**	**2.4**	**73**
AFR	59 574	49	11	10	2.4	14	7.7	6.7	59
AMR	7 635	64	6.8	5.8	4.3	12	4.3	2.3	71
EMR	8 825	51	23	4.4	3.5	10	5.3	3.2	74
EUR	12 551	42	12	10	12	11	2.6	10	54
SEAR	106 423	68	4.3	7.1	5.6	13	1.3	0.8	72
WPR	57 071	81	5.6	3.1	4.0	2.3	1.8	1.9	87 †
Global	**252 079**	**64**	**7.2**	**6.9**	**4.7**	**11**	**3.2**	**3.1**	**72**

– Indicates not available.
† Treatment success ≥85%.
[a] See notes for Table 7.

regions. Third, the regional distribution of adverse re-treatment outcomes resembled the pattern observed for new cases. Thus, countries in the African Region reported high death rates (10%), and many patients were lost to follow-up (28%). Countries in the European Region reported high rates of death (10%) and treatment failure (12%).

Trends in case detection and treatment success: overview of national DOTS programmes

Data on both treatment success and case detection were provided by 177 DOTS countries. Case detection exceeded 50%, and treatment success exceeded 70%, in 75 countries (Figure 20). They include the HBCs Cambodia, the Democratic Republic of the Congo, Myanmar, the Philippines, Thailand and Viet Nam. Of these countries, 22 appear to have reached the WHO targets, but together the 75 countries accounted for only 17% of all new smear-positive cases in 2003. Viet Nam was still the only member of the current group of HBCs to have reached targets for both case detection (>70%) and treatment success (>85%), although Myanmar and the Philippines are close to these targets (Figure 21). Three HBCs – Brazil, the Russian Federation and Uganda – had low rates of both case detection (<50%) and treatment success (<70%). More details of progress in each of the 22 HBCs can be found in the profiles (Annex 1).

Of 161 countries that provided data for both the 2001 and 2002 cohorts, 91 (57%) showed higher treatment success rates for the 2002 cohort, and 68 of 172 (40%) improved case detection by more than 5%. Annex 2 tabulates case detection and treatment success rates by country over the nine years for which there are data.

Trends in prevalence and death rates

The trends in prevalence and mortality for each region are calculated from the trend in incidence (Figure 6) and from estimates of the duration of illness (e.g. time smear-positive) and the case-fatality rate. Summing estimates from across the regions gives the global trends in prevalence and

FIGURE 20

DOTS status in 2003: countries close to targets. 75 countries reported treatment success rates 70% or over and DOTS detection rates 50% or over. 22 countries (including Kiribati, Wallis & Futuna Islands and Marshall Islands, out of range of graph) have reached both targets.

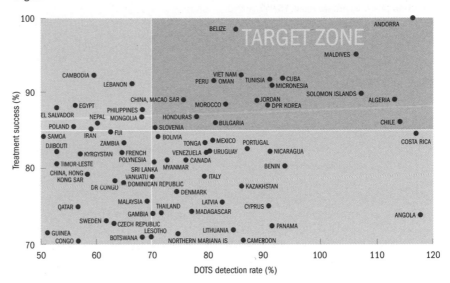

FIGURE 21

DOTS progress in high-burden countries, 2002–2003. Treatment success refers to cohorts of patients registered in 2001 or 2002, and evaluated by the end of 2002 or 2003, respectively. Countries in AFR, AMR, EMR and EUR are shown in blue; those in SEAR and WPR are shown in black.

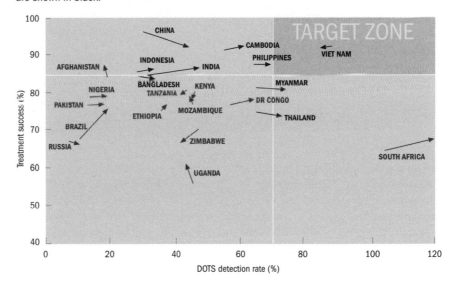

FIGURE 22

(a) Estimated global TB incidence (per 100 000 population per year; grey), prevalence (per 100 000 population; blue), and mortality rates (per 100 000 population per year; black), 1990–2003, including (thin lines) or excluding (thick lines) TB patients coinfected with HIV. (b) As for (a), but for African countries with high rates of HIV infection (≥4% in adults aged 15–49 years).

(a)

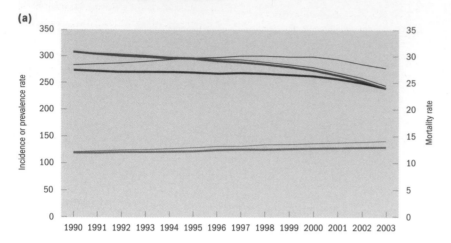

(b)

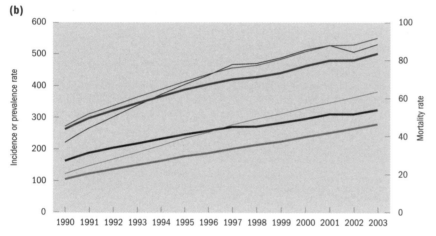

deaths, which are shown in Figure 22a with and without the contribution of HIV-positive TB patients, and in comparison with the trends in incidence (Figure 7). Although the global incidence rate was still increasing in 2003, prevalence and death rates had already begun to fall. Excluding HIV-positive TB patients, the incidence rate increased 0.6% between 2002 and 2003, prevalence fell by 5.7% and mortality by 3.5%. When TB patients coinfected with HIV are included, the incidence rate increased by 1.0%, and prevalence and mortality fell by 5.5% and 2.5%, respectively. The differential effects of HIV on incidence, prevalence and mortality are also visible, and magnified, in the trends for countries of eastern and southern Africa, where all three indicators were still

increasing in 2003 (Figure 22b). Among the nine regions defined in Figure 6, TB prevalence and death rates increased between 2002 and 2003 only in the two African regions; as for incidence rates, prevalence and deaths were falling or stable in the other seven regions.

Planning and DOTS implementation

TB control in the context of the health-care system
Country profiles incorporate information from the summary planning tables that were prepared for the 2004 DEWG meeting and from the questionnaires submitted by all 22 HBCs. The health systems of many countries are still undergoing reform and restructuring. However, all HBCs except the Rus-

sian Federation and Thailand reported that TB control functions are fully integrated with essential national health services. The MoH generally provides support for TB control through a specific technical unit, although in Bangladesh, South Africa and Thailand this function needs to be strengthened. All HBCs have a national plan for TB control and many will conduct, during 2005, a new planning exercise for the next five years. A total of 15 HBCs have prepared, or are developing, a plan for human resource development (HRD) reflecting their specific needs in the context of the health system.

Constraints and remedial actions
In summary tables and questionnaires, countries reported the following constraints:

1. Shortage or inadequate capacity of staff. This remains a major constraint identified by 18 HBCs. The problem is being addressed by various means: situation assessments, development of HRD plans, intensification of training and supervision, redistribution of staff and appointment of new staff. All HBCs except Brazil, Nigeria, South Africa and Zimbabwe plan to implement projects funded by the GFATM in 2005; a shortage of managers, or inadequate managerial capacity, will almost certainly hinder these projects.

2. Inadequate central management capacity. Insufficient capacity at the highest levels delays the implementation of national plans, as reported in Bangladesh, Mozambique, South Africa, Uganda, the United Republic of Tanzania and Zimbabwe. Support from technical partners has been the main temporary remedial action.

3. Inadequate infrastructure. Lack of transportation infrastructure (roads and vehicles), poor communication networks, unreliable or non-existent electricity supplies, inadequate buildings and equipment, and weak primary health-care systems all impede TB control. A total of 12 HBCs reported deficiencies in at least one of these areas.

4. Weak political commitment. Ethiopia, Mozambique, Nigeria, South Africa, Thailand and Zimbabwe reported limited commitment to TB control from central and peripheral levels. Remedial actions include providing better support to local government following decentralization, forming provincial task forces, expanding international support through high-level advocacy missions and advocacy for TB control in civil society, especially in support of patients infected with HIV. Brazil, China and the Russian Federation reported significant progress on legislation to support TB control.

5. Weak laboratory services. The main obstacles are summarized in Table 11.

6. Nearly all HBCs had a secure supply of anti-TB drugs in 2003, thanks in large part to the Global TB Drug Facility (GDF). Mozambique reported drug shortages, but these will be rectified following a successful application to the GDF. South Africa experienced drug shortages due to the phasing in of the new drug combinations and a complete stock-out of streptomycin when the sole supplier stopped production.

7. Poor monitoring and evaluation. Timely and reliable data are essential for monitoring trends and for planning corrective actions. The Russian Federation and South Africa have addressed problems reported in 2003[13] by establishing standardized recording and reporting systems. China has introduced a new Internet-based reporting system, but the data being collected need validation.

8. Insufficient funds. A lack of money is no longer one of the major constraints identified by most HBCs. The governments of the wealthier HBCs make large contributions to TB control, international donors have increased their investments and the GFATM has begun to bridge financial gaps. As a result, some NTPs now have sufficient funding to expand DOTS programmes. However, some of the HBCs did report shortfalls in their 2004 budgets. Some of these countries still report gaps (see section on Financing DOTS Expansion), and others have problems in distributing funds from local or central governments to programmes (e.g. Nigeria). Mozambique has inadequate funds to pay salaries, and Zimbabwe is heavily affected by the country's general financial crisis.

9. Poor access to remote areas. Access to geographically remote and politically unstable areas is a challenge in Afghanistan, Bangladesh, the Philippines and Uganda. The NTP in Viet Nam, having reached the targets for DOTS implementation, has made service provision in remote areas an important part of consolidating programme success.

10. Low public awareness. Limited knowledge about TB and its treatment, and the stigma of having TB (and perhaps also HIV infection), both hamper efforts to detect and treat TB suspects. A

TABLE 11

Status of TB laboratory services, high-burden countries, 2003–2004

	POPULATION PER DIAGNOSTIC FACILITY	INSUFFICIENT EQUIPMENT OR SHORTAGE OF SUPPLIES	SHORTAGE OF STAFF (OR EXISTING STAFF IN NEED OF TRAINING)	QUALITY ASSURANCE	CULTURE	DRUG SUSCEPTIBILITY TESTING (DST)	NATIONAL REFERENCE LABORATORY (NRL)
1 India	100 000		Y	limited, planned	Y	Y	Y
2 China	500 000		Y	limited	Y	Y	Y
3 Indonesia	80 000		Y	limited	Y	Y	N, one acting
4 Nigeria	150 000	Y	Y	limited, planned			Y
5 Bangladesh	230 000			limited	limited	limited	Y
6 Pakistan	100 000	Y	Y	N	limited	limited	Y
7 Ethiopia	180 000		Y	limited	Y	Y	Y
8 South Africa	unknown[a]			Y	Y	Y	private
9 Philippines	75 000		to be trained	limited	limited	limited	Y
10 Kenya	54 000		Y	Y	Y	Y	Y
11 DR Congo	70 000	Y	Y	limited	limited	limited	Y
12 Russian Federation	25 000		to be trained	Y	Y	Y	N
13 Viet Nam	125 000			Y	limited	limited	Y
14 UR Tanzania	65 000		Y	weak	limited	limited	Y
15 Brazil	45 000		to be trained	limited	Y	Y	Y
16 Uganda	60 000		Y	planned	Y	Y	Y
17 Thailand	65 000		to be trained	Y	Y	Y	Y
18 Mozambique	60 000	Y	Y	N	limited	limited	Y
19 Zimbabwe	120 000	Y	Y	limited	limited	limited	Y
20 Myanmar	200 000		Y	weak	limited	limited	Y
21 Afghanistan	100 000	Y	Y	N	limited	limited	N
22 Cambodia	75 000		to be trained	limited	Y	N	Y

"Y" or "N" indicates whether the problem exists or the activity is undertaken.
"Limited" indicates that the activity is restricted to certain areas of the country.
[a] Laboratory services contracted out to National Health Laboratory Service in eight of nine provinces.

FIGURE 23

The number of TB cases that were tested for HIV for every 100 TB cases that were notified in 2003 for countries that reported more than 1000 cases and tested more than 1% of notified cases. The countries are: ARM Armenia; AUS Australia; AZE Azerbaijan; BOT Botswana; BRA Brazil; CAM Cambodia; CNG Congo; CUB Cuba; DJI Djibouti; ELS El Salvador; GEO Georgia; GHA Ghana; GUT Guatemala; HOK Hong Kong SAR; HON Honduras; IVC Côte d'Ivoire; KOR Republic of Korea; LIY Libyan Arab Jamahiriya; LVA Latvia; MAL Malawi; MEX Mexico; NAM Namibia; NIC Nicaragua; PAN Panama; PNG Papua New Guinea; POR Portugal; SOA South Africa; SUD Sudan; SYR Syrian Arab Republic; UZB Uzbekistan; VTN Viet Nam.

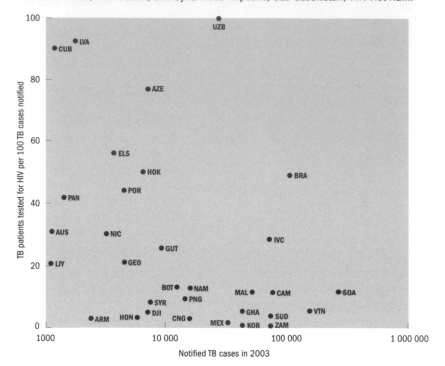

FIGURE 24

The number of TB patients tested for HIV (blue), assessed for ART (grey) and starting ART (pale blue) for every estimated 100 HIV-positive TB patients in each WHO region

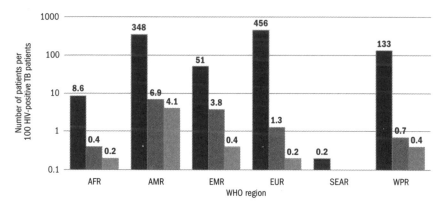

total of 13 HBCs have plans to launch or intensify advocacy and communication campaigns.

Intensified support and action in countries

During 2004, the DEWG launched ISAC, an emergency initiative to reach targets for DOTS implementation by 2005 and to generate further momentum towards the MDG targets for 2015. The goal of ISAC is to rapidly increase managerial capacity for TB control at central and intermediate levels of administration. Participating countries include China, India, Indonesia, Kenya, Pakistan, Romania, the Russian Federation and Uganda.

Partnerships, coordination and advocacy

All HBCs have some mechanism for coordinating TB control activities. Most countries have an NICC that meets regularly to share information on planning and progress. This has served as a model for the creation of Global Fund Country Coordination Mechanisms (CCMs). However, in some countries (e.g. Ethiopia, Viet Nam) the CCM has become the main coordinating body. During 2004, Indonesia, Pakistan and Uganda formed and launched national partnerships to Stop TB, in order to establish collaborations among various stakeholders (NTP, WHO, technical and financial partners, NGOs, and patients' associations), and to share human and financial resources to address more effectively some of the constraints hindering NTP performance. NGOs are actively collaborating with NTPs to improve service coverage in 20 HBCs (Annex 1).

Most of the HBCs recognize the need for improved advocacy and communication on TB control. Ethiopia, India, Kenya, Pakistan, South Africa and Viet Nam reported that such activities were intensified in 2004. Cambodia, the Democratic Republic of the Congo, Indonesia, Nigeria, the Philippines, the United Repbulic of Tanzania and Uganda are planning advocacy and communication campaigns for 2005.

Management of drug resistance

Among the HBCs, Kenya (pilot site in Nairobi), the Philippines (pilot site in Manila) and the Russian Federation (Archangelsk, Ivanovo, Orel and Tomsk oblasts) have DOTS-Plus pilot projects approved by the GLC. The projects in Kenya and the Philippines are supported financially by the GFATM, as is one of the four projects in the Russian Federation (Tomsk). In 2005, applications to the GLC are expected from Bangladesh, Myanmar, the Philippines, the United Republic of Tanzania and Viet Nam.

By December 2004, the GLC had approved 30 DOTS-Plus pilot projects for a total of 10 133 MDR-TB patients in 23 countries.[25] However, only three HBCs – Brazil, the Russian Federation and South Africa – have national policies for the diagnosis and treatment of MDR-TB, and manage MDR-TB under the NTP. Even in the few countries that do have policies, MDR-TB treatment often fails to meet acceptable standards in practice. Second-line drugs are available in almost all HBCs, and are locally produced in Bangladesh, Brazil, China, Kenya, India, Indonesia, the Philippines, Pakistan, the Russian Federation, South Africa, Thailand and Viet Nam. In many countries, substandard MDR-TB treatment is available in the private sector or at specialized health centres, often for a fee.

The planning of activities related to MDR-TB is described in the individual profiles of the 22 HBCs (Annex 1).

Collaborative TB/HIV activities

Among the 199 countries that completed the WHO data collection form, 49% have a national policy of offering HIV testing to TB patients, the first step in accessing appropriate prevention and care services for HIV-positive TB patients. However, in 2003, only 3% of 4.4 million notified TB cases were reported to have been tested for HIV. Of these 199 countries, 46 (23%)

[25] Bolivia, Costa Rica, El Salvador, Egypt, Estonia, Georgia, Haiti, Honduras, Jordan, Kenya, Kyrgyzstan, Latvia, Lebanon, Malawi, Mexico, Nepal, Nicaragua, Peru, Philippines, Romania, Russian Federation, Syrian Arab Republic and Uzbekistan.

FIGURE 25

Progress in developing national policy on collaborative TB/HIV activities, 2002 (blue bars) and 2003 (grey bars). Data are for the 32 countries with high numbers of people with TB who are also HIV-infected which returned the supplementary questionnaire. The bars show the number of countries that have a coordinating body, carry out joint planning for TB and HIV control activities, have a policy of testing TB patients for HIV, have a system for referring TB patients for HIV care and support and that provide ART in the public sector. The numbers in each bar give the percentage of the countries that fall into each category.

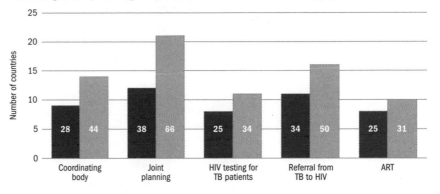

indicated that HIV-positive TB patients were routinely assessed for their eligibility for ART. Only 1349 TB patients were reported to have started ART in 2003.

Figure 23 shows the breakdown of HIV testing rates among TB patients by country, for all countries that notified more than 1000 TB patients in 2003 and tested more than 1% of them for HIV. Even in Brazil, where ART is provided free of charge in the public sector, only half of the notified TB patients were reported to have been tested for HIV. Among other countries that notified more than 10 000 cases each year, Côte d'Ivoire tested less than 30%. Botswana, Cameroon, Malawi, Namibia and South Africa tested about 10%. For other high-incidence countries, the proportions tested were still lower. Some countries with low TB incidence rates, including Cuba and Latvia, tested most of their TB patients.

Regional differences in HIV testing, and in assessment for and provision of ART, are shown in Figure 24, where the denominator is the estimated number of new HIV-positive TB patients in 2003. Under normal circumstances, several TB patients would have to be tested in order to detect one HIV-positive patient. Thus the number of patients tested for HIV should be several times greater than the number estimated to be HIV positive, but the number tested exceeded the estimated number only in the Re-

gion of the Americas, European Region and Western Pacific Region.

By region, as by country, the number of HIV-positive TB patients who were assessed for ART is much smaller than the number who were tested for HIV. In the Region of the Americas, seven HIV-positive TB patients were assessed for ART for every 100 estimated to be HIV-positive, and most of these were in Brazil. In the African Region, the region worst affected by HIV/AIDS, only four patients were assessed for ART for every 1000 HIV-positive TB patients. The percentage of HIV-positive TB patients reported to have started ART was still lower. The Region of the Americas performed better than other regions, but fewer than four out of 1000 HIV-positive TB patients started ART.

Of the supplementary questionnaires sent to 41 high-incidence countries, 32 were returned to WHO. The data show that, between 2002 and 2003, TB/HIV collaboration had improved (Figure 25). However, implementation and recording and reporting remain weak. For example, few countries were able to report the exact numbers of TB patients or HIV-infected people that were benefiting from these activities.

Additional strategies for DOTS expansion

Public public and public private mix for DOTS (PPM). During 2004, 13 HBCs reported improved links between the

TABLE 12

Additional strategies for DOTS expansion planned or implemented, high-burden countries

	PPM (PUBLIC-PUBLIC AND PUBLIC-PRIVATE MIX)	COMMUNITY TB CARE	PRACTICAL APPROACH TO LUNG HEALTH (PAL)
1 India	scale-up	nationwide	
2 China	referral, planned	some areas	
3 Indonesia	pilot	pilot, scale-up	planned
4 Nigeria	planned	planned	planned
5 Bangladesh	scale-up	nationwide	
6 Pakistan	pilot		
7 Ethiopia	pilot	pilot	
8 South Africa	with mining companies	community health workers	
9 Philippines	scale-up	some areas, scale-up	
10 Kenya	scale-up	pilot, scale-up	
11 DR Congo	planned	pilot, scale-up	planned
12 Russian Federation		through NGOs	planned
13 Viet Nam	planned	IEC, scale-up	planned
14 UR Tanzania	pilot	nationwide	planned
15 Brazil			
16 Uganda	planned		
17 Thailand	pilot	some areas, scale-up	planned
18 Mozambique		some areas, scale-up	planned
19 Zimbabwe	pilot	some areas, with TB/HIV	
20 Myanmar	pilot		
21 Afghanistan	planned	Kabul only	
22 Cambodia	planned	pilot	planned

NTP and other health-care providers (Table 12); 14 have established better collaborations with medical colleges; 10 have PPM pilot projects in various stages of implementation. Seven more HBCs are planning PPM initiatives for 2005, and four (India, Kenya, Myanmar and the Philippines) are attempting to implement PPM initiatives nationally. China, India, Indonesia, Kenya and Pakistan have specific plans to scale-up collaborations between NTP and non-NTP public hospitals.

Community TB care. A total of 17 HBCs reported some form of community contribution to TB care. In Bangladesh, India and Uganda, NGOs and community groups have played a vital part in expanding access to TB treatment. Communities are involved in TB care in limited parts of Afghanistan, Cambodia, China, the Democratic Republic of the Congo, Ethiopia, Indonesia, Kenya, Mozambique, the Philippines, South Africa, the United Republic of Tanzania and Viet Nam. Nigeria is planning to carry out a pilot study in 2005.

TABLE 13

Budget and expenditure data received, all countries, 2005

	NUMBER OF COUNTRIES	REPORTS RECEIVED	BUDGET DATA			EXPENDITURE DATA			NO. PATIENTS TO BE TREATED QUANTIFIED
			COMPLETE	PARTIAL	NONE	COMPLETE	PARTIAL	NONE	
AFR	46	35	26	6	3	23	5	7	33
AMR	44	29	15	6	8	12	6	11	21
EMR	22	17	5	7	5	6	5	6	15
EUR	52	16	5	9	2	8	5	3	16
SEAR	11	8	7	1	0	7	0	1	7
WPR	36	29	12	10	7	13	9	7	28
Global	**211**	**134**	**70**	**39**	**25**	**69**	**30**	**35**	**120**

TABLE 14

Budget and expenditure data received, high-burden countries, 2005

	NUMBER OF COUNTRIES	REPORTS RECEIVED	BUDGET DATA			EXPENDITURE DATA			NO. PATIENTS TO BE TREATED QUANTIFIED
			COMPLETE	PARTIAL	NONE	COMPLETE	PARTIAL	NONE	
AFR	9	8	8	0	1	6	0	3[a]	8
AMR	1	1	1	0	0	1	0	0	1
EMR	2	2	1	1[b]	0	1	1[b]	0	2
EUR[c]	1	1	1	0	0	1	0	0	1
SEAR	5	5	4	1[d]	0	4	1[d]	0	4
WPR	4	4	4	0	0	4	0	0	4
Global	**22**	**21**	**19**	**2**	**1**	**17**	**2**	**3**	**20**

[a] Kenya, South Africa and Uganda.
[b] Afghanistan.
[c] Data for the Russian Federation were prepared by WHO staff (Moscow office). See country profile for further details.
[d] Thailand.

Practical Approach to Lung Health (PAL). Cambodia, the Democratic Republic of the Congo, Indonesia, Mozambique, Nigeria, Russian Federation, the United Republic of Tanzania, Uganda and Viet Nam are planning to investigate the feasibility of implementing PAL in 2005. These studies will investigate how the syndromic approach to diagnosis and treatment can influence TB case detection and the rationalization of drug prescription practices.

Financing DOTS expansion

Data received

Financial data were received from 134 out of 211 (64%) countries (Table 13), more in total than for 2004 (123 countries), but with fewer reports from the European Region. Complete budget data were provided by 70 countries (compared with 77 in 2004), and 69 provided complete expenditure data (down from 74 in 2004). Fewer complete reports were provided by the European Region and the Western Pacific Region, perhaps because more data were requested for the present report (in particular, two years of budget data rather than one). The main improvement in reporting was in the African Region, where the number of complete budget and expenditure forms increased by 37% and 44% respectively, probably because WHO

regional office staff intensively followed up on data collection with NTPs.

Data were received from all 22 HBCs except South Africa (Table 14), providing the most complete set of data since financial monitoring was introduced by WHO in 2002. Complete budget data were provided for 19 countries (up from 17 in 2004); data were missing for South Africa and only partially complete for Afghanistan and Thailand. Complete expenditure data were provided for 17 countries (up from 15 in 2004); Kenya, South Africa and Uganda provided no data, and Afghanistan and Thailand provided incomplete data. A total of 20 countries made projections of the number of cases they would treat in 2004 and 2005, compared with the 16 countries that provided projections for 2004 in last year's report. Again, the main improvement in reporting was in the African Region. Countries in the Western Pacific Region as well as India submitted, on time, exemplary data that required minimal follow-up.

Total NTP budgets and funding in HBCs
NTP budgets in 18 of the 22 HBCs have increased during the period 2002–2005, sometimes by substantial amounts (Figure 26, Figure 27, Table 15 columns 3 and 4). The total combined budgets for 2004 and 2005 are US$ 684 million and US$ 741

million, respectively, compared with around US$ 400 million in both 2002 and 2003. The main reason why the budgets for 2004 and 2005 are higher than in previous years is that countries are aiming to detect and treat more patients. This is associated with large proposed spending increases on initiatives to increase case detection and cure rates (US$ 160 million 2002–2005, of which US$ 39 million is in China), investment in buildings and equipment (US$ 63 million 2002–2005), and dedicated NTP staff (US$ 57 million 2002–2005). Important increases are also budgeted for first and second-line drugs (both up by about US$ 30 million 2002–2005). Relatively small budgets were reported for collaborative TB/HIV activities.

The countries with by far the largest budgets for 2005 (Table 15 column 2) are the Russian Federation (US$ 316 million) and China (US$ 158 million), followed by India and Indonesia (both around US$ 45 million). Other countries reported budgets of around or less than US$ 20 million. In absolute terms, China reported the largest budgetary increase between 2002 and 2005 (an additional US$ 60 million; Table 15, column 3). China is committed to achieving the 70% case detection target in 2005, and the budgetary increases reflect plans to achieve this.

FIGURE 26

Total NTP budgets by line item 2002–2005, 21 high-burden countries,[a] 2002–2005

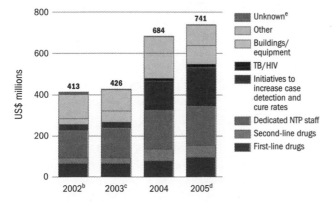

^a Data not available for South Africa.
^b Estimates assume budget 2002 equal to expenditure 2002 (Ethiopia), budget 2003 (Afghanistan, Bangladesh, Mozambique and Uganda) and expenditure 2003 (Russian Federation and Zimbabwe).
^c Estimates assume budget 2003 equal to expenditures 2003 for Mozambique, Russian Federation and Zimbabwe.
^d Budget data for UR Tanzania based on 2004 data.
^e "Unknown" applies to Mozambique in 2002 and Afghanistan 2002–2005, as breakdown by line item not available.

FIGURE 27

Total NTP budgets by source of funding, 21 high-burden countries,[a] 2002–2005

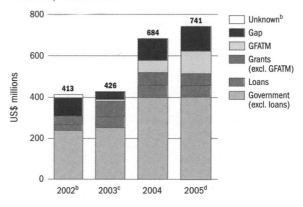

^a Data not available for South Africa.
^b Estimates assume budget 2002 equal to expenditure 2002 (Ethiopia), budget 2003 (Afghanistan, Bangladesh, Mozambique and Uganda) and expenditure 2003 (Russian Federation and Zimbabwe). "Unknown" applies to DR Congo and Nigeria, as breakdown by funding source not available.
^c Estimates assume budget 2003 equal to expenditures 2003 for Mozambique, Russian Federation and Zimbabwe.
^d Budget data for UR Tanzania based on 2004 data.

TABLE 15
NTP budgets and available funding, high-burden countries, 2005

	TOTAL NTP BUDGET (US$ MILLIONS)	CHANGE FROM 2002 (US$ MILLIONS)	CHANGE FROM 2002 (%)	AVAILABLE FUNDING (US$ MILLIONS)					CHANGE IN AVAILABLE FUNDING SINCE 2002, BY SOURCE (US$ MILLIONS)				
				GOVERNMENT (EXCL. LOANS)	LOANS	GRANTS (EXCL. GFATM)	GFATM	GAP	GOVERNMENT (EXCL. LOANS)	LOANS	GRANTS (EXCL. GFATM)	GFATM	GAP
1 India	46	10	29	5	11	6	8	15	-1	-13	0.7	8	15
2 China	158	60	61	98	14	4	21	21	45	14	2	21	-22
3 Indonesia	43	9	25	24	0	4	15	0	17	0	1	15	-25
4 Nigeria[a]	12	3	35	2	0	3	0	7	0.5	0	-2	0	-0.05
5 Bangladesh[b]	22	15	210	3	6	3	8	1	-0.1	6	-0.6	8	1
6 Pakistan	19	14	257	8	0	3	0	9	5	0	2	0	7
7 Ethiopia[c]	7	2	40	0.6	0	1	5	0	-0.6	0	-3	5	0
8 South Africa[d]	–	–	–	–	–	–	–	–	–	–	–	–	–
9 Philippines	8	0.5	6	3	0	4	2	0	-0.7	0	4	2	-4
10 Kenya	14	9	177	3	0	0	3	8	2 [e]	0	-3	3	7
11 DR Congo[a]	11	4.2	64	0.6	0	5	2	3	-0.4	0	-0.3	2	-0.8
12 Russian Federation[f]	316	178	129	220	25	2	30	39	90	25	-6	30	39
13 Viet Nam	12	0.4	4	9	0	0.9	2	0.3	0.5	-2	-0.1	2	0.3
14 UR Tanzania[g]	9	3	59	1	0	5	0.2	2	1	0	0.6	0.2	1
15 Brazil	21	8	59	19	0	2	0	0	6	0	2	0	0
16 Uganda[b]	6	1	22	0.7	0	0.8	0.9	4	0.6	-1	0.3	0.9	0.7
17 Thailand	5	-1	-23	3	0	0	2	0	-3	0	0	2	0
18 Mozambique[b]	7	-1	-10	0.8	0.2	2	4	0.1	0.5	0.2	-0.5	4	-5
19 Zimbabwe[f]	11	9	536	0.5	0	2	0	9	0.4	0	0.04	0	9
20 Myanmar	5	2	86	0.4	0	1	3	0.6	-0.03	0	1	3	-2
21 Afghanistan[b]	3	-0.3	-10	0.3	0	2	0.7	0	0	0	0.5	0.7	-2
22 Cambodia	7	3	60	0.7	0	4	1	1	-0.6	-0.7	3	1	0.01
High-burden countries	**741**	**328**	**59** [h]	**402**	**56**	**55**	**109**	**119**	**161**	**28**	**3**	**109**	**20**

– Indicates not available.

[a] Available funding compared with 2003, as no funding breakdown was provided in 2002; thus total of changes in available funding by source (US$ 321 million) does not equal the total shown in column 3 (US$ 328 million).

[b] Comparisons are with budget for 2003, as budget data for 2002 not available.

[c] Comparisons are with expenditure for 2002, asf budget data for 2002 not available.

[d] No data were provided by the NTP.

[e] May include some loan funding.

[f] Comparisons are with expenditure for 2003, as budget data for 2002 or 2003 not available. Figures for Russian Federation for 2005 based on estimates prepared by WHO staff (Moscow office). See country profile for further details.

[g] Latest available data are for 2004.

[h] Median value.

The increase in the Russian Federation could be larger (US$ 178 million), if it is assumed that the 2002 budget was similar to reported expenditures (budget data were not reported for 2002). In 2003, the Russian Federation developed an ambitious five-year plan to expand DOTS and to upgrade TB control in general, covering the period 2003–2007. For other countries, the budget differences between 2002 and 2005 are all US$ 15 million or less.

In relative terms, the biggest budget increases are for Bangladesh and Pakistan (both more than 200%), followed by Kenya at 177% (Table 15, column 4). Six countries reported changes of 50–100% (Brazil, Cambodia, China, the Democratic Republic of the Congo, Myanmar, the United Republic of Tanzania), and four of 25–50% (Ethiopia, India, Indonesia, Nigeria). When compared with expenditures rather than budgets, the increases since 2003 are enormous for Zimbabwe (536%) and large for the Russian Federation (129%).

These large budget increases have been accompanied by big improvements in available funding for NTPs (Table 15 columns 5–8 and 10–13; Figure 27). For all HBCs, available funding has increased by about US$ 300 million since 2002, reaching US$ 622 million in 2005. In 2005, HBC governments will provide 62% of the required funding (including loans); the GFATM 15% and grants from other sources 7%, leaving a gap equivalent to 16% of the reported budgets. However, sources of funding vary among the 22 HBCs (Figure 28), with a few countries relying mostly on govern-ment funding but most relying extensively on grants from the GFATM and other sources. Most of the increased funding since 2002 is from governments (an increase of US$ 189 million since 2002, including loans, almost all of which is in China and the Russian Federation) and the GFATM (US$ 109 million for 17 HBCs in 2005 compared with no contribution in 2002). There has been virtually no change in grant funding from sources other than the GFATM.

Despite this progress in securing additional funding, there is a large funding gap of US$ 119 million in 2005 (Table 15 column 9), which is higher than the gaps reported for 2003 and 2004. In absolute terms, the largest funding gaps are those reported by China, India, Pakistan, the Russian Federation and Zimbabwe

(US$ 93 million, or 78% of the total gap). The shortfall in India is associated with the end of the existing World Bank credit (1998–2004), but the balance is expected to be made up through additional grants and a new World Bank credit to be negotiated in 2005. Gaps in the other four countries are linked to the development in 2003 and/or 2004 of much more ambitious plans to expand and improve TB control. Proportionally, the largest gaps are in Kenya, Nigeria, Uganda and Zimbabwe (all more than 50% of the total NTP budget; Figure 28). These gaps are large enough to seriously constrain progress in TB control in these countries.

Further details, including charts showing trends in NTP budgets by funding source and line item for each year 2002–2005, are provided in the country profiles (Annex 1).

Total costs of TB control and funding in HBCs

NTP budgets include only part of the resources needed for TB control. In particular, they do not include the costs associated with general health services staff and infrastructure, which are used when TB patients are hospitalized or make outpatient clinic visits for directly observed treatment (DOT) and monitoring. For the 22 HBCs combined, the total costs of TB control are projected to be US$ 1.2 billion and US$ 1.3 billion in 2004 and 2005, respectively, compared with actual costs of around US$ 900 million in 2002 and 2003 (Figure 29, Figure 30, Table 16). These increases in projected costs are because of the large increases in planned NTP spending (described above) and because of the higher costs of clinic visits and hospitalization that are associated with treating more patients.

The largest costs are for the Russian Federation and South Africa,

FIGURE 28

Sources of funding for NTP budgets, 21 high-burden countries,[a] 2005

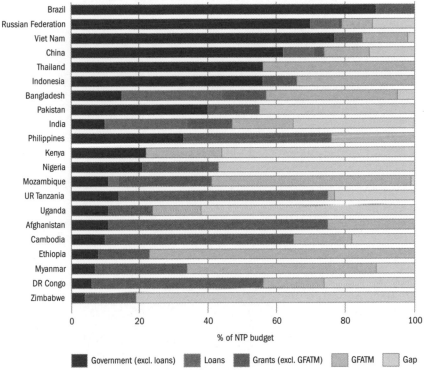

[a] No data available for South Africa. Figures for Russian Federation based on estimates prepared by WHO staff (Moscow office). See country profile for further details.

FIGURE 29

Total TB control costs by line item, 22 high-burden countries, 2002–2005

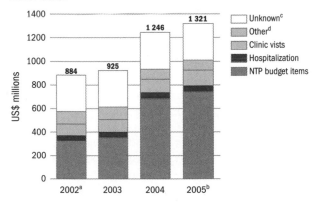

[a] Costs assumed to be as for 2003 for Afghanistan, Bangladesh, Mozambique, Russian Federation, Uganda and Zimbabwe.
[b] Estimate for UR Tanzania is based on 2004 data.
[c] Total TB control costs for Thailand and South Africa could not be broken down as for other countries, so the total is presented as "Unknown". Estimates for South Africa are based on recent costing studies.
[d] "Other" includes costs for hospitalization and fluorography in the Russian Federation not reflected in the NTP budget.

FIGURE 30

Total TB control costs by funding source, 22 high-burden countries, 2002–2005

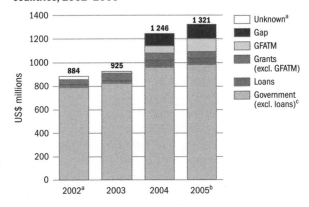

[a] Costs assumed to be as for 2003 for Afghanistan, Bangladesh, Mozambique, Russian Federation, Uganda and Zimbabwe. "Unknown" applies to DR Congo and Nigeria, as breakdown of NTP budget by funding source not available.
[b] Estimate for UR Tanzania is based on 2004 data.
[c] Estimates of total TB control costs (2002–2005) for South Africa are based on costing studies and all costs are assumed to be funded by the government.

TABLE 16
Total TB control costs and available funding, high-burden countries, 2005

	TOTAL COST (US$ MILLIONS)	CHANGE FROM 2002[a] (US$ MILLIONS)	CHANGE FROM 2002 (%)	AVAILABLE FUNDING (US$ MILLIONS)					CHANGE IN AVAILABLE FUNDING SINCE 2002,[b] BY SOURCE (US$ MILLIONS)				
				GOVERNMENT (EXCL. LOANS)	LOANS	GRANTS (EXCL. GFATM)	GFATM	GAP	GOVERNMENT (EXCL. LOANS)	LOANS	GRANTS (EXCL. GFATM)	GFATM	GAP
1 India	89	28	45	48	11	6	8	15	5	-13	0.7	8	15
2 China	158	97	159	98	14	4	21	21	45	14	2	21	-22
3 Indonesia	50	28	125	31	0	4	15	0	20	0	1	15	-25
4 Nigeria	21	10	90	12	0	3	0	7	4	0	-2	0	-0.05
5 Bangladesh	27	17	169	9	6	3	8	1	2	6	-0.7	8	1
6 Pakistan	26	21	434	15	0	3	0	9	9	0	2	0	7
7 Ethiopia[c]	9	1	12	3	0	1	5	0	-1	0	-3	5	0
8 South Africa[d]	300	–	–	300	–	–	–	–	–	–	–	–	–
9 Philippines	30	9	41	25	0	4	2	0	6	0	4	2	-4
10 Kenya	18	11	170	6	0	0	3	8	-0.7	0	-3	3	7
11 DR Congo	34	14	70	24	0	5	2	3	7	0	0	2	-0.8
12 Russian Federation[e]	399	154	63	303	25	2	30	39	66	25	-6	30	39
13 Viet Nam	28	3	13	25	0	0.9	2	0.3	0.2	-2	-0.1	2	0.3
14 UR Tanzania[f]	21	5	31	13	0	5	0.2	2	2	0	0.6	0.2	1
15 Brazil	46	9	25	44	0	2	0	0	7	0	2	0	0
16 Uganda	7	5	198	1	0	0.8	0.9	4	0.7	-1	0.3	0.9	0.7
17 Thailand	11	3	31	9	0	0	2	0	0.6	0	0	2	0
18 Mozambique	9	5	139	3	0.2	2	4	0.1	0.7	0.2	-0.5	4	-5
19 Zimbabwe[e]	15	9	158	5	0	2	0	9	0.4	0	0.04	0	9
20 Myanmar	6	4	232	1	0	1	3	0.6	0.3	0	1	3	-2
21 Afghanistan	3	-1	-34	0.3	0	2	0.7	0	0	0	0.5	0.7	-2
22 Cambodia	12	4	63	5	0	4	1	1	0.3	-0.7	3	1	0.0
High-burden countries	**1321**	**437**	**70** [g]	**982**	**56**	**55**	**109**	**119**	**175**	**28**	**3**	**109**	**20**

– Indicates not available.

[a] TB control costs in 2002 were estimated using expenditure rather than budget data wherever possible. For countries that did not provide expenditure data for 2002 (Kenya and UR Tanzania), available funding was used as a proxy. Where neither budget nor expenditure data were available for 2002 (Afghanistan, Bangladesh, Mozambique, Russian Federation, Uganda and Zimbabwe), comparisons are with 2003.

[b] The sum of changes in available funding is different from the total change in TB control costs (column 3) when expenditures are lower than available funding. A further reason is that changes are calculated with respect to 2003 when a breakdown of funding was not available for 2002 (DR Congo and Nigeria).

[c] Comparisons are with expenditure data for 2002.

[d] No data were provided by the NTP; the cost per patient was estimated using recently published costing studies and multiplied by the number of patients notified in 2003 to give the estimated total cost.

[e] Comparisons are with expenditure data for 2003. Figures for Russian Federation for 2005 based on estimates prepared by WHO (Moscow office). See country profile for further details.

[f] Latest available data are for 2004.

[g] Median value.

which together account for US$ 700 million of the total cost of US$ 1.3 billion estimated for 2005. South Africa is a middle-income country, and the high costs are mainly explained by the higher prices for items such as hospitalization and outpatient visits, compared with those typical in low-income countries. The Russian Federation staffs and runs an extensive network of TB hospitals for treatment, has a large budget for second-line drugs to treat many MDR-TB patients and still carries out mass population screening by fluorography. China and India have the third and fourth highest costs, estimated at US$ 158 million and US$ 89 million respectively in 2005. Seven additional countries have total costs of US$ 25–50

million in 2005, three have costs of around US$ 20 million and the rest have costs of US$ 15 million or less.

The countries with the largest projected absolute increases in annual costs are the Russian Federation (US$ 154 million since 2003) and China (US$ 97 million since 2002). Increases of around US$ 20–30 million since 2002 are estimated for Bangladesh, India, Indonesia and Pakistan. The changes for other HBCs are around or below US$ 10 million. The biggest proportional increases are for Myanmar and Pakistan (both more than 200%), while increases are in the range 100–200% for seven additional countries.

Funding for the general health services staff and infrastructure used by

TB patients during clinic visits and hospitalization is assumed to be funded by governments. This assumption, together with the implicit assumption that health systems have sufficient resources to support the treatment of growing numbers of patients in 2004 and 2005, means that the resources available for TB control are estimated to have increased from almost US$ 900 million in 2002 to US$ 1.2 billion in 2005 (Figure 30). The contribution by HBC governments to the total cost of TB control in 2005 is 79% on average, which is larger than their contribution to NTP budgets (Figure 31). This high average figure conceals important variation among countries; many HBCs are dependent on grants to cover more than one third of the total costs of TB control, or to close large funding gaps. The share of the total costs provided by HBC governments is closely related to average income levels (Figure 32), although Viet Nam stands out as a low-income country with a very high government contribution (90%).

For all HBCs, the estimated gap between the funding already available and the total cost of TB control is US$ 119 million in 2005, i.e. the NTP budget gap reported above. Further details, including charts that show trends in total TB control costs by line item for each year 2002–2005, are provided in the country profiles.

Per patient costs and budgets

There is much variation among countries in budgets and costs per patient (Table 17). The budgets for first-line drugs are lowest in India, Myanmar and the Philippines (US$ 11–17 per patient). In most countries, the budget is in the range US$ 20–35, but higher in Bangladesh, Brazil, Indonesia, Mozambique and the Russian Federation. Higher budgets in Bangladesh and Mozambique are explained by the creation of large buffer stocks, which distort the average value in 2005. In Indonesia, the drug budget has increased to allow use of fixed-dose combinations (FDCs).

The budget per patient, including all line items, is lowest in India, at US$ 34. The budget is also relatively low in Ethiopia and the Philippines (both around US$ 50) and in Myanmar (US$ 68). Most other countries (*n* = 13) have budgets in the range US$ 100–200 per patient. The only low-income country with a budget above US$ 200 per patient is Mozambique. The Russian Federation has by far the highest budget per patient, for reasons explained above (the figure for South Africa may also be high, but no data are available).

The total cost per patient treated in 2005 is lowest in India (US$ 66), below US$ 100 in Ethiopia and Myanmar, and below US$ 150 in Bangladesh and Uganda. It is in the range US$ 150–300 in 11 countries,[26] and

[26] This assumes that if data for Afghanistan were available, the cost would be in this range.

FIGURE 31

Sources of funding for total TB control costs, 22 high-burden countries,ᵃ 2005

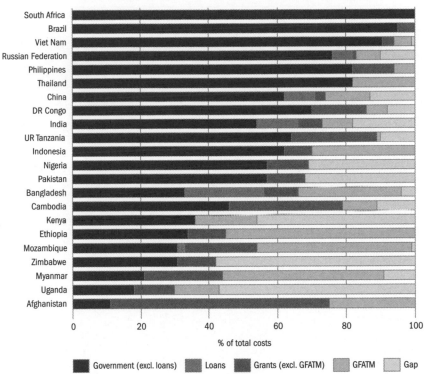

ᵃ Figures for Russian Federation based on estimates prepared by WHO staff (Moscow office) and recent costing studies. See country profile for further details.

FIGURE 32

Government contribution to total TB control costs by GNI per capita, 20 high-burden countries,ᵃ 2005

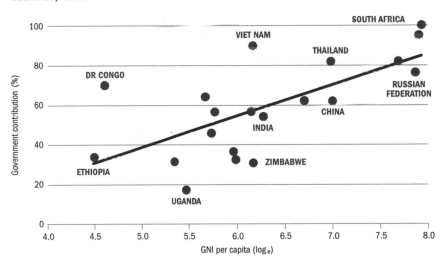

ᵃ No information on GNI per capita available for Afghanistan or Myanmar. Figure for Russian Federation based on estimates prepared by WHO staff (Moscow office) and recent costing studies. See country profile for further details.

TABLE 17
Total costs and NTP budgets per patient, high-burden countries, 2005

	2005 (US$)			CHANGES FROM 2002 (FACTOR[a])		
	FIRST-LINE DRUGS BUDGET	NTP BUDGET	TOTAL COST	FIRST-LINE DRUGS BUDGET	NTP BUDGET[b]	TOTAL COST
1 India	11	34	66	1.1	1.0	1.1
2 China	20	188	188	1.2	1.4	1.4
3 Indonesia	47	155	182	1.5	1.3	1.3
4 Nigeria	29	159	291	0.5	1.2 [c]	1.0
5 Bangladesh[c]	45	116	146	2.2	1.5	1.3
6 Pakistan	23	153	213	0.4	3.3	2.3
7 Ethiopia	34	49	68	1.3	1.1	0.9
8 South Africa	–	–	1320 [d]	–	–	–
9 Philippines	17	48	174	0.7	0.9	1.0
10 Kenya	31	142	173	0.8	2.7	2.1
11 DR Congo	14	94	297	0.4	1.0	1.0
12 Russian Federation[e]	70	2748	3472	1.0	2.5 [c]	1.8
13 Viet Nam	31	129	299	0.9	1.1	1.2
14 UR Tanzania[f]	21	133	320	0.5	1.6	1.2
15 Brazil	47	239	516	1.0	1.4	1.1
16 Uganda[c]	20	111	120	0.4	2.3	2.1
17 Thailand	25	72 [g]	173	0.3	0.6	1.0
18 Mozambique[c]	75	241	311	3.4	3.3	2.2
19 Zimbabwe[c]	35	192	266	1.1	5.8	2.4
20 Myanmar	13	68	80	0.7	3.2	2.5
21 Afghanistan[c]	–	104	–	–	0.3	–
22 Cambodia	27	186	311	0.7	1.4	1.1
High-burden countries (median value)	**28**	**133**	**213**	**0.9**	**1.4**	**1.2**

– Indicates not available.

a Calculated as 2005 value divided by 2002 value.

b Calculated as NTP budget per patient projected in 2005 divided by NTP expenditure per patient notified in 2002. Available funding was used as a proxy for expenditures for India, Kenya, Thailand, Uganda, UR Tanzania and Viet Nam.

c Comparisons are with 2003 data.

d Estimate is based on notifications for 2003, as no projections for 2005 available.

e Figures for 2005 based on estimates prepared by WHO staff (Moscow office). See country profile for further details. Comparison for first-line drugs is with 2004.

f Latest available data are for 2004. Thus comparison is of 2004 with 2002.

g This figure is artificially low because it is based on the central level budget only (see country profile).

FIGURE 33

Cost per patient treated by GNI per capita, 20 high-burden countries,[a] 2005

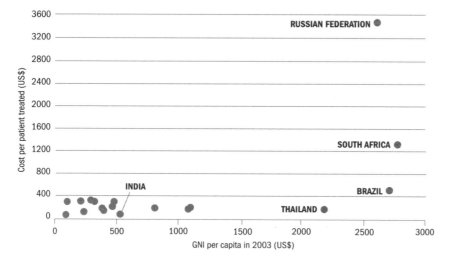

a No information on GNI per capita available for Afghanistan or Myanmar. Figure for Russian Federation based on estimates prepared by WHO staff (Moscow office) and recent costing studies. See country profile for further details.

slightly more than US$ 300 in three countries. There are three countries with much higher costs: Brazil, the Russian Federation and South Africa. Their higher costs are not surprising given their middle-income status and associated higher prices for inputs such as staff (Figure 33), as well as the extensive use of hospitalization in the Russian Federation.

Budgets and costs are generally stable (notably during a period of rapid DOTS expansion in India) or increasing.

Further details, including charts that show five per patient indicators (costs, budgets, available funding, expenditures and first-line drugs budget) for each year 2002–2005, are provided in the country profiles (Annex 1).

Expenditures in comparison with budgets and available funding

For countries that have received large increases in funding, the challenge now is to spend the extra money, and to translate extra spending into improved case detection and treatment success rates. The ability to spend available money can be assessed by comparing expenditures with available funding and budgets (Table 18). Complete sets of data on budgets, funds and expenditures are available for 15 HBCs in 2003 (the most recent year for which expenditure data are currently available). Expenditures were generally less than available funding. In India, costs proved to be lower than anticipated, and all planned activities were implemented. The capacity of the Tanzanian NTP to spend available money is discussed in Annex 1. For other countries, more work is needed to understand the reasons why expenditures are lower than available funding. The findings will have implications for programmes that are now benefiting from large influxes of new money. It is too early to say if large increases in spending can be translated into improved programme performance.

Budgets, funds and targets

Countries can be categorized according to whether the number of patients to be treated is consistent with meeting the 2005 targets, treatment success rates, the extent to which the budget for the projected number of patients is funded, how the budget per patient has changed through time and whether there is evidence that the additional funding can be effectively absorbed (Table 19). India, Myanmar, the Philippines and Viet Nam are in the best financial position to reach the targets (or to maintain the programme at target levels in the case of Viet Nam). Cambodia and China are well placed to do so if they can make up the remaining funding shortfalls. Indonesia appears to have the funding required to achieve targets, and Bangladesh may come close. However, it is unclear how many more cases will actually be detected and successfully treated as a result of the additional funds now available in these two countries. For the remaining 14 HBCs, the planned programmes of treatment are less than required to meet the targets for case detection (11 countries) and/or it is not clear if they are sufficient to meet the target for treatment success, although five of these countries report no or negligible shortfalls in funding.

GFATM contribution to TB control
High-burden countries. The GFATM is the single most important source of grant funding for HBCs, and several countries are relying on the GFATM to fund more than one third of their budgets. After four rounds of proposals, the total value of approved proposals (which, with four exceptions, cover five years) is US$ 818 million (Table 20). The amounts included in the two-year grant agreements[27] total US$ 218 million, and are sometimes lower than the amounts in years 1 and 2 of the original proposals (75% for those proposals for which both the original request for years 1 and 2 and the grant agreement amount are available; the biggest discrepancy is for Indonesia).

By the end of 2004, US$ 116 million had been disbursed. For each country, we can compare the actual and expected rates of disbursal, where the expected rate assumes that disbursements should be spread evenly

[27] Signature of grant agreements is needed before any disbursements can take place.

TABLE 18
Budgets, available funding and expenditures (US$ millions),
15 high-burden countries, 2003

	BUDGET	AVAILABLE FUNDING	EXPENDITURES
1 India	42	42	25
2 China	95	87	80
3 Indonesia	32	29	21
4 Nigeria	13	6	6
5 Bangladesh	7	7	7
6 Pakistan	6	6	3
7 Ethiopia	11	11	8
8 Philippines	7	6	4
9 DR Congo	10	7	5
10 Viet Nam	11	11	11
11 UR Tanzania	5	5	4
12 Brazil	16	16	14
13 Mozambique	8	3	2
14 Myanmar	5	1	1
15 Cambodia	6	3	2
Total	**273**	**239**	**193**

TABLE 19
Categorization of high-burden countries according to financial criteria, 2005

CATEGORY	CRITERIA	COUNTRIES
I	Projected number of cases to be treated in 2005 sufficient to meet 70% case detection target Treatment success rate achieved or close to being achieved for 2002 cohort Budget per patient treated stable or increasing No or minor funding gap, or funding gap likely to be filled Demonstrated ability to absorb any additional funds required to achieve targets	India Myanmar Philippines Viet Nam
IIa	As for I, except that funding gap needs to be filled	Cambodia China
IIb	As for I, except that ability to absorb large increases in funding and translate them into improved detection and treatment success rates is currently unproven	Indonesia
IIc	As for IIb, but projected number of cases treated only within 10% of case detection target	Bangladesh
III	Projected cases not in line with case detection target, and/or unclear if treatment success target can be achieved, but no (or negligible) reported funding gap	Brazil Ethiopia Mozambique South Africa Thailand
IV	Projected cases not in line with case detection target (all except DR Congo) and/or treatment success, and large funding gap	Afghanistan DR Congo Kenya Nigeria Pakistan Russian Federation Uganda UR Tanzania Zimbabwe

TABLE 20
GFATM financing, high-burden countries, as of end 2004

	GRANT	TOTAL BUDGET APPROVED [a] (US$ MILLIONS)	TOTAL YEAR 1 AND 2 BUDGETS (AS IN PROPOSALS) (US$ MILLIONS)	FIRST 2-YEAR GRANT AGREEMENT (US$ MILLIONS)	TOTAL DISBURSEMENTS BY END 2004 (AS OF 20-DEC-2004) (US$ MILLIONS)	TOTAL DISBURSEMENTS BY END 2004 AS % OF GRANT AGREEMENT — ACTUAL RATE OF DISBURSAL	EXPECTED RATE OF DISBURSAL	DATE BOARD APPROVAL	DATE GRANT AGREEMENT SIGNATURE	TIME BETWEEN BOARD APPROVAL AND SIGNATURE OF GRANT AGREEMENT (MONTHS)	TIME BETWEEN GRANT AGREEMENT SIGNATURE AND FIRST DISBURSEMENT (MONTHS)
1 India	G1[b]	9	6	6	4	76	96	22-Apr-02	30-Jan-03	9	6
	G2[c]	29	13	7	2	27	42	13-Jan-03	12-Feb-04	13	2
	G3[c,d]	15	3	3	0	0	8	15-Oct-03	15-Oct-04	12	2+
	G4	27	7	Not signed yet				28-Jun-04		6+	
2 China	G1	48	25	25	25	100	96	22-Apr-02	30-Jan-03	9	2
	G2	56	28	Not signed yet				28-Jun-04		6+	
3 Indonesia		70.7	55	22	16	73	96	22-Apr-02	27-Jan-03	9	2
4 Bangladesh	G1[c]	42	17	11	5	41	21	15-Oct-03	07-Jul-04	9	0.6
	G2[c]	18	8	5	2	44	13	15-Oct-03	24-Aug-04	10	0.2
5 Pakistan	G1[c]	4	2	2	0.7	31	67	13-Jan-03	06-Aug-03	7	4
	G2[c]	13	7	6	2	33	8	15-Oct-03	12-Oct-04	12	1
6 Ethiopia[c]		21	–	11	7	59	88	22-Apr-02	18-Mar-03	11	5
7 South Africa	G1[d]	70	14	2	2	100	67	22-Apr-02	08-Aug-03	16	4
	G2[c,d]	–	–	12	9	76	67	22-Apr-02	08-Aug-03	16	4
	G3[c,d]	72	27	27	13	48	67	22-Apr-02	08-Aug-03	16	4
	G4[d]	25	8	Not signed yet				13-Jan-03		23+	
8 Philippines		11	3	3	3	77	75	13-Jan-03	11-Jun-03	5	0.6
9 Kenya		11	5	5	2	50	75	13-Jan-03	23-Jun-03	5	2
10 DR Congo[b,c]		8	6	6	6	90	75	13-Jan-03	18-Jun-03	5	1
11 Russian Federation	G1(Tomsk)[c]	11	6	6	2	28	8	15-Oct-03	14-Oct-04	12	2
	G2	92	54	Not signed yet				28-Jun-04		6+	
12 Viet Nam[c]		10	3	3	0.4	16	58	13-Jan-03	15-Oct-03	9	5
13 UR Tanzania	G1[c,d]	88	25	24	7	30	13	15-Oct-03	06-Sep-04	11	2
	G2 (Zanzibar)[c]	2	1	1	0.7	70	95	13-Jan-03	07-Sep-04	20	2
14 Uganda[c]		6	7	5	1	25	38	13-Jan-03	15-Mar-04	14	1
15 Thailand		13	7	7	3	45	79	22-Apr-02	18-May-03	13	2
16 Mozambique[c]		18	12	9	0	0	38	13-Jan-03	02-Apr-04	15	9+
17 Myanmar[c]		17	7	7	2	34	17	13-Jan-03	13-Aug-04	19	1
18 Afghanistan[b]		3	2	Not signed yet				28-Jun-04		6+	
19 Cambodia		7	3	3	1	45	58	13-Jan-03	14-Oct-03	9	2
Total		**818**	**361**	**218**	**116**	**45[e]**	**67[e]**			**11[e]**	**2[e]**

– Indicates not available.

[a] Total budget requested is for five years, unless otherwise stated.

[b] Total budget requested is for three years.

[c] Assessment of principal recipient pending.

[d] TB/HIV grant.

[e] Median value.

over the two years following the date on which the agreement is signed (Table 20, column 7). China is the only country where all funds in the two-year grant agreement have been disbursed within the expected period of two years. For eight countries and 10 grants, disbursements are better than expected.[28] For five countries, disbursements are within 20% of the expected value, and for nine countries disbursements are around 25% or more below the expected value. One example is Ethiopia, a country that is largely dependent on GFATM funds. Another is Mozambique, which is also highly dependent on the GFATM, but

which has to date received no funds at all, even though the grant agreement was signed in April 2004. The GFATM web site notes that initial disbursements are often small, given the need for strengthening programme capacity and preparation of procurement plans.[29] Furthermore, low disbursement rates appear to be associated with the principal recipient; for eight countries and nine grants where the disbursements are below the expected value, the GFATM web site notes that assessments of the principal recipient are pending.

The initial delay in disbursement is caused mainly by the time taken to

sign the grant agreement after proposal approval. Once grant agreements are signed, disbursements are usually made within 2 months (the exception is currently Mozambique), compared with delays of between 5 and 23 (median value 11) months between grant approval and signature.

Other countries. After four rounds of proposals, 60 non-HBCs have ap-

[28] However, the figure for Myanmar is misleading, because the NTP is a sub-recipient that had not received any funds by the end of 2004.

[29] http://www.theglobalfund.org/en/funds_raised/commitments/.

proved proposals with a total value of US$ 400 million. The amounts included in the two-year grant agreements[30] total US$ 153 million, of which US$ 65 million had been disbursed by the end of 2004. Disbursements are generally similar or higher than expected values, except in the European and South-East Asia Regions. A summary table with the same indicators as those shown for the HBCs is available upon request.

The regional distribution of GFATM grants for HBCs and other countries is shown in Figure 34.

NTP budgets by WHO region, HBCs and other countries

NTP budgets and sources of funding by WHO region in 2005 are shown for both HBCs and non-HBCs in Figure 35, based on the 55 countries that submitted data of sufficient quality. Total budgets and sources of funding are dominated by the HBCs in the South-East Asia Region and the Western Pacific Region, because the HBCs account for almost all TB cases in these regions. While non-HBCs account for a large share of cases in the European Region, Eastern Mediterranean Region and Region of the Americas, we received insufficient data to make an assessment of total budgets and funding sources, or to make any useful comparisons between HBCs and non-HBCs. For the African Region, we had budget data for countries that account for 79% of TB cases.[31] Non-HBCs add substantially to the HBC budget totals (US$ 128 million versus US$ 77 million for HBCs alone). Proportional to budgets, funding gaps are smaller in non-HBCs in the African Region, with relatively higher funding contributions from the GFATM and governments.

FIGURE 34

Regional distribution of GFATM lifetime budgets, as of end 2004

Total TB and TB/HIV: US$ 1.2 billion
Total TB/HIV: US$ 296 million

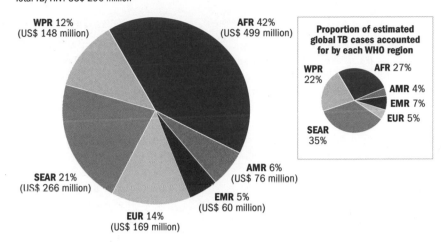

FIGURE 35

Regional distribution of total NTP budgets by source of funding, 20 high-burden and 35 non high-burden countries, 2005[a]
Figures in parentheses show the percentage of all estimated global TB cases in the region accounted for by the countries included in the bar.

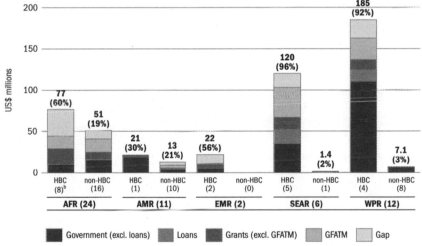

[a] The European Region is excluded because the much higher budget in the Russian Federation makes it difficult to illustrate patterns in other regions. Complete data were received from three countries other than the Russian Federation: Estonia, Latvia and Republic of Moldova. For these three countries funds come entirely from the government with the exception of a GFATM grant for the Republic of Moldova.
[b] Excludes South Africa.

---

[30] Signature of grant agreements is needed before any disbursements can take place.
[31] If data for South Africa were available, the figure would be 89%.

Discussion

Progress towards the Millennium Development Goals

Within the framework of the United Nations MDGs, TB control is guided by five principal indicators, two that quantify DOTS implementation (case detection, treatment success) and three that could measure the impact of DOTS on the epidemic (incidence, prevalence, mortality). The MDG framework is a stimulus to think beyond the 2005 targets for DOTS implementation, and to consider the benefits of TB control up to and beyond 2015. Long-term thinking underpins sustainable TB control, and is vital for planning the trajectory towards TB elimination.

This is the first in this series of annual reports to evaluate changes in incidence, prevalence and deaths from 1990, the MDG reference year, through to 2003. Based primarily on trends in case notifications, the TB incidence rate was, by 2003, falling or stable in seven out of the nine regions of the world defined in Figure 6. Incidence rates in eastern Europe (mostly countries of the former Soviet Union) and Africa (countries with low and high HIV rates) increased during the 1990s, but appear to have peaked in Europe around 2001, and have since fallen. There is no persuasive method of predicting when peak incidence rates will be reached, and at what levels, in Africa, but the rates of increase slowed markedly during the 1990s.

Because these adverse regional effects are diminishing, the rate of increase in global incidence is also slowing, after growing most rapidly in the mid 1990s. The global incidence rate reached 140 per 100 000 population in 2003 (8.8 million new cases, including those who are HIV-positive), but was still increasing at 1.0% annually. This assessment is, however, dependent on the assumptions we have made about trends in HBCs. For example, the series of case notifications for India suggest that the incidence rate is falling, but the preferred assumption, until further evidence becomes available, is that incidence is stable (this is conservative with respect to case detection and the impact of DOTS). If the incidence rate is actually falling in India at 2.4% per year, as indicated by case notifications in 1992–2003, then the global incidence rate would also be falling, albeit slowly.

The trend in global TB incidence has been little affected, so far, by DOTS programmes. Chemotherapy is more likely to have reduced TB prevalence and deaths, but neither of these indicators is measured routinely in HBCs. The calculations presented here, which are derived from estimates of incidence, duration and case fatality, suggest that the global prevalence rate fell from 309 to 245 per 100 000 between 1990 and 2003 (including HIV-positive TB patients), and was falling at 5% per year in 2003. The TB death rate (including deaths among HIV-positive TB patients) was also falling in 2003, but more slowly at 2.5% per year. Prevalence and deaths, like incidence, have been rising in Africa, and most steeply in African countries with the highest rates of HIV infection. In our assessment, incidence, prevalence and death rates are falling or stable in five out of the six WHO regions, and in seven of the nine regions of the world shown in Figure 6.

Treatment success in the 2002 cohort was reported to be 82% of 1.4 million registered cases, close to the 85% target, but no higher than in previous two annual cohorts. The overall rate of treatment success is strongly influenced by data from the three countries that have the largest numbers of new cases annually – China, India and Indonesia. All three submitted data indicating that the 85% target had been exceeded in 2002. These are impressive results, achieved while treating hundreds of thousands of patients, but success rates reported to be higher than 90% (e.g. China) need to be kept under review.

Of greater concern are the low cure rates in the European Region and the African Region in 2002. The European Region reported the highest rate of treatment failure, probably linked to the high levels of drug resistance in countries of the former Soviet Union. It also reported the second highest death rate on treatment, which is likely to be associated both with drug resistance and with the high proportion of elderly patients in Western Europe. The African Region reported the highest death rates in TB patients, undoubtedly associated with HIV coinfection. But the success rate of African DOTS programmes was also low because they lost 19% of patients through default, transfer between treatment centres or by failing to record any outcome of treatment (patients "not evaluated"). Such losses to follow-up were also high in the Region of the Americas, Eastern Mediterranean Region and European Region.

The target for treatment success under DOTS refers only to new smear-positive cases, but information about patients presenting for re-treatment, including the outcomes of treatment for these patients, is also indicative of programme performance. The WHO data collection form for the 2002 cohort asked DOTS programmes to distinguish between re-treatment after relapse, default and failure, both for cases reported in 2003 and for patients undergoing re-treatment during 2002. Although it is probable that the case definitions (Table 2) are not strictly observed (and many re-treated patients were not classified in data submitted to WHO), some of the findings deserve comment. First, the comparative success of treatment for different classes of patients was consistent with expectations: lower on average for re-treated than for new cases; and among re-treated patients, higher for relapses, intermediate for defaulters and lowest for failures. Moreover, patients who defaulted during their first course of treatment tended to default from a second or subsequent course of treatment.

Third, the regional distribution of adverse re-treatment outcomes resembled the pattern observed for new cases: African countries reported high death rates and many patients were lost to follow-up; European countries reported high rates of death and treatment failure. The accuracy of reporting needs to be verified, but these data should help to identify TB patients who, for example, are less likely to comply with treatment (persistent defaulters) and those who are more likely to be infected with HIV (especially in Africa), or who are carrying drug-resistant bacilli (especially in eastern Europe).

Although DOTS programmes have diagnosed and treated more than 17 million cases since 1995, the global DOTS case detection rate was still only 45% in 2003, well below the 70% target. However, the detection rate increased by 8% between 2002 and 2003, faster than at any time since recording began in 1995. If detection continues to increase at this rate, the estimated global case detection rate will be approximately 60% by 2005.

While the acceleration in case-finding during 2003 exceeded expectations, most of the additional patients (63%) were reported by just two countries: China and India. If this pace of expansion is to be maintained or accelerated, other HBCs must contribute more. Approximately 1.8 million smear-positive cases were notified by DOTS programmes in 2003. According to our estimates, another 1.4 million new patients, undetected by DOTS programmes in 2003, were living in just eight HBCs, including China and India. Together, these 3.2 million patients account for more than 70% of new cases arising in 2003. Therefore, intensive case-finding in these countries would contribute greatly to meeting the global target of 70% case detection.

In some regions of the world, large numbers of patients are reported from outside DOTS areas. The 70% target could be reached in the Region of the Americas by ensuring that more than 43 000 smear-positive patients currently reported by non-DOTS programmes are diagnosed and treated under DOTS, the majority in Brazil. In

the European Region, the Russian Federation reported more than 100 000 patients from the 75% of the country not yet covered by DOTS, 23 000 of which were new smear-positive patients. China and India reported an additional 70 000 new smear-positive patients from non-DOTS areas in 2003.

By contrast, DOTS programmes in other HBCs including Bangladesh, Ethiopia, Indonesia, Nigeria and Pakistan will have to recruit patients that are not yet seen and reported by public health surveillance systems. These unreported patients undoubtedly exist because they are found, for example, during population-based prevalence surveys. Some never receive TB treatment; some are treated in public and private clinics and hospitals that are not linked to ministries of health. To ensure that these patients have access to DOTS services, TB control programmes will need to embark on new activities and establish new collaborations, many of which will be specific to the structure of local health services.

Considering both of the targets for DOTS implementation, Viet Nam was still the only member of the current group of HBCs to have reached 70% case detection and 85% treatment success by 2003. However, Cambodia, Myanmar and the Philippines were all close to achieving the targets. Although these Asian countries have different problems to solve, they should, with China and India, be able to meet the targets by 2005.

Smear-positive patients are the focus of the DOTS strategy, but many DOTS programmes also routinely treat smear-negative patients, with pulmonary or extrapulmonary disease. For the countries that report smear-negative patients, the numbers may be less accurate than for smear-positive disease because diagnosis is more difficult. In this context, the remarkable differences between regions in the proportions of patients reported with extrapulmonary disease need further investigation. The exceptionally high extrapulmonary case-load in the Eastern Mediterranean Region (20–30%) might be due to over-diagnosis, but it might also be a real and unex-

plained epidemiological phenomenon.

The establishment of the MDGs presents a challenge, not just for the implementation of DOTS and other means of TB control, but also for the measurement of epidemiological impact. Ideally, all countries would count new cases and deaths via a comprehensive routine system of surveillance and vital registration, and estimate the prevalence of disease and infection by population-based surveys. In reality, countries will have to select some methods of measurement in preference to others. Some guidance on the advantages and disadvantages of different epidemiological measurements is given in Table 21.

Planning and DOTS implementation

All HBCs have a strategic plan for DOTS expansion and, during 2005, many will begin a new planning cycle for the next five years. However, the transition from planning to implementation, and then to the improvement of coverage, case detection and treatment success has been slower than anticipated in several countries. The success of some NTPs in raising funds for TB control (and particularly from the GFATM) has not been followed by productive spending.

Among the obstacles to DOTS expansion, five are of overriding importance: shortages of trained staff, lack of political commitment, weak laboratory services, and the inadequate management of MDR-TB and of TB in people infected with HIV.

The acute shortage of adequately trained staff affects the distribution and quality of services. This workforce crisis is felt particularly in the underperformance of central management, and through failings in the laboratory network. To remedy the problem, the HBCs need, at the very least, strong and clear policies for recruiting, retaining and motivating staff. One way to secure political commitment to solve this and other problems is by strengthening national and international partnerships. A consistent message about the importance of TB control, delivered from various constituencies, is a basis for effective advocacy and communication.

TABLE 21

Advantages and disadvantages of various epidemiological measurements for TB control
Text in blue refers to attributes of the indicator; regular text refers to attributes of the measurement technique.

MEASURE	ADVANTAGES	DISADVANTAGES
Prevalence of infection	**Risk of infection changes relatively quickly in response to control (but prevalence, from which risk is calculated, changes slowly).**	**Measures infection, not disease burden; not an MDG indicator.**
From tuberculin surveys	Relatively cheap and logistically straightforward.	Results often hard to interpret where infection rates are low and where BCG coverage is high or where exposure to environmental mycobacteria is high; measures average risk of infection over past 5–10 years; Stýblo 1:50 rule for indirectly estimating disease incidence may not be applicable under chemotherapy, or where HIV infection rates are high.
Prevalence of disease	**Component due to duration of illness changes relatively quickly in response to control; MDG indicator.**	**Component due to incidence changes slowly in response to control.**
From population-based surveys	Accurate measure of bacteriologically confirmed disease; should change quickly in response to control; surveys useful where routine surveillance data are poor, and are a platform for related investigations e.g. of interactions between patients and health system.	Costly; logistically complex (especially with radiography), therefore cannot be measured annually; does not easily lead to an estimate of TB incidence (denominator of WHO case detection rate), because duration is hard to assess.
Incidence of disease	**Direct measure of denominator of WHO case detection rate; MDG indicator.**	**Changes slowly following reductions in transmission.**
From case notifications	Direct measure of incidence; absolute incidence can be assessed from routine case reports where case detection judged to be high; trends can be judged from series of routine case reports, if measured consistently; every country now has a surveillance system, reporting annually or sub-annually.	Case detection mostly low in high-burden countries (underestimates incidence), and may vary through time (inaccurate trends).
From consecutive prevalence surveys	Direct measure of incidence.	Costly; logistically complex; requires ≥2 surveys with carefully judged survey interval and follow-up of individual patients.
TB mortality	**Direct measure of TB burden accounting for a high proportion of DALYs; case fatality falls quickly in a new control programme; MDG indicator.**	**Component due to incidence changes slowly in response to control; hard to reduce case fatality further in low-burden countries.**
From observations on patient cohorts	Direct observation of number of patients dying.	Deaths observed are those in cohort only, not in the population at large, and not beyond the period of cohort follow-up; deaths among defaulters and transfers usually unknown; TB not always the cause of death for patients on TB treatment.
From product of incidence and case-fatality rate	Simple and widely applicable.	Relies on accurate measures of incidence (above) and case fatality; case fatality measurable in observed DOTS cohorts, but not among patients treated elsewhere or untreated. Approximate at best.
From vital (death) registrations (VR)	Direct measure of TB deaths and trends; can be reported annually or sub-annually.	VR does not yet exist in many high-burden countries (notably in Africa and Asia); typically underestimates TB deaths; sensitivity and specificity untested.
From verbal autopsy (VA)	Review of registered deaths can improve accuracy of cause of death statistics.	Sensitivity and specificity of VA not fully evaluated; where no death registration system exists, laborious to compile deaths from a rare disease, and requires large sample sizes.

Besides the staff shortages, many laboratories participating in DOTS programmes have insufficient equipment and supplies, and limited procedures for quality assurance. All these essential elements need to be in place before laboratories take on the larger tasks of culturing *M. tuberculosis* and testing for drug sensitivity, as will be required to integrate DOTS-Plus projects within DOTS programmes. To help improve capacity in HBCs, the DEWG has established a subgroup concerned with laboratory strengthening.

In addition to the deficiencies in laboratories, the lack of national policies on MDR-TB management, the widespread availability of drugs of uncertain quality and the large numbers of MDR-TB patients treated outside the NTP together suggest that the treatment of drug-resistant TB is often inadequate. The high proportions of re-treatment cases reported by NTPs are also a signal that drug-resistant forms of TB could be common in some populations where no surveys have yet been done. There are several remedies. WHO is in the process of expanding drug resistance surveillance and DOTS-Plus components within the context of regular TB control programmes. WHO is also working to establish a long-term competitive market for quality-assured drugs by leading a project to pre-qualify second-line drugs worldwide. GFATM grants are also being used to stimulate demand for drugs from reliable manufacturers. The Fund has selected the GLC as the mechanism for second-line drug procurement, and for monitoring approved projects.

The management of drug-resistant TB will be aided by a better understanding of the scale and distribution of the problem. Surveillance of drug resistance must be expanded to the five HBCs for which no data are yet available,[8] and to other countries suspected to have high prevalence rates of MDR-TB. Information about new TB patients will be supplemented by data on patients presenting for re-treatment, including the systematic notification of all categories of re-treatment cases, the reporting of treatment outcomes and representative drug resistance surveys.

During 2003, very few TB patients had access to VCT and to ART. The numbers that actually have access to these services are probably somewhat higher than reported, but cannot be accurately known until TB/HIV monitoring systems are substantially improved. HIV/AIDS programme staff are increasingly aware of the fact that people infected with HIV are at high risk of developing active TB, while their counterparts in TB control programmes are seeing the impact of HIV on TB case-load, and on death rates in cohorts of TB patients on treatment. There has, until now, been little collaboration between TB and HIV/AIDS control programmes, but many such programmes are beginning to adopt elements of the WHO interim policy on collaborative TB/HIV activities.[15] Even with the imperfect data presented in this report, it is clear that

much closer collaborations of this kind are needed to develop and improve access to prevention, treatment and support services, for both TB and HIV/AIDS patients.

Notwithstanding these weaknesses, this report has also identified a series of positive developments in DOTS implementation. The contributions to TB control of NGOs and community groups are clear expressions of the growing commitment of civil society. The work of these groups puts patients at the centre of the DOTS strategy, and improves access to TB services in remote areas and among disadvantaged and marginalized populations. NGOs are increasingly recognized as essential members of national partnerships for TB control. This recognition is helping not only to coordinate routine activities but also to develop a collaborative approach to solving the problems faced by NTPs. Some African countries are planning to involve community groups in collaborative TB/HIV activities. PPM projects are showing a measurable impact on case detection in several Asian countries, and may prove to be a mechanism for expanding TB control services in African cities.

With the significant influx of resources for TB control (from the GFATM, banks and bilaterals), especially to HBCs, some additional, catalytic funding is needed to ensure that NTPs have the technical capacity to make the best use of the new grants and loans. To satisfy this need, Stop TB partners launched a new initiative in 2003 – ISAC – an extraordinary effort to push towards the 2005 targets in selected countries, including China, India and Indonesia. The technical work under way aims to facilitate the access of patients to DOTS services, for example by expanding the geographical coverage of DOTS, by involving a greater diversity of public and private health-care providers, by strengthening in-country advocacy and social mobilization, and through partnership building and collaborative TB/HIV activities.

Financing DOTS expansion

There has been a big increase in NTP budgets and a big improvement in the

funding available for TB control since 2002, with particularly large increases between 2003 and 2004. The total reported NTP budgets for the 22 HBCs in 2005 are US$ 741 million, of which US$ 622 million is available and US$ 119 million is a funding gap. The total estimated costs of TB control[32] are projected to be US$ 1.3 billion, of which US$ 1.2 billion is already available. With the exception of large additional government contributions in China, Indonesia and the Russian Federation, almost all of the extra funding for TB control since 2002 is from GFATM grants. The GFATM now plays a major role in the financing of TB control, contributing more than one third of the budget in several HBCs, and over half in a few.

As usual, the summary statistics conceal important variations among countries. Our analyses suggest that in 2005, the HBCs fall into four categories. In the first are four countries (India, Myanmar, the Philippines and Viet Nam) that have budgets consistent with reaching the 2005 targets, and which are likely to have minimal or no funding shortfall. India has continued to expand rapidly with fully-funded budgets over the period 2002–2004, which, in 2003, provided more than enough money for planned activities. The Indian Revised National TB Control Programme has also maintained a constant budget per patient treated during the rapid expansion of DOTS. In the second are four countries that are close to being in this group, but which need to make up funding shortfalls (China, Cambodia), or where it is unclear how many more cases will actually be detected and successfully treated as a result of the substantial additional funds now available (Bangladesh, Indonesia). China stands out as having developed much larger budgets for 2004 and 2005 compared with previous years, for mobilizing a substantial increase in domestic and external financing to fund these budgets and for being the first HBC to secure full disbursement of a

---

[32] i.e. NTP budgets plus the cost of hospitalization and outpatient clinic visits of TB patients that are usually not included in NTP budgets.

two-year GFATM grant. In the third group are five countries that report no, or negligible, funding gaps for 2005, but whose plans are not sufficient to reach the targets for case detection (e.g. Ethiopia) or there are doubts about whether existing plans will ensure achievement of the treatment success target (e.g. South Africa). The nine countries in the final group need special attention because they report large funding gaps and, in addition, do not expect to treat enough patients to reach the case detection target (eight countries) and/or there are doubts about whether they can reach the treatment success target. Among these nine countries, Nigeria and Zimbabwe are the only low-income HBCs not to have secured GFATM funding to date. Pakistan's funding shortfall is a consequence, in large part, of planning for accelerated DOTS expansion in 2005.

The funding gap of US$ 119 million identified by all NTPs for 2005 is higher than reported in 2003 and 2004, but may still be an underestimate. The budget gap is the difference between the funds needed to carry out planned activities and the funds actually available. If the activities planned by NTPs for 2005 are a realistic assessment of what can achieved, the budget gaps reported are arguably an accurate reflection of the funding gap. However, the activities required to meet the 2005 case detection target are greater than planned in 12 countries, and while Brazil and South Africa may already detect more than 70% of all TB cases it is unclear whether they are budgeting sufficient resources to reach the target for treatment success. In this sense, the funding gaps are underestimates, although Brazil and South Africa are relatively wealthy middle-income countries that should be able to find any necessary resources from domestic budgets (Brazil has already increased its NTP budget by 50% since 2002). Apart from the question of whether NTPs are budgeting enough to meet targets, further reasons why the NTP budgets and associated funding gaps could be considered too low are the generally limited budgets for collaborative TB/HIV activities, especially in African countries, and the typically small or non-existent budgets for second-line drugs to treat MDR-TB patients (the Russian Federation is a notable exception).

For NTPs to carry out their activities as planned, they must actually receive the funds promised or anticipated. The establishment of the GFATM has not so far caused a decline in grant funding from other sources, and the Fund is thus apparently providing additional money. Nevertheless, its central financing role in several countries, and its smaller but nonetheless important contribution in others, means that the rate at which funds are made available in countries is of considerable importance. If these funds are not received by the NTP, gaps will replace expected GFATM contributions. This is a concern for some countries, where delays in receiving expected disbursements are already evident. The most important example is Mozambique, which had not received funds by the end of 2004, even though its proposal was approved in January 2003. Removing the obstacles to disbursement should be a priority, particularly in countries where GFATM grants contribute a large share of planned budgets.

For those countries that have secured large additional grants or loans, the key question now is whether the NTP can spend the money effectively. In 2003, expenditures were lower than the funding available, and in that year the total amount of money available was much lower than in 2004 or 2005. The most obvious need is for additional staff, particularly those with general and financial management skills. This need has already been recognized in several countries, and additional funds have been sought through the ISAC initiative. For example, China's ISAC proposal includes a budget to support the recruitment of new staff at provincial level. Bangladesh has also identified a need for additional staff at central level, following its successful application to the GFATM.

When countries succeed in mobilizing additional funds, the new money must be translated into better programme performance. For most countries it is too early to say whether or not this is happening, because the biggest budgetary and funding increases have mostly been in 2004. However, it is striking that India's TB control programme is both relatively low cost and very effective. As data become available for more years, it will be possible to assess the relative cost-effectiveness of TB control in the 22 HBCs, and the reasons for variation among countries.

Some HBCs still have difficulties in providing financial data. South Africa has not yet been able to complete the financial section of the WHO data collection form. A major part of the explanation is that budgeting for TB control is decentralized in South Africa. Decentralization has also affected the completeness of data available for Afghanistan and Thailand. Most NTPs find it more difficult to provide data on expenditures than budgets. Similarly, expenditures are not yet available on the GFATM web site, although the Fund does provide an impressive volume of data on budgets, grant agreements and disbursements. Efforts to follow up data were intensified in the African Region in 2004, and resulted in major improvements in the quantity and quality of data collected. Similar efforts are now needed in other regions, both for the HBCs and other countries.

In summary, financing for global TB control has improved since 2002, dramatically in some countries. Some HBCs now have sufficient funds, but must show that they can spend them effectively; some have no apparent shortfall, but should verify that their budgets are sufficient to meet targets; some have an obvious funding gap, and must focus on raising the money needed to improve programme performance.

Profiles of high-burden countries

Afghanistan

Afghanistan has undertaken a programme of health service reconstruction. With help from international partners, funds have been mobilized to create an NTP and to start DOTS activities. The DOTS strategy is included in the country's basic package of health-care services (BPHS). Afghanistan has brought together many NGOs in a common effort to deliver DOTS services, and their involvement has been critical in carrying out programme activities. Along with the general health system, TB control services face several impediments, notably an inadequate number of health facilities, continuing insecurity in many areas and staff shortages at all levels. Nevertheless, the NTP has made substantial progress in recent years. DOTS coverage has increased slowly and treatment success rates have been close to or above the global target for four consecutive years. Improving the currently low case detection rate will

require improvements in the security situation. In Afghanistan, more women than men seek treatment from the public TB control programme; it is possible that more men than women are treated by private practitioners. Private physicians and other health-care providers including community volunteers are being encouraged to engage in DOTS.

System of TB control

Over the past two decades, the health service infrastructure collapsed; reconstruction is hampered by the dangers of working in regions where the central government is not fully in control. Nevertheless, progress has been made in rebuilding the general health system, including TB services. The DOTS strategy is a component of the BPHS, and since 2002 the NTP has been strengthened at all levels.

The NTP consists of a central unit under the MoPH General Directorate

of Health Care and Promotion, which is responsible for the overall implementation and management of the NTP, and for policy development. The National TB Institute (NTI) at the central level in Kabul supports training, technical assistance, operational research and laboratory activities. In provinces and districts, TB coordinators supervise and monitor DOTS activities in general health service facilities on four levels: health posts, basic health centres, comprehensive health centres and district hospitals.

There is no national reference library (NRL) in Afghanistan, but the NTI is upgrading its activities so that it can function as an NRL. Additionally, there are eight regional and 144 district laboratories for diagnostic activities.

Surveillance and monitoring

Surveillance was improved with the introduction of the DOTS strategy in the late 1990s and, although the 2003 estimate of 53% DOTS coverage is probably optimistic, there was a steady rise in the number of smear-positive cases diagnosed between 1997 and 2002. With these improvements, the estimated case detection rate was 19% in 2002 and 18% in 2003. Although the case detection rate is not expected to be much higher than this, a tuberculin skin-test survey carried out in Kabul in 2000[1] suggests that the national incidence rate of 150 smear-positive cases per 100 000 population could be an overestimate. This is one aspect of case detection that needs further scrutiny in Afghanistan. Another is the unusual finding, noted in *Global Tuberculosis Control 2004*, that many more women seek treatment from the DOTS programme than men, especially among young adults. Operational research to address this issue is almost complete,

PROGRESS IN TB CONTROL IN AFGHANISTAN

indicators

DOTS treatment success, 2002 cohort	87%
DOTS detection rate, 2003	18%
NTP budget available, 2004	100%
Government contribution to NTP budget, including loans, 2004	8%
Government contribution to total TB control costs, including loans, 2004	NA
Government health spending used for TB control, 2004	NA

Major achievements

— Formation of the organizational structure and terms of reference of the central NTP unit under the General Directorate of Health Care and Promotion of the MoPH

— Definition of the structure and roles of the TB laboratory network, including the National TB Institute and provincial and district laboratories

— Revision of the national TB guidelines and translation into Dari and Pashtu languages

— Training of over 900 health personnel on DOTS implementation and expansion

Major planned activities

— Expand DOTS and integrate TB control activities into the basic package of essential health services

— Improve capacity of NGOs and other partners, and involve the private sector and the community in TB activities

— Provide adequate supplies and equipment for laboratories throughout the country in a timely manner

Establish an EQA system for smear microscopy

NA indicates not available.

[1] Dubuis M et al. A tuberculin skin test survey among Afghan children in Kabul. *International Journal of Tuberculosis and Lung Disease* 2004, 8:1065–1072.

LATEST ESTIMATES[a]		TRENDS	2000	2001	2002	2003
Population	23 896 943	DOTS coverage (%)	15	12	38	53
Global rank (by est. number of cases)	21	Notification rate (all cases/100 000 pop)	33	46	60	58
Incidence (all cases/100 000 pop/year)	333	Notification rate (new ss+/100 000 pop)	14	21	28	27
Incidence (new ss+/100 000 pop/year)	150	Detection of all cases (%)	10	14	18	17
Prevalence (all cases/100 000 pop)	671	Case detection rate (new ss+, %)	9.0	14	19	18
TB mortality (all cases/100 000 pop/year)	93	DOTS case detection rate (new ss+, %)	9.0	14	19	18
TB cases HIV+ (adults aged 15–49, %)	0.0	DOTS case detection rate (new ss+)/coverage (%)	60	117	50	34
New cases multidrug resistant (%)	7.3	DOTS treatment success (new ss+, %)	86	84	87	–

Notification rate (per 100 000 pop)

— = ss+ cases   — = all cases (13 808 in 2003)

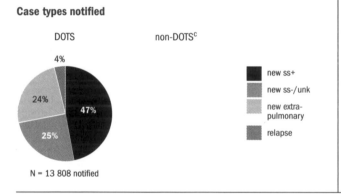

Notification rate by age and sex (new ss+)[b]

— = female   — = male

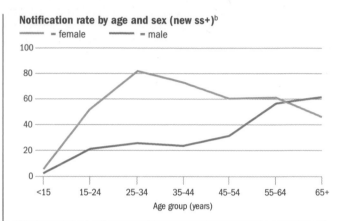

Case types notified

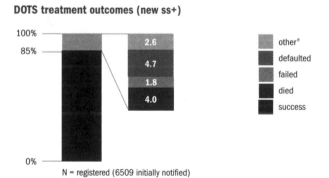

N = 13 808 notified

DOTS progress towards targets[d]

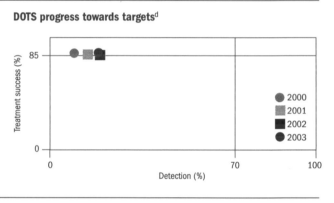

DOTS treatment outcomes (new ss+)

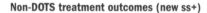

N = registered (6509 initially notified)

Non-DOTS treatment outcomes (new ss+)

Notes

ss+ indicates smear-positive; ss-, smear-negative; pop, population; unk, unknown.

Absence of a graph indicates that the data were not available or applicable.

[a] See Methods for data sources. Prevalence and mortality estimates include patients with HIV.

[b] The sum of cases notified by age and sex is less than the number of new smear-positive cases notified for some countries.

[c] Non-DOTS is blank for countries which are 100% DOTS, or where no non-DOTS data were reported.

[d] DOTS case detection rate for given year, DOTS treatment success rate for cohort registered in previous year.

[e] "Other" includes transfer out and not evaluated, still on treatment, and other unknown.

and the results will be available in early 2005.

Treatment success among DOTS patients registered in 2002 was 87%, and has exceeded the 85% target in three of the last four annual cohorts. With respect to monitoring progress towards the Millennium Development Goals, the focus in Afghanistan is still on assessing TB burden and trends, and on evaluating DOTS implementation.

Improving programme performance

Given the dangers of working in some provinces, national and international experts are sometimes unable to carry out supervision and monitoring visits. Nevertheless, a network of 46 national TB experts has been established, including an NTP manager, a deputy NTP manager, a National Surveillance Officer, a National Logistics Officer, the NTI director and a deputy, eight regional coordinators and 32 provincial coordinators. National TB guidelines have been revised and translated into the Dari and Pashtu languages.

More than 900 health personnel have been trained to provide DOTS services since early 2002. Once the organization of the NTP is complete, the priorities will be to further develop the HR development strategy and to increase training of staff at all levels. A national workshop on HR development for TB control was conducted by the NTP and WHO in March 2004 to revise the basic curricula for all health personnel through the development of appropriate learning materials and training schedules. Five medical schools are preparing training material and courses for all disciplines and are introducing DOTS into the undergraduate curriculum.

Reconstruction of health services has taken place through contracting NGOs to provide basic health services, including TB control, in geographically defined areas. Contracts have been made with 30 NGOs.

In September 2003, the NTP and WHO, in agreement with other partners, procured anti-TB drugs in bulk through the GDF; this supply should cover the needs for 2004 and part of 2005. To maintain regular supplies to all regions, a national warehouse of anti-TB drugs and laboratory consumables was set up at the NTI, and a computer programme for calculating drug needs and requests has been developed. There are no data on drug resistance, DST is not performed and second-line drugs are not available.

Other areas in which programme performance needs to be improved include diagnostic and laboratory services, links with other health-care providers and links with the community. The need for collaborative TB/HIV activities is unclear, given the lack of information about the prevalence of HIV.

Diagnostic and laboratory services

Diagnostic and laboratory services in Afghanistan face major difficulties because of inadequate laboratory equipment and supplies, limited numbers of trained staff and high staff turnover. In 2004, microscopes, reagents and other laboratory materials, including microscopy slides and sputum containers, were purchased and distributed with support from donors. Once basic infrastructure is developed, the priorities will be training of staff, the establishment of an EQA system, and regular monitoring and supervision.

TB/HIV coordination

No data are available on the prevalence of HIV in the general population or in TB patients. A rapid appraisal of the HIV situation is planned, which will provide an estimate of the prevalence of HIV in the general population and among various vulnerable groups.

Links with other health-care providers

The NTP regards the involvement of private sector providers as an important component of DOTS implementation and expansion. Many patients are treated privately, but private physicians are not yet involved in DOTS services. The NTP plans to establish a PPM-DOTS task force and to develop PPM guidelines. Progress in including all relevant public sector providers in DOTS has been made, and public hospitals, medical colleges, prison health-care services and army health facilities are now involved in many areas.

Links with the community

There is community involvement in TB control activities in Kabul City, where around 10 000 widows have been trained to assist with health education. In Nemruz Province, local people help with TB case referral.

Partnerships

An interagency coordination committee (ICC) for TB control has been established and holds regular meetings in Kabul. A country coordination mechanism (CCM) to facilitate support from the GFATM also exists, and meets monthly to address technical and operational issues. WHO and JICA are the main technical partners, and several NGOs including the Anti-TB Association, CARE International, COOPI, GMS, LEPCO, MEDAIR and MSF are providing additional technical assist-

NTP budget by source of funding

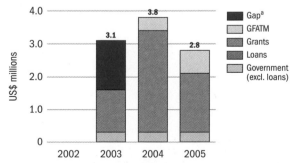

a Funding gaps exist in 2004 and 2005. However, they have not been quantified due to the rapidly changing social, economic and security situation and are therefore not shown in the graph. See text for further details.

ance. CIDA, the Government of Italy and USAID are the major funding partners.

Budgets and expenditures

Budget and expenditure data are limited for Afghanistan. The NTP budget has been approximately US$ 3–4 million in each year 2003–2005. Almost all funding is provided by grants, including from the GFATM. It is extremely difficult to estimate either the total funds needed or the funding gap because of the highly volatile situation in the country. Although a funding gap of US$ 1.5 million was reported for 2003 (see *Global Tuberculosis Control 2004*), the general situation has deteriorated and it is likely that in 2004 and 2005 the funding gap is much greater. This is illustrated by the funding gap for the BPHS, which includes TB control. For the years 2004 and 2005, the funding gap for the BPHS is US$ 49 million and US$ 43 million respectively, and is expected to increase to US$ 70 million in 2006.

A breakdown of the NTP budget by line item is not available for any year 2003–2005, although expenditures on drugs were reported to be about US$ 1 million in 2003 (equivalent to about US$ 74 per patient treated), and relatively large investments in infrastructure were made in the same year.

Bangladesh

Bangladesh adopted the DOTS strategy in 1993. Since then, the NTP has expanded to cover nearly all of the country. For many years, NGOs have been largely responsible for delivering DOTS services and have had a formal involvement in the NTP since 1994. Their collaboration has been instrumental in promoting DOTS and achieving high DOTS coverage. Participation of NGOs in programme delivery continues to be an enormous asset, while the government ensures coordination and sustainability of TB control. With TB control a government priority, recognized as an essential service to be delivered by the health system, the NTP needs to build capacity and strengthen programme management. This is now a matter of urgency as there has been a large increase in funding, mainly from the GFATM, and the amount of money available for TB control almost tripled in 2004 and 2005. Thanks to this encouraging financial position, ambitious plans have been made to dramatically increase case detection and to accelerate a comprehensive programme to strengthen laboratories. With many and diverse partners from the public and private sectors, clear central leadership will be crucial to ensure coordination, to maintain momentum and to undertake the expanded activities now made possible through the additional funding.

System of TB control

The NTP is recognized as a priority in the revised Health, Nutrition and Population Sector Programme. Under the guidance of the Director-General of Health Services, the NTP manager is responsible for the NTP at central level. At the subnational level, the NTP is integrated into the divisional, district and upazila (subdistrict) general health services. Chest disease clinics, located in district capitals and metropolitan cities, support the NTP by offering diagnostic and treatment services for surrounding areas and serving as referral centres for entire districts. NGOs provide NTP services at upazila level in collaboration with the government; some have their own health-care infrastructure. At the peripheral level, health inspectors and assistants, medical assistants, village doctors and NGO community health workers provide basic services such as identification and referral of TB suspects, provision of DOT, tracing of defaulters and various behaviour-change communication activities.

The NTP has established a network of nearly 600 sputum microscopy centres, each one covering a population of about 230 000, on average. There is one NRL, which is part of the central public health laboratory, and 45 intermediary laboratories in chest disease clinics. Peripheral laboratories are found in upazila health complexes, in private urban facilities, medical colleges and in health services for special population groups including health services in prisons, the police and industry.

Surveillance and monitoring

The incidence rate of TB in Bangladesh is uncertain because the estimate is based on a 40-year-old tuberculin survey and on local prevalence surveys that may not be nationally representative. Between 1980, when WHO records began, and the introduction of DOTS in 1993, the case notification rate appeared to be in slow decline, despite some variation. Since 1994, there has been a significant rise in the average age of TB patients, allowing for demographic changes, and the notification rates for men are higher in older age groups. Together, these observations suggest that the TB incidence rate is falling, and this assumption underpins the projected year-on-year changes in the estimated smear-positive incidence rate for Bangladesh.

The smear-positive case detection rate increased rapidly after the introduction of DOTS, stabilized between 1998 and 2001 at around 23%, but has recently increased again, reaching 33% in 2003. Most of these gains have been made as the role of upazila health complexes in case-finding has increased, in addition to chest

---

PROGRESS IN TB CONTROL IN BANGLADESH

Indicators

DOTS treatment success, 2002 cohort	84%
DOTS case detection rate, 2003	33%
NTP budget available, 2004	94%
Government contribution to NTP budget, including loans, 2004	28%
Government contribution to total TB control costs, including loans, 2004	43%
Government health spending used for TB control, 2004	3%

Major achievements
— Expansion of DOTS and initiation of PPM-pilot projects in Dhaka City
— Introduction of DOTS in prisons, academic institutions and workplaces
— Sustained strong collaboration between the government and NGOs
— Revision of national guidelines, incorporating new treatment regimens with FDCs, and laboratory guidelines
— Expansion of EQA for smear microscopy to most microscopy centres

Major planned activities
— Create new microscopy centres in populations of more than 300 000
— Provide basic training for newly appointed technicians and refresher training for all laboratory staff
— Implement activities according to GFATM project proposal, in order to improve case detection

NA indicates not available.

LATEST ESTIMATES[a]		TRENDS	2000	2001	2002	2003
Population	146 736 131	DOTS coverage (%)	92	95	95	99
Global rank (by est. number of cases)	5	Notification rate (all cases/100 000 pop)	55	54	57	60
Incidence (all cases/100 000 pop/year)	246	Notification rate (new ss+/100 000 pop)	28	29	33	37
Incidence (new ss+/100 000 pop/year)	111	Detection of all cases (%)	22	22	23	24
Prevalence (all cases/100 000 pop)	490	Case detection rate (new ss+, %)	25	26	29	33
TB mortality (all cases/100 000 pop/year)	57	DOTS case detection rate (new ss+, %)	23	25	29	33
TB cases HIV+ (adults aged 15–49, %)	0.1	DOTS case detection rate (new ss+)/coverage (%)	26	26	30	33
New cases multidrug resistant (%)	1.4	DOTS treatment success (new ss+, %)	83	84	84	–

Notification rate (per 100 000 pop)

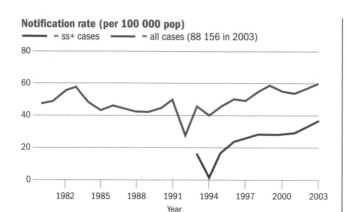

Notification rate by age and sex (new ss+)[b]

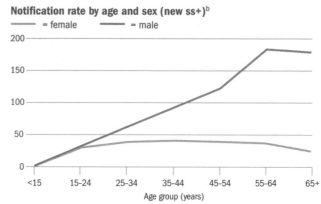

Case types notified

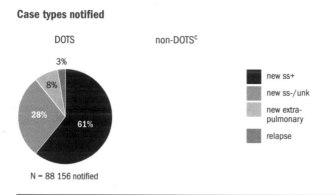

DOTS progress towards targets[d]

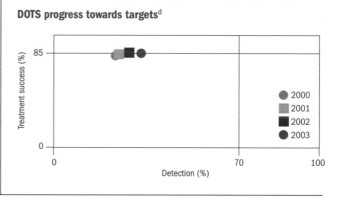

DOTS treatment outcomes (new ss+)

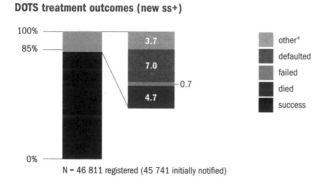

Non-DOTS treatment outcomes (new ss+)

Notes

ss+ indicates smear-positive; ss-, smear-negative; pop, population; unk, unknown.

Absence of a graph indicates that the data were not available or applicable.

[a] See Methods for data sources. Prevalence and mortality estimates include patients with HIV.

[b] The sum of cases notified by age and sex is less than the number of new smear-positive cases notified for some countries.

[c] Non-DOTS is blank for countries which are 100% DOTS, or where no non-DOTS data were reported.

[d] DOTS case detection rate for given year, DOTS treatment success rate for cohort registered in previous year.

[e] "Other" includes transfer out and not evaluated, still on treatment, and other unknown.

disease clinics, which were the dominant source of patients in 1995. Since 2000, the DOTS programme has also reported more patients from metropolitan areas. Despite these improvements, and notwithstanding uncertainty concerning the true incidence rate, case detection by the DOTS programme is still low. Treatment success was 84% for the 2002 cohort and has been 80% or more since 1998. Default (7%) was the most important reason why treatment success was still below the 85% target in 2002. Stimulated by the need to make a better assessment of the scale of the TB problem, and to provide a baseline for evaluating the epidemiological impact of DOTS, the NTP has drawn up plans to carry out a national disease prevalence survey.

Improving programme performance

In 2002, DOTS was expanded to Dhaka city. In 2003, national guidelines were updated to strengthen the implementation of DOTS, including the control of childhood TB. Laboratory manuals have been revised and distributed throughout the country; specific guidelines for involving private practitioners and delivering DOTS services in workplaces are being developed. In view of proposed DOTS expansion activities funded by the GFATM, there is a need to strengthen capacity at the central level. Additional management capacity and technical assistance are urgently needed if the planned activities are to be implemented on schedule.

Collaboration with NGOs and additional partners in the metropolitan city centres has been expanded. With the increasing number of partners, strong supervision and standardized systems for referral, recording and reporting need to be developed. With different NGOs working in the same area, the supervision, structure and accountability between NGOs, the NTP and the Chief Health Officer in metropolitan city areas also need to be addressed.

A TB control steering committee was established to support, direct and monitor procedures and activities to ensure that NTP and global targets are

reached. In late 2003, as noted above, international partners assisted the government in developing a plan for a national prevalence survey in Bangladesh.

Short-course treatment for all TB cases has been further standardized with the introduction of new treatment regimens and FDCs. The new treatment regimens follow WHO recommendations and are more consistent with private sector prescription practices, which may facilitate increased referral of patients. They also simplify drug management at all levels. The difficulties of ensuring drug quality and an uninterrupted drug supply have been alleviated by the successful application for funding by the NTP to the GDF. There is no national policy on the management of MDR-TB, and MDR-TB cases are not treated within the NTP. However, the Damien Foundation Bangladesh (DFB) treats all confirmed MDR-TB cases in the areas it covers. The National Institute of Diseases and Chest Hospitals also treats MDR-TB. Some second-line drugs are produced in the country.

A budget for both DRS and DOTS-Plus will be included in the country's application to the fifth round of the GFATM. Should the GFATM application be approved, Bangladesh will apply to the GLC for reduced-price quality-assured second-line drugs and for technical assistance in implementing sound MDR-TB control measures.

Three other areas in which programme performance needs to be improved are diagnostic and laboratory services, TB/HIV coordination and links with other health-care providers.

Diagnostic and laboratory services

EQA is becoming a routinely accepted standard in many NGO-supported areas in Bangladesh, and NGOs are offering their services to the government to expand EQA. A major challenge for the NTP is to refocus the NRL on training, EQA, expansion of culture services and drug susceptibility testing, in addition to routine microscopy work. Future laboratory priorities include basic training for newly appointed technicians and refresher training for all laboratory staff on smear microscopy and quality assurance.

Diagnostic services will be expanded by establishing new microscopy centres in upazilas with population coverage greater than 300 000. By 2005, EQA for smear microscopy should be available in all urban and rural diagnostic centres.

TB/HIV coordination

The HIV prevalence in the adult population (aged 15–49 years) and the proportion of HIV-positive patients among adult TB cases are still low at 0.01% and 0.1%, respectively, according to the latest UNAIDS and WHO estimates. A similar figure for HIV prevalence among TB cases was found in Dhaka in 1999. There is as yet little collaboration between the NTP and the national HIV/AIDS programme.

Links with other health-care providers

Most DOTS implementation in Bangladesh has been done by NGOs, and during 2004 their involvement has increased. The main NGO partners include the Bangladesh Rural Advancement Committee (BRAC) and DFB, who together cover most of the rural districts in the country; urban areas are covered mainly by other NGOs. There are a number of PPM-DOTS initiatives in Bangladesh. Several private chest physicians in Dhaka have become involved in DOTS services, and the participation of more private practitioners is needed. DFB is expanding its cadre of private "village doctors", who are currently responsible for the detection of about 10% of patients and the provision of DOT to 45% of patients in DFB areas. BRAC has started similar initiatives in periurban areas, while in rural areas they deliver DOT through a network of community workers. Recently, the NTP and collaborating NGOs have begun to include medical colleges, prison health services and the private corporate sector in DOTS activities.

Partnerships

Several technical partners participate in TB control activities in Bangladesh, led by BRAC and the DFB. Thanks to the joint efforts of the partners, the CCM has made a successful application for funding from the GFATM. Financial support is also provided by

(a) NTP budget by source of funding

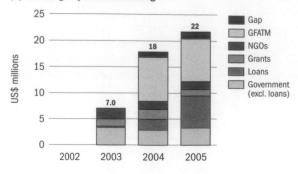

Legend: Gap, GFATM, NGOs, Grants, Loans, Government (excl. loans)

(b) NTP budget by line item

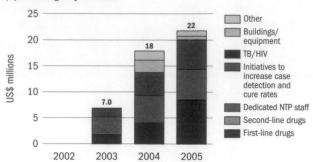

Legend: Other, Buildings/equipment, TB/HIV, Initiatives to increase case detection and cure rates, Dedicated NTP staff, Second-line drugs, First-line drugs

(c) Total TB control costs by line item[a]

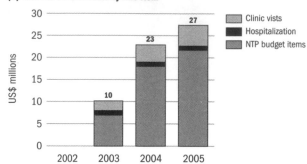

Legend: Clinic vists, Hospitalization, NTP budget items

(d) Per patient costs, budgets, available funding and expenditures

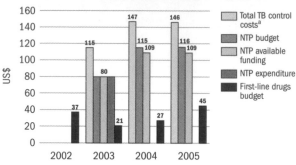

Legend: Total TB control costs[a], NTP budget, NTP available funding, NTP expenditure, First-line drugs budget

[a] Total TB control costs for 2002 and 2003 are based on expenditures, whereas those for 2004 and 2005 are based on budgets. Estimates of the costs of clinic visits and hospitalization are WHO estimates based on data provided by the NTP and from other sources. See Methods for further details.

CIDA, the World Bank and other partners through general funding for the health sector.

Budgets and expenditures

The TB control budget data reported to WHO include both a budget for the NTP and the budgets for the two major NGOs that are responsible for DOTS implementation in most of Bangladesh (i.e. BRAC and DFB). The budgets for both 2004 and 2005 are substantially higher than in previous years, at about US$ 20 million compared with US$ 7 million in 2003. This reflects an ambitious plan to more than double the number of patients treated between 2003 and 2005. Most of the budget is funded for both 2004 and 2005, mainly because of increased funding from a World Bank

credit and a substantial GFATM grant. There is a funding gap of US$ 1–2 million in both 2004 and 2005; this money is needed to cover the national prevalence survey, to recruit staff in order to strengthen management at the central level and to carry out additional activities to increase case detection and treatment success rates. The substantially improved funding position means that spending on TB control by the NTP and the major NGOs could almost triple between 2003 and 2005. The larger budgets in 2004 and 2005 will allow for increased spending on first-line drugs, in line with projected increases in the number of patients treated as well as the development of a buffer stock in 2005 (this buffer stock is the reason for the relatively high budget for first-line drugs

in 2005). They will also allow for some investment in infrastructure, and increased spending on initiatives aimed at improving case detection. The NTP budget per patient is projected to increase from US$ 80 in 2003 to US$ 116 in 2005; if this happens, the total cost of TB control, including visits to health clinics for observation of treatment and monitoring, and limited hospitalization, is projected to increase from US$ 10 million in 2003 to US$ 27 million in 2005 (from US$ 115 to US$ 146 per patient treated). It remains to be seen whether the increased funding can be absorbed effectively and whether increased expenditures result in improved case detection.

Brazil

Brazil is one of the largest countries in the WHO Region of the Americas and it has the highest TB burden in the region. Providing TB control and other health services throughout the country poses immense organizational and logistic challenges. However, the data from recent years indicate a steady downward trend in TB incidence in Brazil. Although DOTS is currently available to only some 35% of the population, a concerted effort is being made to include all of the 315 high-burden municipalities by 2007. There is increasing awareness of the public health importance of TB by the new Brazilian health authorities, who have recognized the DOTS strategy as the best solution to Brazil's TB control problems. The Brazilian MoH has now prioritized the DOTS strategy in its new programme for TB control. TB and leprosy were declared national priority diseases in 2004 and increased government funds were assigned to control them. In addition, 2004 saw the launch of Brazil's Stop TB Partnership involving numerous technical and do-

nor agencies and other public and private sector partners in TB control.

System of TB control

Brazil adopted the DOTS strategy in 1998, establishing it in four states as demonstration areas. Brazil has a massive and complex decentralized health-care system. At the state and municipal levels, the TB control programme is represented by local TB coordinators who are responsible to the respective state and municipal health secretaries. Recently, the government created the position of Secretary of Health Surveillance (SVS) within the new structure of the MoH, which has given added priority to TB control. The SVS has also facilitated collaboration of the NTP with the national laboratory and the HIV/AIDS programmes. TB patients are treated in the out patient facilities of the public health service and only a few complicated cases require hospitalization.

TB laboratory services are carried out by the National Public Health Labo-

ratories Network. There is one NRL, 27 central public health laboratories (one per state) and more than 4000 local laboratories.

Surveillance and monitoring

Among the HBCs, Brazil has a relatively comprehensive TB surveillance system, and the observed downward trend in the case notification rate probably represents a real decline in incidence. The rate of fall is about 3% per year both for smear-positive and for all TB cases, but a faster rate of decline should be achievable by an expanded DOTS programme. DOTS coverage increased to 34% in 2003 and the case detection rate to 18%, giving a detection rate of 55% within DOTS areas. However, an estimated 81% of all new smear-positive TB cases are found nationally (by DOTS and non-DOTS services), suggesting that Brazil could meet and even exceed the target of 70% case detection simply by ensuring that patients already notified are correctly diagnosed and treated by DOTS services.

As DOTS coverage increases, the monitoring of patients on treatment needs to be carried out more rigorously. The treatment success rate under DOTS in 2002 was 75%, with 18% of patients lost through default or transfer to other treatment centres without follow-up. A large proportion of patients (29%) completed treatment without evidence of smear conversion. Among patients registered for re-treatment, only 36% were cured. An additional 24% completed treatment, but the demonstration of smear conversion is vital for re-treatment patients, who could be carrying drug-resistant bacilli. Treatment success rates were even lower among the subset of patients receiving re-treatment after default (51%) or failure (42%). As control efforts intensify, Brazil's system of routine surveillance should be strengthened as the main instrument for monitoring trends in TB cases and deaths and for evaluating the future impact of control measures.

PROGRESS IN TB CONTROL IN BRAZIL

Indicators

DOTS treatment success, 2002 cohort	75%
DOTS case detection rate, 2003	18%
NTP budget available, 2004	100%
Government contribution to NTP budget, including loans, 2004	86%
Government contribution to total TB control costs, including loans, 2004	94%
Government health spending used for TB control, 2004	0.3%

Major achievements

— Approval of TB national plan (2004–2007) by the government
— Launch of the Stop TB Partnership in October 2004
— Organization of 15 regional meetings to discuss the national TB plan and strategies for DOTS expansion, attended by all 27 state TB control coordinators and by the municipal TB control coordinators of all 315 priority municipalities
— Creation of a Task Force Group to monitor and assist the states and priority municipality in DOTS implementation

Major planned activities

— Establish a TB/HIV coordination body in 2005 to implement strategies to increase provision of VCT to TB patients
— Increase microscopy coverage in all 315 priority municipalities and improve quality control of existing microscopy centres
— Implement a national workplan involving different sectors of civil society and the community for TB control

LATEST ESTIMATES[a]		TRENDS	2000	2001	2002	2003
Population	**178 470 430**	DOTS coverage (%)	7.0	32	25	34
Global rank (by est. number of cases)	15	Notification rate (all cases/100 000 pop)	45	43	46	45
Incidence (all cases/100 000 pop/year)	62	Notification rate (new ss+/100 000 pop)	24	22	23	22
Incidence (new ss+/100 000 pop/year)	28	Detection of all cases (%)	67	65	72	73
Prevalence (all cases/100 000 pop)	92	Case detection rate (new ss+, %)	79	75	82	81
TB mortality (all cases/100 000 pop/year)	8.2	DOTS case detection rate (new ss+, %)	7.5	8.0	9.6	18
TB cases HIV+ (adults aged 15–49, %)	3.8	DOTS case detection rate (new ss+)/coverage (%)	108	25	38	55
New cases multidrug resistant (%)	0.9	DOTS treatment success (new ss+, %)	73	67	75	–

Notification rate (per 100 000 pop)

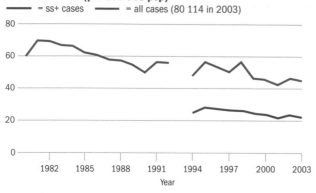

Notification rate by age and sex (new ss+)[b]

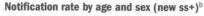
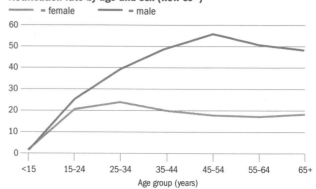

Case types notified

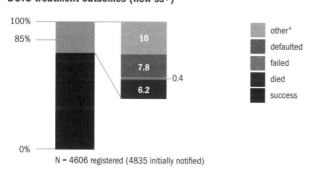

N = 16 560 notified   N = 63 554 notified

DOTS progress towards targets[d]

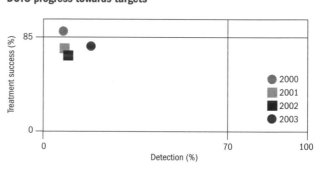

DOTS treatment outcomes (new ss+)

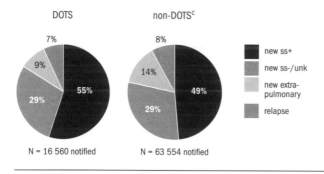

N = 4606 registered (4835 initially notified)

Non-DOTS treatment outcomes (new ss+)

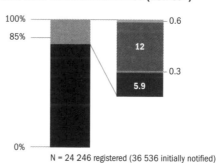

N = 24 246 registered (36 536 initially notified)

Notes

ss+ indicates smear-positive; ss-, smear-negative; pop, population; unk, unknown.

Absence of a graph indicates that the data were not available or applicable.

[a] See Methods for data sources. Prevalence and mortality estimates include patients with HIV.

[b] The sum of cases notified by age and sex is less than the number of new smear-positive cases notified for some countries.

[c] Non-DOTS is blank for countries which are 100% DOTS, or where no non-DOTS data were reported.

[d] DOTS case detection rate for given year, DOTS treatment success rate for cohort registered in previous year.

[e] "Other" includes transfer out and not evaluated, still on treatment, and other unknown.

The creation of the SVS will strengthen Brazil's TB surveillance system by integrating TB with surveillance and control of other endemic diseases and improving coordination; however, it is also important to optimize Brazil's information system (SINAN) for TB surveillance and DOTS monitoring.

Improving programme performance

The MoH, together with health authorities at state and municipal levels, is working hard to strengthen TB control and to reorganize primary health-care services for DOTS implementation. It is important to ensure better integration and coordination of activities at the primary health-care level, particularly those included in the Family Health Programme (Programa de Saúde da Família – PSF) and the Community Outreach Programme (Programa de Agentes Comunitários – PAC). Training in DOTS TB control is currently being provided to other public and private health-care professionals. However, appropriate training and continuous good quality supervision and monitoring activities from the state to the municipal and from the

municipal to the local levels are indispensable for effective DOTS implementation. Training for 20 000 Family Health Teams is planned for 2005. Another important area for improving programme performance is the provision of TB control services in high-risk populations such as the indigenous groups and prison populations.

A national TB control plan for 2004–2007 was approved by the government in 2004. It aims to strengthen the NTP and to reach 100% DOTS coverage in the 315 priority municipalities that account for an estimated 70% of the country's TB burden. The plan includes the creation of a training task force to improve HR capacity for TB control, with the goal of offering DOTS services in all basic health-care facilities in all the priority municipalities by the end of 2007. During 2004, five regional meetings were organized to discuss the national TB plan and strategies for DOTS expansion in the first quarter; two more cycles of five regional meetings each were conducted to monitor this plan in the second and third quarter. All 27 state TB control coordinators and the municipal TB control coordinators of

the priority municipalities attended one of these meetings. A Task Force Group was created in 2004 to monitor and assist the states and priority cities in DOTS implementation.

Diagnostic and laboratory services

As DOTS services expand to the 315 priority municipalities, laboratory capacity needs to be increased, and quality assurance must be introduced. The TB laboratory manual is under revision and the task force organizing training has begun the strengthening of laboratory services; this will continue in 2005. Laboratory information systems and monitoring and supervision will also be improved. During 2004, three regional managerial courses, with the support of an international consultant, were developed to increase the capacity for sputum smear microscopy and quality assurance. More than 800 laboratory personnel countrywide were trained on those topics.

TB/HIV coordination

Brazil is a country with a concentrated HIV epidemic. In 2003, the estimated HIV seroprevalence in the general

(a) NTP budget by source of funding

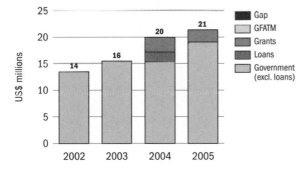

(b) NTP budget by line item

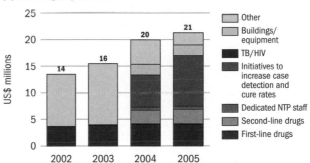

(c) Total TB control costs by line item[a]

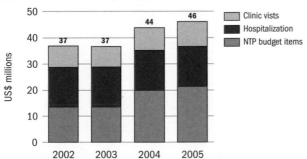

(d) Per patient costs, budgets, available funding and expenditures

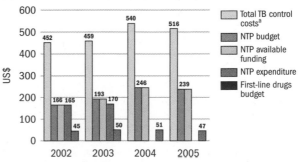

[a] Total TB control costs for 2002 and 2003 are based on expenditures, whereas those for 2004 and 2005 are based on budgets. Estimates of the costs of clinic visits and hospitalization are WHO estimates based on data provided by the NTP and from other sources. See Methods for further details.

population was 0.65%. The NTP estimates that the prevalence of HIV among new TB patients was 8%. This is substantially higher than the WHO estimate of 3.8%, which may underestimate the effect of shared risk factors for TB and HIV. ART is available to all HIV-infected individuals (including TB patients) through the public health system. The recently created SVS has contributed to the collaboration between the NTP and the National AIDS Programme, and to better coordination between them. A national TB/HIV plan is now in place and includes the establishment of a TB/HIV coordination body in 2005, plus strategies to increase the provision of VCT to TB patients and to provide DOTS services to HIV-positive individuals suffering from TB.

Links with other health-care providers
Private hospitals and clinics are required to refer TB suspects and cases to government TB facilities. A small number of NGOs are involved in DOTS provision, and the NTP is planning to host a meeting of national NGOs in 2005 to formulate a collaborative agreement. Brazil has no PPM-DOTS

taskforce or guidelines, but plans to strengthen ties with the Brazilian Society of Pulmonology and Phthisiology through a collaborative agreement. There are also plans to enhance the involvement of the Brazilian research network in the 2004–2007 national plan for DOTS expansion, particularly in the area of operational research.

Partnerships

Brazil has established effective international technical partnerships with agencies such as PAHO, WHO, IUATLD and CDC to support adequate DOTS implementation and expansion. Funding partners include USAID (two TBCTA projects), DFB and GLRA. The launch of the Stop TB Partnership in Brazil in October 2004 signifies another important step towards involving different sectors of civil society and the community in TB control, as does the launch of a national advocacy plan to disseminate TB and DOTS information.

Budgets and expenditures

The NTP budget has been steadily increasing, from US$ 14 million in 2002 to US$ 21 million in 2005 (a 50% in-

crease in four years). As would be expected in an upper-middle income country, the budget is fully funded and most financing is provided by the government, although grant funding was received in 2004 and is expected in 2005. This sound funding situation reflects the commitment of both the government and the international community to TB control. The budget for first-line drugs has been consistently around US$ 4 million and around US$ 50 per patient. In 2004 and 2005, there has been an increase in the budget for activities aimed at improving case detection and cure rates, including an extensive training programme and upgrading of the laboratory network. NTP expenditures were US$ 14 million, equivalent to about US$ 170 per patient treated, in both 2002 and 2003. When costs not covered by the NTP budget are included (i.e. 2509 dedicated TB hospital beds and visits to clinics for DOT and monitoring during treatment), the cost per patient treated is estimated at US$ 450–550 during the period 2002–2005. The total cost of TB control is estimated at US$ 37–46 million.

Cambodia

Cambodia achieved nationwide DOTS coverage at district level in 1998, at a time when the health services were still relatively centralized. Since then, a policy of progressive decentralization has been followed, designed to improve the access of the population to health care. With the establishment of peripheral health centres, the NTP has gradually introduced its activities in these settings, resulting in substantially improved access to TB control services. By the end of 2004, the remaining health centres will be included. A national TB prevalence survey in 2002 yielded a great deal of valuable information, which continues to be applied in strengthening the programme. Results will be published and will serve as an important basis for the assessment of the burden of TB and the impact of DOTS services on the TB epidemic. The shortage of staff to support the expanding programme is now being addressed, and there are plans to tackle the urgent need for better coordination between the TB and HIV control programmes.

System of TB control

Cambodia's NTP operates under the responsibility of the National Center for Tuberculosis and Leprosy Control (CENAT) and within the overall national health system. It comprises TB referral hospitals, provincial TB centres and district TB units. In 1994, TB control was decentralized from provincial hospitals to district hospitals, and in 1999 to health centres. As of 2003, more than 145 TB units and 700 health centres are implementing the DOTS strategy.

There are 180 laboratories in the country including the TB reference laboratory of CENAT, which is responsible for the development of training materials, training of laboratory technicians, and supervision and quality assurance of the provincial laboratories. The reference laboratory carries out culture of mycobacteria and HIV testing but not regular drug susceptibility testing, which will be started in the near future. There are 24 provincial laboratories with responsibility for the supervision and training of health centre staff in sputum smear microscopy and quarterly reporting to CENAT.

Surveillance and monitoring

Cambodia's case detection rate under DOTS was 60% in 2003, after the noticeable upturn in case detection since 2001. This assessment of the case detection rate is based on an estimate of incidence that pre-dates the 2002 prevalence survey. Analysis of the results of that survey will allow a reassessment of the burden of TB in the country and of the case detection rate. The proportion of all cases diagnosed as smear-positive in 2003 was 67%, falling from the highest recorded level of 82% in 1999, possibly because of improvements in diagnosis (fewer false-positives).

The treatment success rate reported among new smear-positive cases has exceeded 90% since 1995, which is unusually high given that 13% of TB patients were thought to be coinfected with HIV in 2003. The success rate for re-treatment patients in 2002 was also remarkably high (89%). Despite some uncertainty about case detection and treatment success, Cambodia is in a strong position to evaluate the future impact of the expanding DOTS programme on TB prevalence, incidence and deaths. As found in population-based surveys in other countries, the 2002 survey in Cambodia has yielded much more than an estimate of prevalence, including data that suggest numerous ways improving routine diagnosis and treatment.

Improving programme performance

The strong commitment of the Cambodian government to poverty elimination and health infrastructure development will have a positive effect on the control of TB in the future. Capacity building for DOTS expansion in all areas of the NTP continues to be a leading priority for the programme. In response to the low ac-

---

PROGRESS IN TB CONTROL IN CAMBODIA

Indicators

DOTS treatment success, 2002 cohort	92%
DOTS case detection rate, 2003	60%
NTP budget available, 2004	81%
Government contribution to NTP budget, including loans, 2004	10%
Government contribution to total TB control costs, including loans, 2004	44%
Government health spending used for TB control, 2004	NA

Major achievements
— Implementation of DOTS in 320 additional health centres during 2003, for a total of 706 out of 856
— Community-based DOTS introduced in collaboration with NGOs in four operational districts
— Introduction of six-month short-course treatment regimen in three operational districts

Major planned activities
— Implement DOTS in an additional 150 health centres to reach 100% coverage by end 2004
— Conduct follow-up study of TB suspects detected during the national TB prevalence survey conducted in 2002
— Continue to train health-care workers on community DOTS and six-month short-course treatment regimen

NA indicates not available.

LATEST ESTIMATES[a]		TRENDS	2000	2001	2002	2003
Population	14 143 527	DOTS coverage (%)	99	100	100	100
Global rank (by est. number of cases)	23	Notification rate (all cases/100 000 pop)	144	142	178	199
Incidence (all cases/100 000 pop/year)	508	Notification rate (new ss+/100 000 pop)	113	107	125	134
Incidence (new ss+/100 000 pop/year)	225	Detection of all cases (%)	27	27	35	39
Prevalence (all cases/100 000 pop)	762	Case detection rate (new ss+, %)	49	47	55	60
TB mortality (all cases/100 000 pop/year)	95	DOTS case detection rate (new ss+, %)	49	47	55	60
TB cases HIV+ (adults aged 15–49, %)	13	DOTS case detection rate (new ss+)/coverage (%)	49	47	55	60
New cases multidrug resistant (%)	0.0	DOTS treatment success (new ss+, %)	91	92	92	–

Notification rate (per 100 000 pop)

— = ss+ cases   — = all cases (28 216 in 2003)

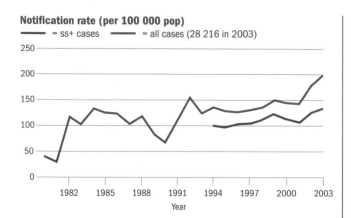

Notification rate by age and sex (new ss+)[b]

— = female   — = male

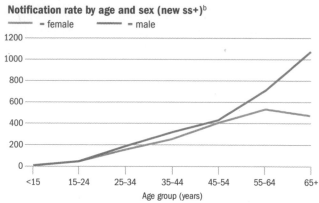

Case types notified

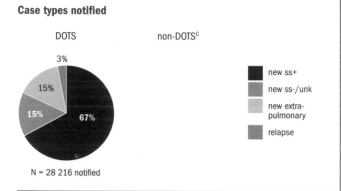

N = 28 216 notified

new ss+
new ss-/unk
new extra-pulmonary
relapse

DOTS progress towards targets[d]

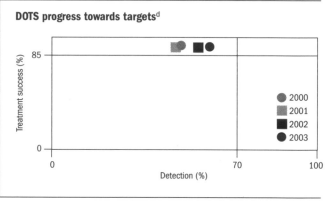

- 2000
- 2001
- 2002
- 2003

DOTS treatment outcomes (new ss+)

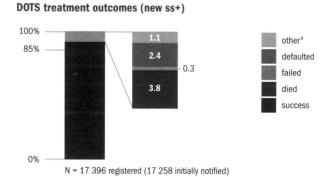

N = 17 396 registered (17 258 initially notified)

other[e]
defaulted
failed
died
success

Non-DOTS treatment outcomes (new ss+)

Notes

ss+ indicates smear-positive; ss-, smear-negative; pop, population; unk, unknown.

Absence of a graph indicates that the data were not available or applicable.

[a] See Methods for data sources. Prevalence and mortality estimates include patients with HIV.

[b] The sum of cases notified by age and sex is less than the number of new smear-positive cases notified for some countries.

[c] Non-DOTS is blank for countries which are 100% DOTS, or where no non-DOTS data were reported.

[d] DOTS case detection rate for given year, DOTS treatment success rate for cohort registered in previous year.

[e] "Other" includes transfer out and not evaluated, still on treatment, and other unknown.

cess to health services and DOTS in some areas, DOTS services were expanded to 320 additional health centres in 2003. There are plans to implement DOTS in the remaining 150 health centres by the end of 2004. A six-month short-course chemotherapy regimen has been introduced in pilot studies in three operational districts, and training in the new regimen for health-care workers will continue into 2005. A follow-up study of TB suspects detected during the 2002 prevalence survey has started and will be completed during 2004. A drug resistance survey conducted in 2000–2001 found that the prevalence of MDR-TB was negligible among new cases and 3% among re-treatment cases.

The lack of human resource capacity remains a challenge for the NTP. At the request of CENAT, a representative from KIT met with key personnel and staff focus groups to assess human resource development needs in 2003. A workshop was subsequently organized to develop an outline for management training; training activities have been intensified and new staff have been recruited. There is still an urgent need for both in-country and international training for staff (including managers), and to recruit more staff. The NTP is planning to address these issues through recruitment of staff from outside the NTP with the aid of partners, making use of additional funding from the GFATM and the World Bank.

Other areas where programme performance needs to be improved are diagnostic and laboratory services, TB/HIV coordination and links with other health-care providers and the community.

Diagnostic and laboratory services

Two of 24 provincial laboratories have been upgraded during 2003 to perform culture and drug susceptibility testing. The EQA system, introduced in 2002, is still under development and must be strengthened and expanded. There are too few staff with sufficient training to run the laboratory and diagnostic services in Cambodia. During 2005, training programmes will improve technical knowledge and enhance staff motivation. Drug susceptibility testing is not available in Cambodia, but its introduction is considered a priority.

TB/HIV coordination

A national TB/HIV prevalence survey in 2003, carried out by the VCT service at CENAT, estimated HIV seroprevalence among TB patients at 12% (similar to the WHO estimate of 13% among adult TB patients). As yet, there are no data on TB incidence or mortality among PLWHA. TB/HIV collaborative pilot studies in four provinces included screening and treatment for TB among PLWHA, isoniazid preventive treatment for PLWHA who are infected with *M. tuberculosis*, surveillance of HIV in TB patients and ART for HIV-infected TB patients. A workshop to assess the pilot projects concluded that TB/HIV collaboration is hampered by the disease-specific focus of the individual programmes, the quality of TB/HIV counselling and lack of joint IEC material. IEC materials and standardized reporting and recording forms for TB/HIV activities are being developed.

Links with other health-care providers

The 2002 prevalence survey showed that among people with TB symptoms who sought any type of health care, 89% went first to the private sector

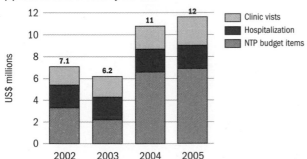

(a) NTP budget by source of funding

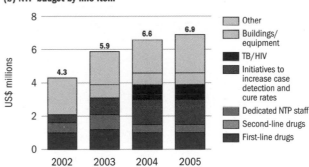

(b) NTP budget by line item

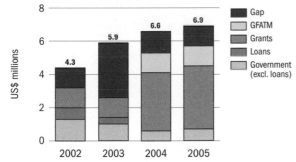

(c) Total TB control costs by line item[a]

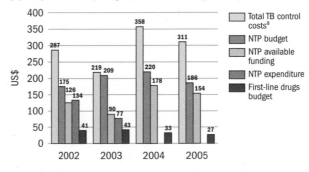

(d) Per patient costs, budgets, available funding and expenditures

[a] Total TB control costs for 2002 and 2003 are based on expenditures, whereas those for 2004 and 2005 are based on budgets. Estimates of the costs of clinic visits and hospitalization are WHO estimates based on data provided by the NTP and from other sources. See Methods for further details.

(pharmacies and doctors). However, the private sector has not yet been formally involved in the NTP in Cambodia. The majority of private providers diagnose and treat TB but the quality of the services provided by them is generally poor, as shown in a study carried out by CENAT in collaboration with the Quality Assurance Project of Cambodia's University Research Corporation. However, many private providers are interested in collaborating with the NTP, and a pilot project involving private practitioners and pharmacies will be launched in 2005.

Links with the community
Community-based DOTS has been introduced in four districts, and training started in 2004 for community-based DOT workers.

Partnerships
Cambodia has a diverse group of technical partners including CDC (TB/HIV pilot programme activities), JICA (training and supervision, laboratory technical support, IEC, procurement, operational research, TB/HIV), KNCV (training and workshops, community DOTS) and WHO (training and supervision, laboratory technical support, IEC, procurement, TB/HIV). The main financial partners are CIDA, GFATM, JICA, USAID, WHO and the World Bank.

Budgets and expenditures
The NTP budget has increased from about US$ 4 million in 2002 to almost US$ 7 million in 2005, in line with planned increases in case detection. Available funding almost doubled between 2002 and 2005, from about US$ 3 million in 2002 to almost US$ 6 million in 2005. This improvement is becasue of a large increase in grant funding, including from the GFATM. However, funding gaps have persisted in each year from 2002 to 2005. In both 2004 and 2005, the gap is about US$ 1 million, equivalent to about 15% of the total budget requirement. The increased budgets in 2004 and 2005 are mainly a result of higher proposed spending on TB/HIV collaborative activities, and initiatives to increase case detection and cure rates (e.g. implementation of community-based care in remote areas and active case-finding).

Reported expenditures were lower than available funding in both 2002 and 2003. On a per patient basis, the NTP budget has varied from between US$ 175 (in 2002) and US$ 220 (for 2004), while actual expenditures per patient were US$ 134 and US$ 77 in 2002 and 2003, respectively. When costs not covered by the NTP budget are included (i.e. 1200 dedicated TB hospital beds and visits to clinics for DOT and monitoring during treatment), the cost per patient treated is estimated to range from around US$ 220 to US$ 360. The total cost of TB control was about US$ 7 million in 2002. Provided the 2005 budget is fully funded and spent and the projected number of cases are treated, this will rise to almost US$ 12 million in 2005.

China

China has seen a radical change in political commitment to TB control during 2003 and 2004. There has been a clear government decision to meet the global targets for diagnosis and treatment of TB by the end of 2005. This decision was endorsed by the State Council at a meeting on TB control in September 2004, and a pledge was secured to make an eight-fold increase in central government funding for TB control. Following the accelerated DOTS expansion undertaken in recent years, coverage will reach 95% by the end of 2004 and is expected to reach 100% in 2005. Building on the experience of the severe acute respiratory syndrome (SARS) epidemic, China has further recognized the importance of a public health approach to communicable diseases and has set up a new national Internet-based reporting system, under which all cases of several specified communicable diseases, including TB, must be notified. The recently revised law on infectious diseases also strengthens the mandatory reporting of TB, and this is expected to improve TB case reporting substan-

tially. The main challenge is to ensure the quality of TB services during a phase of rapid expansion and to address the shortages of staff and laboratory services needed to support the expanding programme.

System of TB control

China introduced DOTS on a wide scale in 1992 by expanding DOTS to 13 of 31 mainland provinces, municipalities and autonomous regions ("provinces" hereafter) using funds from a World Bank loan. By 2000, most counties (1132 of 1208) in these 13 provinces had been using DOTS for at least five years. Further expansion of DOTS activities in other parts of China followed in 2002. By 2003, 91% of the population lived in areas covered by the DOTS strategy. Nationwide coverage is planned for the end of 2005.

The government is increasing its investment in public health substantially, and the MoH has put the control of TB among its top priorities. In 2004, an eight-fold increase in funding for the NTP has been pledged for TB control activities. A recent evalua-

tion of the progress towards the 10-year national TB control plan carried out by the MoH, Ministry of Finance, and the National Development and Reform Commission has resulted in further government commitment to TB control at all levels.

The TB laboratory network operates under the guidance of the NTP manager and consists of one national reference laboratory, 31 provincial TB reference laboratories, 336 TB laboratories at the prefecture/city level and 2683 peripheral laboratories. Microscopy is performed by all laboratories, while 16% carry out culture and less than 2% do drug susceptibility testing. Culture is occasionally performed in 5–10% of county laboratories, except in some major cities including Beijing where culture is done routinely for all TB suspects. Drug susceptibility testing is available to diagnose drug resistance at some provincial and prefecture level laboratories.

Surveillance and monitoring

The estimated incidence rate for China was revised during 2004[1] and is believed to be falling by 1% per year, as is the measured rate of decline in the annual risk of TB infection over the decade since 1990. However, on the basis of the currently available data, these assessments of trend should be treated as approximate.

China made the second largest contribution to the increase in global case detection between 2002 and 2003, after India. The case detection rate achieved by the DOTS programme was 30% in 2002, and increased sharply to 43% by the end of 2003 as population coverage reached 91%. A rapidly implemented TB control programme faces the challenging task of maintaining quality as the programme

---

PROGRESS IN TB CONTROL IN CHINA

Indicators

DOTS treatment success, 2002 cohort	93%
DOTS case detection rate, 2003	43%
NTP budget available, 2004	88%
Government contribution to NTP budget, including loans, 2004	74%
Government contribution to total TB control costs, including loans, 2004	74%
Government health spending used for TB control, 2004	0.5%

Major achievements
— A State Council TB control meeting on TB control involving all provinces
— Increased political commitment, especially at local levels, and increased funding from government and partners
— Establishment of a nationwide Internet-based system for the compulsory reporting of infectious diseases, including TB
— Monitoring mission to six priority provinces organized by the MoH

Major planned activities
— Strengthen system of referral of TB patients from hospitals to local TB dispensaries
— Build human resource capacity according to the NTP guidelines
— Expand EQA system to all cities and counties, and drug resistance surveillance in additional provinces

---

[1] Using the annual risk of TB infection (ARTI) measured in 2000, and by applying Stýblo's rule of thumb relating TB incidence to ARTI (smear-positive incidence increases by 50/100 000 population for every 1% increase in ARTI).

LATEST ESTIMATES[a]		TRENDS	2000	2001	2002	2003
Population	1 304 196 022	DOTS coverage (%)	68	68	78	91
Global rank (by est. number of cases)	2	Notification rate (all cases/100 000 pop)	36	37	36	47
Incidence (all cases/100 000 pop/year)	102	Notification rate (new ss+/100 000 pop)	16	16	15	21
Incidence (new ss+/100 000 pop/year)	46	Detection of all cases (%)	34	35	35	46
Prevalence (all cases/100 000 pop)	246	Case detection rate (new ss+, %)	34	34	32	45
TB mortality (all cases/100 000 pop/year)	18	DOTS case detection rate (new ss+, %)	31	31	30	43
TB cases HIV+ (adults aged 15–49, %)	0.7	DOTS case detection rate (new ss+)/coverage (%)	45	45	39	47
New cases multidrug resistant (%)	5.3	DOTS treatment success (new ss+, %)	95	96	93	–

Notification rate (per 100 000 pop)

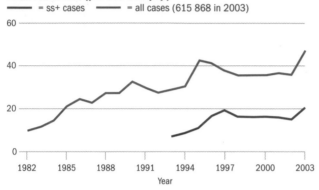

= ss+ cases   = all cases (615 868 in 2003)

Notification rate by age and sex (new ss+)[b]

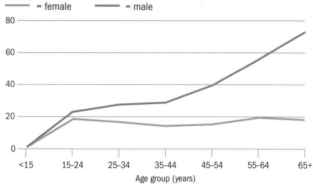

= female   = male

Case types notified

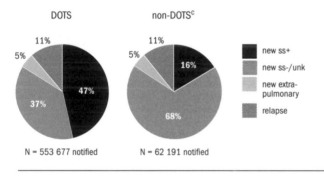

DOTS

non-DOTS[c]

new ss+

new ss-/unk

new extra-pulmonary

relapse

N = 553 677 notified

N = 62 191 notified

DOTS progress towards targets[d]

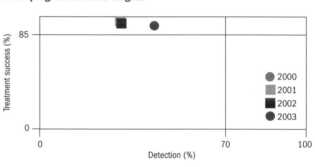

2000
2001
2002
2003

DOTS treatment outcomes (new ss+)

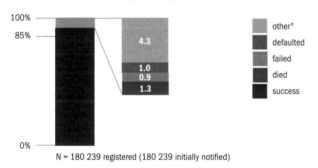

other[e]

defaulted

failed

died

success

N = 180 239 registered (180 239 initially notified)

Non-DOTS treatment outcomes (new ss+)

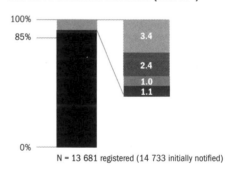

N = 13 681 registered (14 733 initially notified)

Notes

ss+ indicates smear-positive; ss-, smear-negative; pop, population; unk, unknown.

Absence of a graph indicates that the data were not available or applicable.

[a] See Methods for data sources. Prevalence and mortality estimates include patients with HIV.

[b] The sum of cases notified by age and sex is less than the number of new smear-positive cases notified for some countries.

[c] Non-DOTS is blank for countries which are 100% DOTS, or where no non-DOTS data were reported.

[d] DOTS case detection rate for given year, DOTS treatment success rate for cohort registered in previous year.

[e] "Other" includes transfer out and not evaluated, still on treatment, and other unknown.

expands. At least two aspects of the monitoring data from China need closer scrutiny. One is the steady decrease in the proportion of DOTS patients diagnosed as smear-positive from 1996 to 2003; the other is the exceptionally high treatment success rate, reported to be 93% for the 2002 cohort of new smear-positive patients.

A full analysis of the year 2000 prevalence survey has confirmed that, in the 13 World Bank project provinces implementing DOTS between 1991 and 2000, culture-positive TB prevalence fell by 37% more than in other areas of the country, with a 30% decline directly attributable to DOTS.[1] Although the geographical coverage of DOTS increased substantially between 2002 and 2003, the case detection rate within DOTS areas was only 47% in 2003. Case detection will be improved by the new communicable disease surveillance system (implemented by the Chinese Center for Disease Control and Prevention), which has begun to notify TB patients via the Internet from all major hospitals and health centres as well as the TB dispensaries.

Improving programme performance

During 2003, 27 of 31 provinces in China began scaling up existing and new TB control projects, and the country's two largest projects – funded by the World Bank/DFID and GFATM – are now fully operational. With anti-TB drugs provided free of charge by grants from the Government of Japan and the central government, 2003 is the first year that all provinces in China have had sufficient resources to implement the complete DOTS technical package. This is the main reason for the increase in case detection for both old and new DOTS areas and accounts for the increase in the case detection rate in DOTS areas from 35% in 2002 to 47% in 2003.

Insufficient human resources – both the quantity and expertise of staff

– is a major constraint to TB control. China has begun to address this problem by developing a new national TB training plan. With new funding from the GFATM and the ISAC initiative, China plans to recruit and train additional staff at the central and provincial levels.

With the aim of reaching the global targets by 2005, China has developed a national TB health promotion strategy to increase case detection and cure rates, especially among the poor and vulnerable. Special efforts are being made to increase public awareness of TB. The capacity of TB control staff to carry out health promotion activities at national and provincial levels will be enhanced, as will their communication and outreach skills.

Given the size of China, drug resistance surveys are carried out in individual provinces rather than nationally. The first survey began in 1996 in Henan Province, and since then six additional mainland provinces and Hong Kong SAR have reported drug-resistance data. China has an organized DRS plan, and many provinces are in various stages of planning and implementation. Another three provinces have completed drug resistance surveys; four more provinces have surveys in progress. A nationwide survey in 2000 estimated that 10% of prevalent bacteriologically confirmed TB cases have MDR-TB disease. MDR-TB patients are treated on an individual basis and have to pay for the services. Second-line drugs are produced in the country and are widely available.

Diagnostic and laboratory services, TB/HIV coordination and links with other health-care providers are three priority areas in which programme performance needs to be improved.

Diagnostic and laboratory services
With 500 000 people for every microscopy diagnostic unit, diagnostic services offer a challenge to TB control in China. As activities expand, improving the quality of laboratory services is a priority. Rapid expansion of the new internationally recommended EQA system is also a priority for China, and a new national EQA manual for smear microscopy was developed and issued to TB control

institutions at each level. Training courses are being held on EQA implementation. Quality assurance for smear microscopy currently includes a quarterly review, on-site evaluation and panel testing. The national reference laboratories have set an EQA target for 2004 to cover 100% of provincial and prefecture laboratories and 60% of county laboratories. There are, however, no quality assurance systems in place for culture testing.

TB/HIV coordination
The Chinese government estimates that there are currently 840 000 people living with HIV in the country, but by the end of 2003, only around 62 000 had been reported to the authorities, of which nearly 9000 were reported with AIDS; reported AIDS deaths have been rapidly increasing. While less than 0.2% of Chinese adults are currently infected with HIV, high rates of HIV infection have been found among intravenous drug users and among people who sold blood plasma to supplement their incomes in provinces such as Anhui, Henan and Shandong.[2] The Government of China is planning to collect data on HIV prevalence among TB patients in provinces known to have a relatively high HIV prevalence, and to use sentinel surveillance or surveys to determine trends in HIV prevalence among TB patients in provinces where the prevalence of HIV is not known. The MoH plans to establish a national TB/HIV coordinating body.

Links with other health-care providers
TB suspects and patients seek care from public hospitals at all levels. The focus of PPM DOTS in China is to link hospitals to TB dispensaries, which is potentially the most important way to increase case detection and to improve the quality of patient care. Data from the prevalence survey conducted in 2000 indicate that more than 75% of smear-positive cases are initially managed in either county general hospitals or township hospitals in China. In the past, many cases diagnosed and treated in hospitals were not reported to the TB dispensaries. Patients in hospitals should now also be reported through the new surveillance

[1] China Tuberculosis Control Collaboration. The effect of tuberculosis control in China. *Lancet*, 2004, 364:417–422.

[2] *UNAIDS 2004 Report on the global AIDS epidemic*. Geneva, Joint United Nations Programme on HIV/AIDS, 2004.

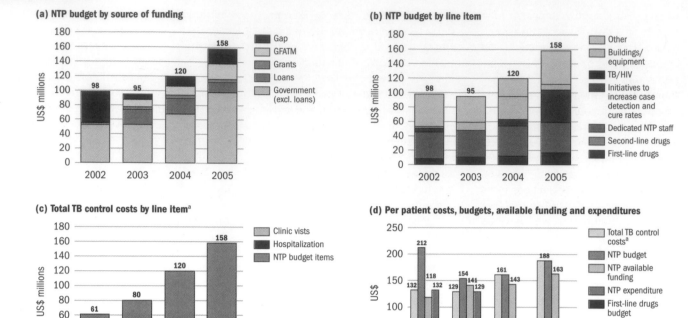

(a) NTP budget by source of funding

(b) NTP budget by line item

(c) Total TB control costs by line item[a]

(d) Per patient costs, budgets, available funding and expenditures

[a] Total TB control costs for 2002 and 2003 are based on expenditures, whereas those for 2004 and 2005 are based on budgets. See Methods for further details.

system. Pilot initiatives to involve hospitals are in place and are showing encouraging results.

Partnerships

In addition to the government funding for TB control, funds are provided for TB control projects from outside sources, with technical assistance from WHO and KNCV. The World Bank/DFID project provides funding for 16 project provinces. The Government of Japan provides funds for anti-TB drugs, microscopes and health promotion materials in 12 provinces. The GFATM has approved US$ 25.4 million for the first two years of a five-year TB project, with initial funds disbursed to 24 provinces. Another GFATM project was approved in July 2004. The Damien Foundation Belgium supports TB control activities in Tibet (since 1995), Inner-Mongolia (since 2001) and Qinghai (since 2003). CIDA began

funding TB control activities through WHO in 2003, and the project now covers a population of 75 million in its second year. FIDELIS, run by IUATLD, is exploring new approaches to improve quality of DOTS services and increase case detection.

Budgets and expenditures

In line with plans to reach the global targets for case detection and treatment in 2005, the budget is projected to increase from around US$ 100 million in 2002 and 2003 to US$ 160 million in 2005. Due to a large funding gap, actual expenditures were only around US$ 60 million in 2002.

Budgets from 2003 onwards have been substantially boosted by increased government funding, a new World Bank loan and successful applications to the GFATM. Despite this progress, a funding gap of US$ 21 million still exists for 2005. This fund-

ing gap reflects faster than expected expansion of DOTS to new areas, greater than anticipated increases in case detection and plans to introduce additional initiatives to increase case detection in 2005 (e.g. tracing of patients reported through the general communicable disease reporting system, an increased number of sputum examinations at subcounty level and more IEC activities). Some of the funding gap may be filled by an increase in local government funding, but the extent to which this will occur is currently unclear. An increasing budget for first-line drugs is planned to meet the increase in treated cases, with the cost per patient treated remaining at about US$ 20 for the period 2002–2005. If expenditures match budgets in 2004 and 2005, the total cost of TB control activities per patient treated will increase from about US$ 130 in 2002 to US$ 190 in 2005.

Democratic Republic of the Congo

The Democratic Republic of the Congo, despite being among the poorest countries in the world, has made substantial progress in TB control in recent years; by 2004, DOTS services were available to approximately 80% of the population. While there is strong government support for the NTP, the provision of adequate TB services throughout the country has been hampered by a combination of difficulties. The country's health infrastructure has suffered in the past from an underdeveloped primary care system, lack of funds and resources as well as from the destructive effects of civil unrest and natural disasters. In spite of these constraints, TB case detection and cure rates have both improved steadily since the early 1990s, and the NTP hopes to reach the global targets by 2005. The likelihood of achieving these objectives has been greatly boosted by an award from the GFATM, as well as increased government funding, which have transformed the financial basis of TB control services and will allow for the extension and strengthening of activities. Furthermore, the special problems posed by the epidemic of TB in people infected with HIV are being addressed in an expanding programme of collaborative TB/HIV activities.

System of TB control

The NTP was officially launched in 1980 (Programme National Antituberculeux Integré, PATI 1) and consists of a central unit, 20 provincial coordination centres, 777 TB diagnosis and treatment centres and a network of health posts (consisting of a nurse or health-care worker) distributed in 515 health districts. Better health coverage resulted from a health mapping exercise carried out in 2004, following which the number of health districts was increased from 306 to 515. TB services follow the expanded health network to improve access by providing services closer to where the patients live and to promote health-seeking behaviour.

The TB laboratory network consists of one NRL, which was significantly upgraded in preparation for the application to the GLC, 20 provincial laboratories implementing EQA and 800 district laboratories, giving 1 laboratory per 70 000 inhabitants. There are no microscopy services in any of the peripheral health posts.

Surveillance and monitoring

As a result of progressive expansion of DOTS services, coverage of approximately 80% was reached in 2004. The TB notification rate for both smear-positive and all forms of TB has increased over the past 20 years, partly as a result of improved case-finding and partly as a result of a rise in TB incidence linked to the spread of HIV. For the Democratic Republic of the Congo, as for some other countries in central Africa, the accuracy of the estimated case detection rate (63% in 2003) is uncertain. The treatment success rate was 78% for the 2002 cohort; 7% of patients died and 13% defaulted or were lost to follow-up after transfer to other treatment centres. Both of the latter indicators were high for patients undergoing re-treatment following relapse, failure or default; the relapse re-treatment success rate was 70%. High HIV prevalence, poor health infrastructure and large numbers of displaced persons contribute to this low treatment success rate. However, preliminary data suggest that the treatment success rate for the first quarter of 2003 was 81%. Improvement of the treatment success rate is a high priority for the NTP.

Improving programme performance

Revised TB control guidelines have been prepared (Programme National Antituberculeux Integré, PATI 4) and will be published soon. These guidelines, which include the introduction of the 6-month regimen for treatment, have already been used as the basis for training sessions on the progressive introduction of the new regimen.

PROGRESS IN TB CONTROL IN THE DEMOCRATIC REPUBLIC OF THE CONGO

Indicators

DOTS treatment success, 2002 cohort	78%
DOTS case detection rate, 2003	63%
NTP budget available, 2004	84%
Government contribution to NTP budget, including loans, 2004	5%
Government contribution to total TB control costs, including loans, 2004	64%
Government health spending used for TB control, 2004	NA

Major achievements

— Review of the national TB control guidelines (Programme National Antituberculeux Integré, PATI 4), including introduction of 6-month treatment regimen
— Extensive training at all levels, including initiation of more than 4000 community health workers
— Establishment of a TB/HIV coordinating body to coordinate activities of the National AIDS Control Programme and the NTP
— Improved capacity of laboratories, including provision of 800 microscopes

Major planned activities

— Host external monitoring mission planned for February 2005
— Prepare five-year strategic plan (2006–2010)
— Implement a national drug resistance survey
— Update and revise NTP technical guidelines
— Expand collaborative TB/HIV activities, following recent award from the President's Emergency Plan for AIDS Relief

NA indicates not available.

LATEST ESTIMATES[a]		TRENDS	2000	2001	2002	2003
Population	**52 771 230**	DOTS coverage (%)	70	70	70	75
Global rank (by est. number of cases)	11	Notification rate (all cases/100 000 pop)	125	134	138	160
Incidence (all cases/100 000 pop/year)	369	Notification rate (new ss+/100 000 pop)	74	84	87	102
Incidence (new ss+/100 000 pop/year)	160	Detection of all cases (%)	39	40	39	44
Prevalence (all cases/100 000 pop)	564	Case detection rate (new ss+, %)	53	58	57	63
TB mortality (all cases/100 000 pop/year)	81	DOTS case detection rate (new ss+, %)	53	58	57	63
TB cases HIV+ (adults aged 15–49, %)	21	DOTS case detection rate (new ss+)/coverage (%)	76	83	81	84
New cases multidrug resistant (%)	1.5	DOTS treatment success (new ss+, %)	78	77	78	–

Notification rate (per 100 000 pop)

■ = ss+ cases ■ = all cases (84 687 in 2003)

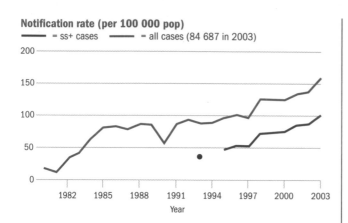

Notification rate by age and sex (new ss+)[b]

= female = male

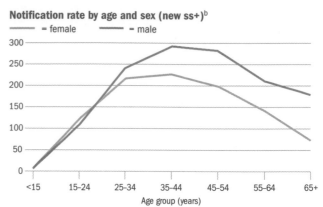

Case types notified

DOTS non-DOTS[c]

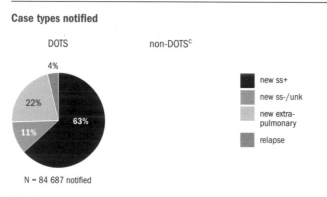

N = 84 687 notified

- new ss+
- new ss-/unk
- new extra-pulmonary
- relapse

DOTS progress towards targets[d]

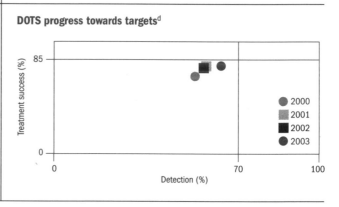

- 2000
- 2001
- 2002
- 2003

DOTS treatment outcomes (new ss+)

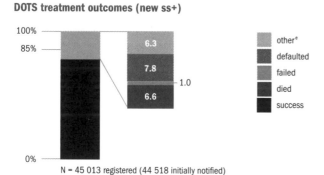

N = 45 013 registered (44 518 initially notified)

- other[e]
- defaulted
- failed
- died
- success

Non-DOTS treatment outcomes (new ss+)

Notes

ss+ indicates smear-positive; ss-, smear-negative; pop, population; unk, unknown.

Absence of a graph indicates that the data were not available or applicable.

[a] See Methods for data sources. Prevalence and mortality estimates include patients with HIV.

[b] The sum of cases notified by age and sex is less than the number of new smear-positive cases notified for some countries.

[c] Non-DOTS is blank for countries which are 100% DOTS, or where no non-DOTS data were reported.

[d] DOTS case detection rate for given year, DOTS treatment success rate for cohort registered in previous year.

[e] "Other" includes transfer out and not evaluated, still on treatment, and other unknown.

A new strategic plan will be prepared for the period 2006–2010.

The supply of anti-TB drugs is adequate, thanks to a second GDF grant approved in 2004 for another three-year period. However, the country's drug policy and system of drug management need to be revised to ensure sustainable supply and better drug distribution, with regular reporting on drug stocks at every level.

A national drug resistance survey is planned for 2005. The protocol has been finalized and implementation should start soon. A national policy for the diagnosis and treatment of MDR-TB is being developed.

Extensive training activities were carried out in 2003 at all levels, including initiation of more than 4000 community health workers.

Supervision of laboratory, medical, financial and administrative functions is carried out on a regular basis, but the time devoted to each visit is inadequate and only half of the planned visits were carried out in 2003. Nonetheless, supervision has resulted in improvements in the procedures for recording and analysis of observations made during patient visits. There has also been a striking improvement in

the management and flow of funds because of a revision of financial and administrative procedures under the guidance of a newly-recruited finance officer at central level.

Data collection is more reliable than in the past, although delays are experienced and data collection forms remain unnecessarily complicated.

The award of a GFATM grant has greatly increased the funding available for TB control in 2004, making it possible to address the problems of staffing, training, medical supplies and equipment. With improvements in the facilities for diagnosis and patient care, case detection and cure rates should continue to rise in the coming years.

Three areas where programme performance particularly needs to be improved are laboratory services for culture and DST, TB/HIV coordination and links with other health-care providers.

Diagnostic and laboratory services
The quality of DOTS implementation relies on an effective laboratory network. New equipment was installed during 2003 and 2004 in most peripheral laboratories, and EQA is imple-

mented in most laboratories. EQA included external laboratory supervision in half of the provinces in 2003. On-the-spot slide reading is carried out in half of the districts visited during the external visits. The link between the NRL and the NTP needs to be strengthened to ensure effective coordination. The central laboratory is poorly equipped and the quality of slide reading is poor in laboratories where microscopes are old and need to be replaced.

TB/HIV coordination
More than 20% of adult TB patients are infected with HIV (WHO estimate). The National AIDS Control Programme and the NTP have established a TB/HIV coordinating body in 2003, and one NPO has been recruited to support these activities. Since 2002, several DOTS centres have started collaborative TB/HIV activities in Kinshasa, with financial and technical support from WHO, MSF and the World Bank. Following a recent award from the President's Emergency Plan for AIDS Relief, collaborative TB/HIV activities will be expanded in 2005.

(a) NTP budget by source of funding

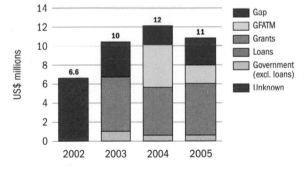

(b) NTP budget by line item

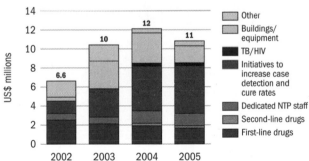

(c) Total TB control costs by line item[a]

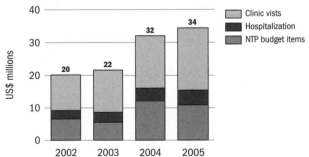

(d) Per patient costs, budgets, available funding and expenditures

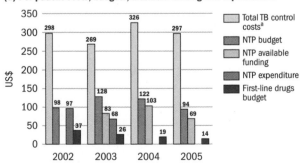

[a] Total TB control costs for 2002 and 2003 are based on expenditures, whereas those for 2004 and 2005 are based on budgets. Estimates of the costs of clinic visits and hospitalization are WHO estimates based on data provided by the NTP and from other sources. See Methods for further details.

Links with other health-care providers

The NTP is collaborating with general hospitals, medical colleges, and military and police health services; specialist TB hospitals and the prison health-care service do not implement DOTS. Limited formal involvement of the private sector has started with the training of private physicians in DOTS activities. These providers are also represented in some provincial and national task force meetings.

Partnerships

The Democratic Republic of the Congo benefits from several financial and technical partnerships for TB control. The GFATM is a principal source of funds, and the national budget for TB control has increased in 2004. Additional support from the Government of Belgium was agreed in 2004. UNDP, the principal recipient of the GFATM funds, has established four public and private recipients for the TB control proposal (the NTP, La Ligue Nationale Antituberculeuse et Antilépreuse du Congo, DFB and the National School of Public Health). Through this arrangement, other partners have been included.

Budgets and expenditures

The NTP budget has been between US$ 10 million and US$ 12 million for the years 2003–2005, compared with about US$ 7 million in 2002. Almost all of the available funding for 2003–2005 comes from grants, with the government contributing less than 10% of the NTP budget (no breakdown of the budget by funding source in 2002 has been provided to WHO). This makes the Democratic Republic of the Congo largely dependent on external financing. Despite the approval of the GFATM grant in round 2, and sustained commitment from other donors, an important funding gap remains: US$ 2.9 million (26% of the NTP budget) in 2005.

The budget for first-line drugs has decreased from US$ 2.5 million in 2002 to US$ 1.7 million in 2005, reducing the first-line drug budget per patient treated from US$ 37 to US$ 14. In contrast, the budget for initiatives to increase case detection and cure rates has grown from US$ 1.3 million in 2002 to US$ 5 million in 2005 and is now the largest single budget item.

The total cost of TB control, which includes the cost of clinic visits and dedicated TB hospital beds, in addition to the NTP budget, is projected to increase from an estimated US$ 20 million in 2002 to US$ 34 million in 2005, in line with anticipated increases in the numbers of patients to be treated (the cost per patient treated is around US$ 300 per patient in both 2002 and 2005). The government contribution to the total cost of TB control is much larger than to the NTP budget, varying from 60% to 76% of total costs.

Ethiopia

Ethiopia has given priority to TB, HIV/AIDS and malaria prevention and control for more than a decade. The DOTS strategy is being implemented in most districts, and almost all hospitals and health centres provide DOTS services. However, basic health services are not yet accessible to about 40% of the population, and intensive efforts are being made to ensure better access throughout the country. Health facilities suffer from a high turnover of staff to deliver TB services; this constraint is being addressed through a comprehensive HRD plan and training programmes. Available data suggest that the incidence of TB has risen in recent years, partly as a result of the impact of the HIV/AIDS epidemic. Special efforts are being made to address the needs of TB patients coinfected withHIV coinfection. Ethiopia has carried out its first national drug resistance survey and found that the rate of MDR-TB is low. The country has successfully maintained an uninterrupted supply of anti-TB drugs for several years. Approval of a grant from the GFATM opened up additional possibilities to expand and improve TB control services in 2004 and 2005.

System of TB control

The health policy in Ethiopia, dating from 1993, gives priority to the control of communicable diseases, including TB, HIV/AIDS and malaria. The health system is being progressively decentralized under the country's primary health-care strategy. Recently, a four-tier health-care delivery structure was established to implement this policy. The primary health-care unit is the basic level of health care for Ethiopia and consists of a health centre with five satellite health posts, each serving 5000 people. In 2005, this network will be extended by the addition of two health extension workers for each subdistrict (kebelle). The health system also includes district (woreda), regional and specialized hospitals, serving 250 000, 1 000 000 and 5 000 000 people, respectively. During the past year, further decentralization to the woredas in major regions of the country has led to an increase in the transfer of health personnel from regions and zones to woredas and a decreasing role of the zone in TB control activities.

In 1994, the NTP (known locally as the TB and Leprosy Prevention Control Team) was established. Since 2000, it has been part of the Disease Prevention and Control Department of the Federal MoH. In 1996, a Project Development Plan (PDP), designed to support TB control through the NTP for five years, was signed by the Government of Ethiopia, WHO and KNCV. In 2001, this plan was extended for an additional year.

The laboratory services in Ethiopia include one NRL, regional reference laboratories in some regions and peripheral laboratories.

Surveillance and monitoring

The steady rise in case notifications since 1993 is because of increasing DOTS coverage, improved reporting and the impact of HIV/AIDS. While the relative contributions of these three factors are uncertain, it has been assumed that the national smear-positive case detection rate by the DOTS programme has remained constant at around 36%, while incidence has increased. The case detection rate within DOTS areas was only 38% in 2003, due largely to the important difference between DOTS coverage as defined in this report (95%) and the proportion of the population thought to have access to health services of any kind, including for TB (50%). The proportion of notified cases diagnosed as smear-positive is low in Ethiopia, and has stayed within the range 27–35% during the period 1995–2003.

Despite the moderately high prevalence of HIV infection (4.4% of adults aged 15–49 years in 2003), it remains difficult to explain the extraordinary proportion of cases that are reported as extrapulmonary TB (>34% in 2003, regional variation 29–54%). The vast majority of extrapulmonary cases are reported as lymph node TB; this phenomenon is currently being investigated through a large operational research study in six sites in four regions.

Treatment success among new patients was only 76% in the 2002

PROGRESS IN TB CONTROL IN ETHIOPIA

Indicators

DOTS treatment success, 2002 cohort	76%
DOTS case detection rate, 2003	36%
NTP budget available, 2004	100%
Government contribution to NTP budget, including loans, 2004	8%
Government contribution to total TB control costs, including loans, 2004	31%
Government health spending used for TB control, 2004	10%

Major achievements

— Provision of DOTS services by 98% of hospitals and health centres
— Uninterrupted drug supply for several years
— Strong HRD plan with up-to-date training material and methodology
— Drug resistance survey completed with relatively low MDR-TB rate reported

Major planned activities

— Commence collaborative TB/HIV activities in pilot sites as well as in hospitals scheduled to provide ART
— Involve communities and private providers in TB control
— Conduct major training activities in all regions and woredas following the recent HRD plan

LATEST ESTIMATES[a]		TRENDS	2000	2001	2002	2003
Population	70 678 002	DOTS coverage (%)	85	70	95	95
Global rank (by est. number of cases)	7	Notification rate (all cases/100 000 pop)	139	141	160	166
Incidence (all cases/100 000 pop/year)	356	Notification rate (new ss+/100 000 pop)	47	49	53	56
Incidence (new ss+/100 000 pop/year)	155	Detection of all cases (%)	45	43	47	47
Prevalence (all cases/100 000 pop)	533	Case detection rate (new ss+, %)	35	35	36	36
TB mortality (all cases/100 000 pop/year)	79	DOTS case detection rate (new ss+, %)	35	35	36	36
TB cases HIV+ (adults aged 15–49, %)	21	DOTS case detection rate (new ss+)/coverage (%)	41	50	38	38
New cases multidrug resistant (%)	2.3	DOTS treatment success (new ss+, %)	80	76	76	–

Notification rate (per 100 000 pop)

— = ss+ cases   — = all cases (117 600 in 2003)

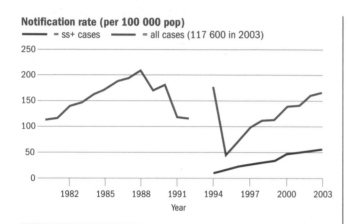

Notification rate by age and sex (new ss+)[b]

— = female   — = male

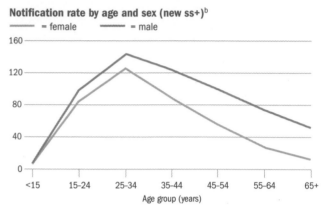

Case types notified

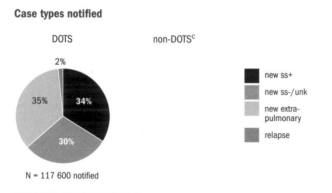

DOTS   non-DOTS[c]

- new ss+
- new ss-/unk
- new extra-pulmonary
- relapse

N = 117 600 notified

DOTS progress towards targets[d]

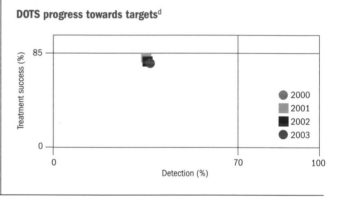

- 2000
- 2001
- 2002
- 2003

DOTS treatment outcomes (new ss+)

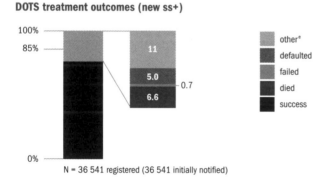

- other[e]
- defaulted
- failed
- died
- success

N = 36 541 registered (36 541 initially notified)

Non-DOTS treatment outcomes (new ss+)

Notes

ss+ indicates smear-positive; ss-, smear-negative; pop, population; unk, unknown.

Absence of a graph indicates that the data were not available or applicable.

[a] See Methods for data sources. Prevalence and mortality estimates include patients with HIV.

[b] The sum of cases notified by age and sex is less than the number of new smear-positive cases notified for some countries.

[c] Non-DOTS is blank for countries which are 100% DOTS, or where no non-DOTS data were reported.

[d] DOTS case detection rate for given year, DOTS treatment success rate for cohort registered in previous year.

[e] "Other" includes transfer out and not evaluated, still on treatment, and other unknown.

cohort, considerably lower than Ethiopia's maximum of 80% reported for 2000. However, this decrease is explained by the fact that the NTP now includes all notified cases in the analysis. Among new patients who were registered for treatment in 2002, the outcome of treatment is not known for 10% following transfer between treatment units; 7% died and 17% completed treatment without evidence of smear conversion.

Improving programme performance

In recent years, the high turnover of staff involved in TB control and the effects of decentralization have resulted in a workforce that is not well trained in the principles of TB control. HRD in the NTP therefore received special emphasis in 2003, with the completion of a comprehensive HRD plan, production of a first edition of TB/leprosy training modules and associated materials for all levels of staff involved in TB control, and the creation of a pool of 53 competent TB and leprosy trainers distributed over all regions. Detailed regional training plans for 2005 have been drafted and funding for their implementation secured. The first phase of the plans focuses on in service training; the second phase will also involve incorporation of TB control principles in the pre-service curricula.

Anti-TB drugs and laboratory supplies are procured by the Pharmaceutical Administration and Supplies Services of the Federal MoH using international competitive bidding, with funding from the GFATM. Despite delays in the procurement process, there has not been any interruption to the availability of drugs, mainly because of the continued maintenance of a one-year buffer stock. NTP training increasingly includes pharmacy staff. Four-drug FDCs have been introduced for the intensive phase of treatment for new patients.

Although almost 95% of the woredas have at least one health facility providing DOTS services, more than half of the smaller health stations/posts do not provide directly observed TB treatment. Covering all

these units is one of the main objectives of the NTP, but implementation has been constrained by a shortage of staff for monitoring and supervision as well as a delay in HRD.

Ethiopia's first drug resistance survey is close to completion, with preliminary results indicating 1.7% MDR among new cases, somewhat lower than the WHO estimate of 2.3%.

Three other areas in which programme performance needs to be improved are diagnostic and laboratory services, TB/HIV coordination and links with other health-care providers and the community.

Diagnostic and laboratory services

All laboratories are supplied with microscopes and reagents by the NTP, and staff are included in TB-related training activities. A system of quality assurance is in place, but implementation is weak. The NTP developed and issued a national laboratory manual for smear microscopy in 2002, which will be revised and re-edited in 2005.

TB/HIV coordination

A national TB/HIV coordinating body has been established and specific terms of reference developed. The committee includes the Federal MoH, academia, bilateral donors and the technical partners of the TB and HIV programmes. Nine pilot sites have been selected to pilot collaborative TB/HIV activities under the guidance of the committee. A national TB/HIV surveillance plan is being finalized. TB/HIV activities are managed by a national TB/HIV coordinator (WHO) based at the Federal MoH.

A national TB/HIV orientation workshop and various training courses have been conducted for the staff of pilot sites, in management of TB and other opportunistic infections in PLWHA and in VCT. Guidelines have been developed for the use of isoniazid preventive therapy in PLWHA infected with *M. tuberculosis* and for the use of co-trimoxazole preventive therapy in HIV-infected TB patients. Isoniazid (through the GDF), co-trimoxazole and HIV test kits (both through the Federal MoH) have been distributed. Ethiopia hosted, facili-

tated and participated in three major international activities: the meeting of the TB/HIV Global Working Group, TB/HIV Surveillance International Workshop (CDC/WHO) and two global TB/HIV managers training courses (WHO/GLRA).

Links with other health-care providers

Observations during monitoring and supervision as well as a small scale study in Addis Ababa have shown that many patients are managed in private clinics. Patient management is generally limited to diagnosis since, officially, anti-TB drugs in Ethiopia are available only in government health facilities. Most patients in whom TB is diagnosed in the private sector are referred to public health centres for registration and treatment. However, anti-TB drugs have been shown to circulate illegally, and treatment of an unknown number of patients is initiated in the private sector, disregarding national treatment guidelines. A pilot project is planned in Addis Ababa so that private providers will be increasingly involved in training activities as well as laboratory quality assurance activities.

Links with the community

Given the sparse distribution of health facilities, and the consequent limited access to DOTS services in Ethiopia, plans are under way to involve the community in TB control. With GFATM funding, pilot projects will start in four districts of four regions. National guidelines for community involvement in DOTS and training modules and materials have been developed and distributed.

Partnerships

For many years, the NTP has been consistently supported by the Royal Netherlands Embassy, GLRA and WHO. More recently, support has been received from the GFATM, with a large grant approved in the first round of applications. Other partners are CDC and USAID. MSF Belgium is providing support in the Somali Region, but this will be discontinued in 2005 when the regional health bureau assumes responsibility for the region.

(a) NTP budget by source of funding

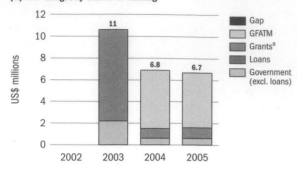

Legend: Gap, GFATM, Grants[a], Loans, Government (excl. loans)

(b) NTP budget by line item

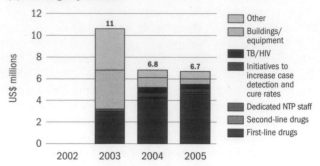

Legend: Other, Buildings/equipment, TB/HIV, Initiatives to increase case detection and cure rates, Dedicated NTP staff, Second-line drugs, First-line drugs

(c) Total TB control costs by line item[b]

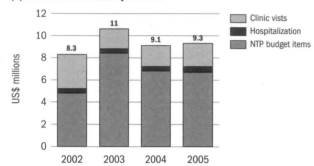

Legend: Clinic vists, Hospitalization, NTP budget items

(d) Per patient costs, budgets, available funding and expenditures

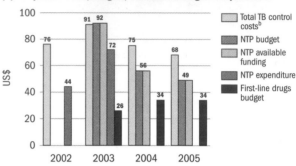

Legend: Total TB control costs[b], NTP budget, NTP available funding, NTP expenditure, First-line drugs budget

[a] The 2003 budget data provided to WHO did not separate the GFATM contribution from other grants.

[b] Total TB control costs for 2002 and 2003 are based on expenditures, whereas those for 2004 and 2005 are based on budgets. Estimates of the costs of clinic visits and hospitalization are WHO estimates based on data provided by the NTP and from other sources. See Methods for further details.

Budgets and expenditures

The total NTP budget was US$ 11 million in 2003, and lower at around US$ 7 million in both 2004 and 2005 (US$ 92 and US$ 49 per patient in 2003 and 2005, respectively). The relatively high total in 2003 was a result of a large budget for capital investments (included in the "buildings and equipment" category) as well as a large budget in the "other" line item category. In practice, only 53% and 34%, respectively, of these budgets were spent. Following approval of a GFATM grant in round 1 of US$ 11 million for the first two years, Ethiopia has not reported any funding gaps for 2003–2005. Grants, including from the GFATM, represent more than 90% of the NTP budget in 2004 and 2005, making the NTP highly dependent on external funding. Programme sustainability is a concern, as grants support key areas such as first-line anti-TB drugs. In addition, continuous funding from the GFATM will depend on NTP performance during the first two years of the grant.

As the expected number of TB patients to be treated is increasing, the first-line drug budget is steadily expanding to reach US$ 4.6 million in 2005, and remains the largest budget item.

The total TB control cost per patient (including the estimated costs of bed-days and clinic visits as well as the costs reflected in NTP budgets and expenditures) has remained relatively low, varying from US$ 68 to US$ 91 between 2002 and 2005.

India

India, the country with the greatest burden of TB, is also the country where the most dramatic advances are being made in DOTS expansion. Thanks to a massive recent scale-up, TB services were available to some 67% of the population by 2003, and full nationwide DOTS coverage is planned for 2005. During 2003 alone, some 250 million additional people were included and treatment provided to more than 900 000 TB patients. At the same time, there has been a considerable improvement in the level of case detection, with India making a greater contribution than any other country to the global increase in case-finding since 2000. Mobilizing all public sector health-care providers, especially medical colleges, as well as many private and other health-care providers outside the government service, has been important to achieving such swift progress, and successful efforts continue to increase their involvement. Maintaining quality during rapid growth is a priority, while addressing the urgent need for addi-

tional staff and laboratory support for the expanded services. The Indian TB control programme is outstanding not only because of the recent progress but also because it has been made at a lower than predicted cost.

System of TB control

India's Revised National TB Control Programme (locally RNTCP, hereafter NTP) was introduced on a pilot scale in 1993 and, after a period of pilot testing, was formally launched by the government in 1997. By mid-1998, the programme had expanded to serve some 20 million people. There followed a phase of rapid expansion from late 1998 so that, by 2003, the areas covered by the DOTS strategy included 778 million people (around 67% of the population).

The laboratory network currently comprises 3 national reference laboratories (these are the LRS Institute of TB and Respiratory Diseases, Delhi; the National TB Institute, Bangalore and the TB Research Centre, Chennai), 15 state laboratories, 522 district

laboratories and nearly 9000 peripheral NTP-designated microscopy centres. The national reference laboratories train state-level laboratory staff, and monitor and oversee the state laboratories. The state laboratories train district laboratory and supervisory staff, and monitor and oversee the peripheral microscopy centres; some of them perform culture and drug susceptibility testing. Sputum smear microscopy services are provided by the district and peripheral level microscopy centres.

Surveillance and monitoring

Coverage was extended by 250 million people during 2003, with more than 900 000 patients placed on DOTS treatment during that year. Based on this remarkable progress, it is planned to cover a total of 850 million people by the end of 2004 and to reach 100% coverage by October 2005. The estimated smear-positive incidence was revised on the basis of a three-year national tuberculin survey that was completed during 2003. There was a striking improvement in the DOTS case detection rate in 2003, with an estimated 47% of all new smear-positive cases in the country detected by the NTP compared with 31% in 2002, and 69% detected in the areas already covered by the DOTS programme. This increase in case detection represents 39% of the increase in cases detected by DOTS programmes worldwide, and India has made a larger contribution than any other country to the acceleration in global case-finding observed since 2000. The reported treatment success has also increased over the past three years (to 87% for 2002), despite the rapid growth of the national DOTS cohort (to more than 37 000 new smear-positive patients in 2003).

In contrast to the upward trend in case notifications seen in the NTP, the notification rate of all TB cases, from all sources in India, has been falling gradually since 1992. It remains unclear whether this downward trend

PROGRESS IN TB CONTROL IN INDIA

Indicators

DOTS treatment success, 2002 cohort	87%
DOTS case detection rate, 2003	47%
NTP budget available, 2004	100%
Government contribution to NTP budget, including loans, 2004	74%
Government contribution to total TB control costs, including loans, 2004	86%
Government health spending used for TB control, 2004	2%

Major achievements

— Expansion of DOTS to cover an additional 250 million population during 2003
— Scaling up of PPM DOTS project in 12 sites
— GFATM round 1 activities started and round 2 agreement signed
— Involvement of medical colleges through national, subnational and state task forces
— Involvement of health facilities under other ministries
— Publication of new guidelines on EQA and development of a DRS protocol for two states
— Development of guidelines for management of paediatric TB

Major planned activities

— Prepare for DOTS expansion in remaining states (laboratories, human resource, procurement) – entire country to be covered by October 2005
— Sustain quality of existing DOTS services by implementing a revised supervision and monitoring strategy
— Continue human resource capacity building through revision of all training material

LATEST ESTIMATES[a]		TRENDS	2000	2001	2002	2003
Population	1 065 462 272	DOTS coverage (%)	30	45	52	67
Global rank (by est. number of cases)	1	Notification rate (all cases/100 000 pop)	110	105	101	101
Incidence (all cases/100 000 pop/year)	168	Notification rate (new ss+/100 000 pop)	34	37	38	41
Incidence (new ss+/100 000 pop/year)	75	Detection of all cases (%)	65	63	60	60
Prevalence (all cases/100 000 pop)	290	Case detection rate (new ss+, %)	46	50	50	54
TB mortality (all cases/100 000 pop/year)	33	DOTS case detection rate (new ss+, %)	12	24	31	47
TB cases HIV+ (adults aged 15–49, %)	5.2	DOTS case detection rate (new ss+)/coverage (%)	42	53	60	69
New cases multidrug resistant (%)	3.4	DOTS treatment success (new ss+, %)	84	85	87	–

Notification rate (per 100 000 pop)

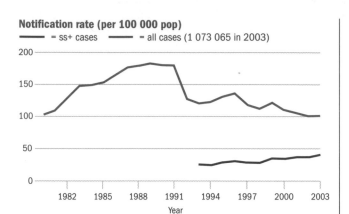

Notification rate by age and sex (new ss+)[b]

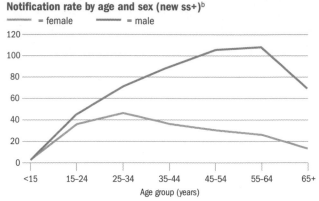

Case types notified

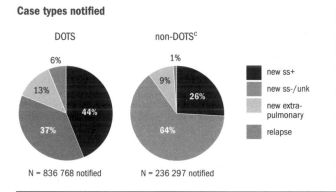

DOTS progress towards targets[d]

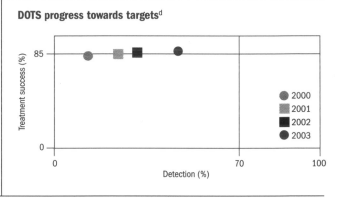

DOTS treatment outcomes (new ss+)

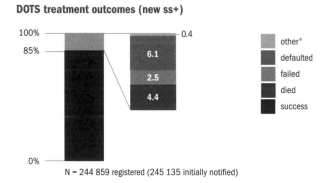

Non-DOTS treatment outcomes (new ss+)

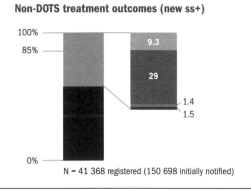

Notes

ss+ indicates smear-positive; ss-, smear-negative; pop, population; unk, unknown.

Absence of a graph indicates that the data were not available or applicable.

[a] See Methods for data sources. Prevalence and mortality estimates include patients with HIV.

[b] The sum of cases notified by age and sex is less than the number of new smear-positive cases notified for some countries.

[c] Non-DOTS is blank for countries which are 100% DOTS, or where no non-DOTS data were reported.

[d] DOTS case detection rate for given year, DOTS treatment success rate for cohort registered in previous year.

[e] "Other" includes transfer out and not evaluated, still on treatment, and other unknown.

reflects a real decrease in incidence, or improvements in diagnosis (eliminating false-positives). National data for the years up to 2003 do not yet provide evidence that the NTP has reduced incidence and prevalence, although it is clear that there are significantly fewer deaths among cases notified (18 deaths averted per 100 patients treated are reported at www.tbcindia.org). The epidemiological evidence for impact is most likely to come from areas where the programme has been operating for longest and where the implementation of DOTS has been studied most intensively, notably in the "model DOTS project" being carried out by the Tuberculosis Research Centre in Chennai.

Improving programme performance

Maintaining the quality of TB services is crucial as the programme moves towards full coverage, and this will be a major challenge in the coming years. To address it, several activities are under way, including the development of guidelines for the management of paediatric TB and the introduction of a revised supervision and monitoring strategy with detailed indicators for activities at all levels.

The most important constraint to the extension of quality TB services is the shortage of staff to manage the rapidly expanding programme, particularly at central and state levels. To improve this situation, additional technical staff have been recruited to assist the NTP manager, the limits on hiring contractual laboratory technicians have been relaxed and efforts are being made to achieve an adequate distribution of laboratory technicians to states where laboratories are understaffed. Subdistrict contracted laboratory supervisors have greatly contributed to the success of the programme, and efforts will be made to sustain capacity over the next few years. Further political commitment at the state level is needed to ensure that the programme is fully staffed with stable management. The capacity of current staff will be increased through training programmes run in part by expert consultants.

It is estimated that 3.4% of previously untreated TB cases are multidrug resistant. Currently, the NTP does not supply second-line drugs for MDR-TB patients. There are plans to build capacity at the state level for DRS and DOTS-Plus. Although MDR-TB patients are not treated under the NTP, second-line drugs are widely available and used by many practitioners, both public and private.

During 2005, priority will be given to preparing the remaining districts for DOTS implementation. The preparatory activities include the improvement of laboratories and stores, recruitment, relocation and training of staff, and procurement of equipment and supplies. Some of the districts are in areas where operations are difficult to access and where intensive monitoring will be required. Funds secured through the GFATM will be used to expand the programme to cover 56 million population in all 47 districts of the three newly-created states of Chhattisgarh, Jharkhand and Uttaranchal (round 1), and 110 million population in 56 districts of the states of Bihar and Uttar Pradesh (round 2). In addition, GFATM funds will be used to maintain DOTS coverage in 110 million population in the states of Andhra Pradesh and Orissa (round 4).

Diagnostic and laboratory services, TB/HIV coordination and links with other health-care providers and the community are three priority areas to improve programme performance.

Diagnostic and laboratory services

The TB laboratory network is being strengthened to meet the needs of the expanding programme, by upgrading existing laboratories, creating new microscopy centres and establishing EQA. Based on new international guidelines, an EQA system for sputum microscopy was adopted at the beginning of 2004 for the NTP smear microscopy laboratory network, and includes a random blinded cross-check of routine slides each month. Panel testing at the district level is done by the state laboratories once a year. Currently, only NTI Bangalore and TRC Chennai are quality assured for both culture and drug susceptibility testing. The national reference laboratories participate in annual proficiency testing coordinated by the Antwerp and Chennai supranational laboratories. Building capacity for DST at the intermediate laboratory level has started in two state-level laboratories in 2004 and is planned for two others by the end of the 2004; a national plan has also been developed to systematically perform DRS surveys in large states of the country.

TB/HIV coordination

An estimated 5.1 million people are infected with HIV in India. HIV is likely to have a significant impact on the TB epidemic in the six states where the prevalence of HIV is greater than 1%, namely Andhra Pradesh, Karnataka, Maharashtra, Manipur, Nagaland and Tamil Nadu. The prevalence of HIV in TB patients has been measured in a number of tertiary care hospital settings, reaching 25% in one such hospital in Pune, Maharashtra, in 2001. However, the results from such studies are not representative of the HIV levels in TB patients in India as a whole. In 2004, HIV surveillance in TB patients has started in four districts in the six high-prevalence states, using a more representative sampling methodology.

Coordination of HIV and TB services has been prioritized in the six states with the highest HIV prevalence. HIV and TB staff have been cross-trained, referral linkages between the district VCT centres of the HIV programme and microscopy centres of the DOTS programme established and a surveillance system to document cross-referrals is currently in the pilot phase. Joint HIV/TB coordination committees will be established at the national and state levels with support from GFATM, and a referral system will be created at the subdistrict level between the existing NTP infrastructure and the VCT centres.

Links with other health-care providers

Private and other health-care providers, including NGOs and medical colleges, play an extremely important role in DOTS implementation in India. The Government of India has formulated and published schemes to promote participation of NGOs (2001) and private practitioners (2002) in implementing DOTS. During the past few years, several local initiatives have emerged in both urban and rural settings; the NTP has provided drugs free of charge and has taken responsibility for supervision and monitoring of laboratory and treatment services. The evaluated initiatives have shown an increase in case notification between 3% and 30%. Most projects have also achieved treatment success greater than the programme target of 85%. Encouraged by the success of these early experiments, the NTP, in collaboration with WHO, has embarked on scaling up PPM DOTS in 14 cities across the country. The strategy is to offer technical support to the city TB control programmes to facilitate partnership development through a full-time PPM consultant assisted by two field supervisors. Future expansion of PPM DOTS will link all public, corporate, voluntary and private individual and institutional providers to the NTP. The programme has adapted the existing recording and reporting system in order to evaluate the PPM-DOTS activities. Monitoring during the two initial quarters showed that PPM-DOTS

providers other than those under the DoH contributed 39% of the cases detected under DOTS in the pilot cities. Public and private medical colleges alone accounted for 18%.

Links with the community
Community volunteers are used as DOT providers all over the country. In some parts, there has been effective involvement of the community through patient–provider–community meetings. IEC campaigns also involve the community at large, especially during events such as World TB Day.

Partnerships
WHO has helped to establish a network of more than 85 field consultants and provides technical support for all aspects of the programme. These field consultants work with the programme managers at state and district level and report directly to the central unit of the NTP. India receives anti-TB drugs for 240 million of its population through the GDF. Financial partners include CIDA, DANIDA, DFID, GFATM, USAID and the World Bank.

Budgets and expenditures
In line with the rapid DOTS expansion taking place in India, the NTP budget has increased from US$ 36 million in 2002 to a projected US$ 46 million in 2005. Most funding is provided by the government, through a World Bank credit and domestic government revenue. With an increase in funding from the GFATM, grants will provide about 30% of the budget in 2005. No budget gaps were reported for 2002–2004; although there is currently a funding gap of US$ 15 million for 2005, it is expected that this will be filled by a combination of additional grants and a new World Bank credit.

The largest budget items are first-line drugs and dedicated staff, which together account for more than 50% of the total budget in each year 2002–2005. The budget per patient treated has remained stable as DOTS has expanded, at about US$ 35–40. The same is true of total TB control costs (which include visits to health facilities and expenditures on dedicated TB hospital beds in addition to items covered by the NTP budget). The total TB control cost per patient treated has consistently remained at about

(a) NTP budget by source of funding

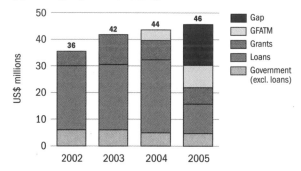

(b) NTP budget by line item[a]

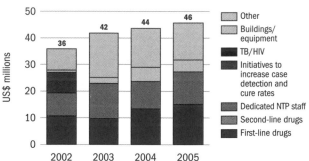

(c) Total TB control costs by line item[b]

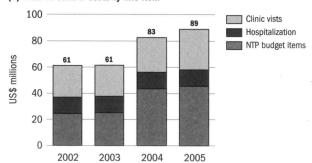

(d) Per patient costs, budgets, available funding and expenditures

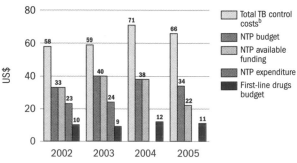

[a] TB/HIV collaborative activities and initiatives to increase case detection and cure rates are not budgeted separately, and are thus included under other budget lines.
[b] Total TB control costs for 2002 and 2003 are based on expenditures, whereas those for 2004 and 2005 are based on budgets. Estimates of the costs of clinic visits and hospitalization are WHO estimates based on data provided by the NTP and from other sources. See Methods for further details.

US$ 60–70, as total TB control costs have increased from about US$ 60 million in 2002 to a projected US$ 89 million in 2005; these figures may be overestimates because they assume that 75% of all DOT is undertaken at health facilities and that about 10 000 dedicated hospital beds are still being used for TB patients. In practice, community workers or volunteers may provide DOT to more than 25% of patients, at no cost to the health system, and increasing numbers of hospital beds previously dedicated to TB patients are being reallocated to other uses. A costing study will be undertaken in 2005 to further refine these estimates. While progress has been made at the planned rate, actual expenditures were lower than budgets in both 2002 and 2003, so the cost of DOTS expansion has been lower than anticipated.

Indonesia

Indonesia is entering a phase of rapid and comprehensive acceleration of its TB activities thanks to a substantial increase in funding for 2004 and 2005. With a fully-funded budget, many opportunities are being taken to improve surveillance, case detection and laboratory services, to extend the involvement of other health-care providers in DOTS and to improve TB/HIV coordination. A population-based TB prevalence survey was carried out in 2004; the data will provide a more accurate estimate of the national burden of TB, and provide a basis for assessing the future impact of the NTP on the TB epidemic. Although Indonesia has achieved a high level of DOTS coverage (98%), this has not yet been matched by high levels of case detection because of several factors, including a backlog of staff to be trained, suboptimal laboratory support and the lack of effective links with the hospi-tal sector and private practitioners. Substantial improvements in the weaker areas of the programme should accrue from the greatly increased investment in the NTP.

System of TB control
In the decentralized primary health-care system, TB control is offered through the district health services. District populations range from under 10 000 to more than 2 million, with the majority between 50 000 and 150 000.

Indonesia does not yet have a designated NRL for TB. A fully functioning national TB laboratory network is currently being developed. The existing laboratory network, which is not formally linked with the NTP, consists of microscopy health centres and independent health centres where trained laboratory staff carry out smear diagnosis. Provincial health laboratories provide some assessments of the quality of smear microscopy, and perform culture and drug susceptibility testing on request.

Surveillance and monitoring
Since the burden of TB has been estimated from old (>20 years) and possibly unreliable data, Indonesia carried out an important national disease prevalence survey during 2004. Analysis of the survey data was still in progress in January 2005, and it is not yet clear whether the best estimate of smear-positive prevalence for 2003 will be significantly different from the WHO estimate of 295 per 100 000 population. Because TB cases have been reported with variable effort and consistency since 1980, the notifications over time give no indication of the underlying trend in incidence. However, the higher notification rates among older men suggest that the epidemic could be in slow decline. The national HIV infection rate remains low (0.1% in adults aged 15–49 years in 2003), but HIV appears to be generating more TB cases among young adults in some parts of Java and Papua.

The very high reported DOTS coverage (98% since 2000) has not been matched by high rates of case detection, although the smear-positive case detection rate has increased markedly between 2000 (19%) and 2003 (33%). Optimizing the functional capacity of health centres plus improved collaboration between the NTP, lung clinics and a limited number of public and private hospitals contributed to this success, and further strengthening of these links is needed. The NTP DOTS programme has been recruiting smear-negative and extrapulmonary cases faster than smear-positive cases since 1995. This may be a result of the heavy reliance on X-ray diagnosis in smear-negative patients, particularly in lung clinics and lung hospitals (involvement since 2002). Among new smear-positive patients, treatment success exceeded the 85% target in

PROGRESS IN TB CONTROL IN INDONESIA

Indicators
DOTS treatment success, 2002 cohort	86%
DOTS case detection rate, 2003	33%
NTP budget available, 2004	100%
Government contribution to NTP budget, including loans, 2004	57%
Government contribution to total TB control costs, including loans, 2004	63%
Government health spending used for TB control, 2004	5%

Major achievements
— Strengthening of management capacity by placing staff at central and provincial level
— Step-wise and cascade training as part of human resource development
— Detailed planning and budgetary exercises conducted at district level for smooth disbursement of donor funds
— Improved supervision and monitoring from central and provincial level
— Involvement of public chest clinics and limited public and private hospitals in PPM DOTS

Major planned activities
— Expand hospital DOTS linkage projects in a phased manner in all provinces and districts
— Develop and implement an advocacy and communications framework for sustaining political commitment and increasing case detection rate
— Strengthen laboratory network and cooperation between NTP and laboratory directorates at all levels, through joint planning, supervision and monitoring activities at district level
— Accelerate HR development activities by accelerating the training backlog of health-centre staff and by training staff from hospitals and other sectors

LATEST ESTIMATES[a]		TRENDS	2000	2001	2002	2003
Population	**219 883 460**	DOTS coverage (%)	98	98	98	98
Global rank (by est. number of cases)	3	Notification rate (all cases/100 000 pop)	40	43	71	81
Incidence (all cases/100 000 pop/year)	285	Notification rate (new ss+/100 000 pop)	25	25	35	42
Incidence (new ss+/100 000 pop/year)	128	Detection of all cases (%)	14	15	25	28
Prevalence (all cases/100 000 pop)	675	Case detection rate (new ss+, %)	19	20	27	33
TB mortality (all cases/100 000 pop/year)	65	DOTS case detection rate (new ss+, %)	19	20	27	33
TB cases HIV+ (adults aged 15–49, %)	0.5	DOTS case detection rate (new ss+)/coverage (%)	19	20	28	34
New cases multidrug resistant (%)	0.7	DOTS treatment success (new ss+, %)	87	86	86	–

Notification rate (per 100 000 pop)

— = ss+ cases — = all cases (178 260 in 2003)

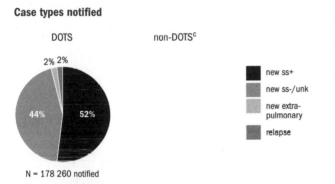

Notification rate by age and sex (new ss+)[b]

— = female — = male

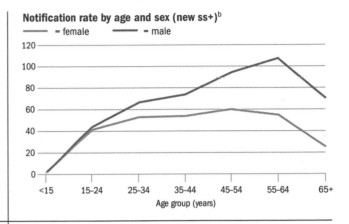

Case types notified

DOTS   non-DOTS[c]

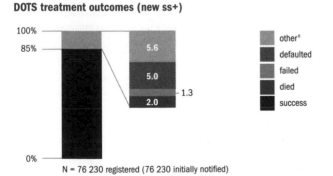

- new ss+
- new ss-/unk
- new extra-pulmonary
- relapse

N = 178 260 notified

DOTS progress towards targets[d]

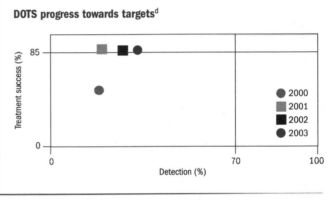

- 2000
- 2001
- 2002
- 2003

DOTS treatment outcomes (new ss+)

- other[e]
- defaulted
- failed
- died
- success

N = 76 230 registered (76 230 initially notified)

Non-DOTS treatment outcomes (new ss+)

Notes

ss+ indicates smear-positive; ss-, smear-negative; pop, population; unk, unknown.

Absence of a graph indicates that the data were not available or applicable.

[a] See Methods for data sources. Prevalence and mortality estimates include patients with HIV.

[b] The sum of cases notified by age and sex is less than the number of new smear-positive cases notified for some countries.

[c] Non-DOTS is blank for countries which are 100% DOTS, or where no non-DOTS data were reported.

[d] DOTS case detection rate for given year, DOTS treatment success rate for cohort registered in previous year.

[e] "Other" includes transfer out and not evaluated, still on treatment, and other unknown.

the 2002 cohort. Treatment results have been consistently good since the NTP began to evaluate outcomes comprehensively in 2000, although many patients complete treatment without evidence of cure (15% in 2002). There is no evidence yet that DOTS is reducing the burden of TB in Indonesia, but the 2004 prevalence survey data will give a baseline against which performance can be assessed towards the end of the decade.

Improving programme performance

The decentralization of health-care delivery has unfortunately had a negative effect on human resource capacity and development. Constraints include a high rotation of staff and hiring restrictions. As of December 2003, only 34% of health centre staff were adequately trained. Steps are being taken to alleviate this situation, and Indonesia was approved for additional funding through ISAC, which will help to reduce the training backlog by intensifying activities through mobile "master trainer's teams". As part of HR development, management capacity has been strengthened at the central and provincial levels during 2004, leading to a considerable improvement in supervision and monitoring by staff at these levels. Closer collaboration between the central, provincial and district health authorities is having a positive impact on TB control activities.

As a result of increased donor support and funding, Indonesia has carried out detailed planning and budgetary exercises at the district level for efficient disbursement of new funds.

Drug resistance surveillance has not yet been instituted in Indonesia. However, laboratory facilities at Surabaya have been upgraded because this laboratory will be used as the reference laboratory for future drug resistance surveys. Limited surveys in Jakarta have found MDR-TB in more than 4% of previously untreated cases; a fully representative survey is needed to determine whether this situation prevails throughout the country (the national WHO estimate is 0.7%). A survey in Central Java is planned for early 2005. There is no national policy

for the management of MDR-TB, and pulmonologists treat MDR-TB cases on an individual basis. Some of the second-line drugs are produced in the country.

Diagnostic and laboratory services

The link between TB laboratories and the NTP remains weak but will be made stronger with the establishment of a central laboratory working group and an NRL. A national assessment caried out in November 2004 evaluated the current laboratory services and will be used to guide planning for future improvements. There is also a need to improve and strengthen the EQA system. Priorities should include training of laboratory staff and preparation of a plan and timetable to carry out training and supervision at the provincial level.

TB/HIV coordination

Indonesia is classified as a country with low HIV prevalence but with concentrated epidemics, primarily among injecting drug users. A TB/HIV workshop was held in 2002 to consider experiences from central and provincial levels and to develop an action plan for tackling the dual epidemic. A national TB/HIV coordinating body was established and a situation analysis undertaken to assess the linkages between the HIV and TB control programmes in four provinces with high HIV burdens. Guidelines on the management of TB in PLWHA have been published and a pilot project on collaborative TB/HIV activities at the district level is in progress, with funding from WHO.

Links with other health-care providers

Indonesia has developed a national strategy for PPM DOTS, focusing primarily on the involvement of public chest clinics and public and private hospitals. Several small-scale pilot projects have been started, and the hospital DOTS linkage project in Yogyakarta has shown a dramatic increase in case detection (>400%) since it began in 2000. Countrywide, very few general hospitals, medical colleges or prison health facilities are involved in DOTS, and there are no treatment providers outside the NTP

that notify cases. However, plans are under way to scale up the successful pilot projects and to start involving private medical practitioners in DOTS.

Partnerships

KNCV and WHO are the lead technical partners in Indonesia and support all aspects of DOTS expansion activities. Other technical partners include Kuis/Johns Hopkins, MSH, NLR, TBCTA and World Vision. Major financial partners are the ADB, CIDA, the Dutch Government, GFATM and USAID. A national TB Partners forum meets three to four times a year to share information with partners and donors and to strengthen collaboration between the various participants in TB control.

Budgets and expenditures

Funding for TB control has improved substantially since 2002, when the NTP reported a funding gap exceeding 50% of the total budget requirement, and expenditures amounting to US$ 18 million. Available funding more than doubled between 2002 and 2003, although a small funding gap remained. The 2004 budget was fully funded, as is the projected budget of US$ 43 million for 2005. If the funds are fully disbursed, spending by the NTP in 2005 will more than double that in 2002. This impressive growth in funding is primarily because of a large grant from the GFATM, which will provide 34% of the NTP budget in 2005, in addition to the increase in government funding. The additional funds allow for an increase in the anti-TB drug budget, as well as more spending on initiatives to improve case detection and cure rates. As projected total case detection and total spending increase, the NTP budget and total TB control costs (i.e. the NTP budget plus estimated spending on health clinic visits not covered by the NTP budget) are expected to remain relatively constant per patient, at about US$ 150–160 and US$ 180, respectively. It remains to be seen whether the increased funding can be absorbed, and whether increased expenditures result in improved case detection.

(a) NTP budget by source of funding

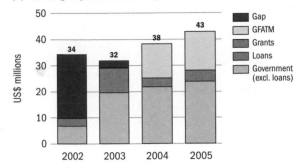

Legend:
- Gap
- GFATM
- Grants
- Loans
- Government (excl. loans)

(b) NTP budget by line item

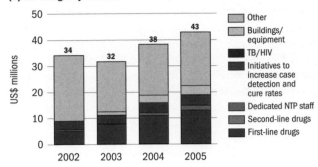

Legend:
- Other
- Buildings/ equipment
- TB/HIV
- Initiatives to increase case detection and cure rates
- Dedicated NTP staff
- Second-line drugs
- First-line drugs

(c) Total TB control costs by line item[a]

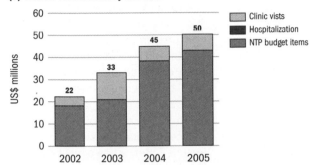

Legend:
- Clinic vists
- Hospitalization
- NTP budget items

(d) Per patient costs, budgets, available funding and expenditures

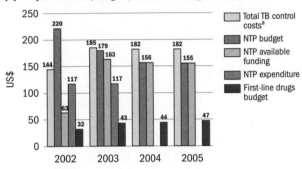

Legend:
- Total TB control costs[a]
- NTP budget
- NTP available funding
- NTP expenditure
- First-line drugs budget

[a] Total TB control costs for 2002 and 2003 are based on expenditures, whereas those for 2004 and 2005 are based on budgets. Estimates of the costs of clinic visits and hospitalization are WHO estimates based on data provided by the NTP and from other sources. See Methods for further details.

Kenya

Kenya adopted the DOTS strategy in the early 1990s and achieved nationwide DOTS coverage in 1996. The diagnosis and treatment of TB are integrated into the Kenyan public health services. TB notification rates have increased five-fold in the past 10 years, the main explanation is probably the impact of the HIV epidemic, although improvements in programme performance may also have contributed; encouraging private physicians to provide DOTS services has increased case-finding in recent years. Furthermore, in collaboration with NGOs, DOTS services are being extended to remote areas, nomadic populations and urban slums. PPM-DOTS initiatives are succeeding but there is still scope to increase the involvement of community workers. An estimated 29% of TB patients are HIV-positive, and TB/HIV coinfection is now a significant problem. Kenya is actively promoting collaboration between the TB and HIV programmes, supported by the "3 by 5" initiative and funding from the President's Emer-gency Plan for AIDS Relief. It is anticipated that up to 35% of those who start ART in the public sector will be TB patients.

System of TB control

The NTP (known locally as the National Leprosy and TB Programme) adopted the DOTS strategy in the early 1990s, and TB diagnosis and treatment are integrated into the public health services at all levels. At the central level, the NTP develops TB control policies and offers technical assistance to health-service providers. Other central level responsibilities include surveillance, training, advocacy and resource mobilization activities.

Kenya's laboratory system includes the Central TB Reference Laboratory based at the Kenya Medical Research Institute, which functions as an NRL, four private medical laboratories in Nairobi that are able to perform culture and susceptibility testing for first-line drugs and 619 laboratories that perform smear microscopy. All public and faith-based hospitals, health centres and some dispensaries carry out sputum microscopy. About three quarters of all registered medical laboratories in Kenya – government, NGO and private – do smear microscopy for the NTP.

Surveillance and monitoring

The TB notification rate increased five-fold between 1980 and 2003, but the rate of increase is declining. In assessing the case detection rate, it has been assumed that the increase in case notifications reflects a real increase in incidence; it is also possible that case detection has improved in recent years. The spread of HIV infection in Kenya has almost certainly been responsible for much of the increase but also makes it difficult to estimate the true case detection rate without more detailed analysis of subnational data. The proportion of notified cases that are diagnosed as smear-positive has fallen steadily since 1995, possibly because HIV-positive people are more likely than HIV-negative people to present with smear-negative TB. A similar pattern is seen in other countries in eastern and southern Africa where the prevalence of HIV is high.

The treatment success rate in 2002 was 79%, still below the 85% target, largely because 15% of patients defaulted or were transferred to other treatment centres without follow-up, and 5% died. The loss of patients from the cohort could be associated with HIV infection but may also reflect weaknesses in programme management. For either or both of these reasons, the treatment outcomes for new smear-positive patients have not improved much since 1994. The treatment outcomes among patients registered for re-treatment following relapse were somewhat worse, and the death rate was 10%. Outcomes are not available for patients treated after failure or default.

As long as the incidence of TB remains high because of the HIV epidemic in Kenya, the epidemiological

---

PROGRESS IN TB CONTROL IN KENYA

Indicators

DOTS treatment success, 2002 cohort	79%
DOTS case detection rate, 2003	46%
NTP budget available, 2004	75%
Government contribution to NTP budget, including loans, 2004	25%
Government contribution to total TB control costs, including loans, 2004	38%
Government health spending used for TB control, 2004	7%

Major achievements
— Significant improvement in human resources capacity in the central unit
— Expansion of PPM DOTS, reinstatement of NRL, establishment of the TB/HIV coordinating body, and development of several guidelines and of the urban TB control strategy
— Secured sufficient drugs and funds for DOTS implementation and expansion
— Increased case-finding through decentralization of TB diagnostic services, coupled with improvement of diagnostic procedures
— Development and implementation of the COMBI plan that is aimed at influencing the health-seeking behaviour of the population to improve early case detection

Major planned activities
— Implement effective TB/HIV collaborative programme: VCT, co-trimoxazole preventive therapy and ART for HIV-infected TB patients
— Improve human resources by recruiting additional staff at central and peripheral levels to boost training and supervision

LATEST ESTIMATES[a]		TRENDS	2000	2001	2002	2003
Population	**31 987 119**	DOTS coverage (%)	100	100	100	100
Global rank (by est. number of cases)	10	Notification rate (all cases/100 000 pop)	210	235	254	286
Incidence (all cases/100 000 pop/year)	610	Notification rate (new ss+/100 000 pop)	94	101	109	119
Incidence (new ss+/100 000 pop/year)	262	Detection of all cases (%)	46	47	46	47
Prevalence (all cases/100 000 pop)	884	Case detection rate (new ss+, %)	48	47	46	46
TB mortality (all cases/100 000 pop/year)	133	DOTS case detection rate (new ss+, %)	44	47	46	46
TB cases HIV+ (adults aged 15–49, %)	29	DOTS case detection rate (new ss+)/coverage (%)	44	47	46	46
New cases multidrug resistant (%)	0.0	DOTS treatment success (new ss+, %)	80	80	79	–

Notification rate (per 100 000 pop)

— = ss+ cases   — = all cases (91 522 in 2003)

Notification rate by age and sex (new ss+)[b]

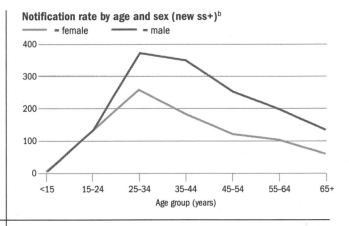

— = female   — = male

Case types notified

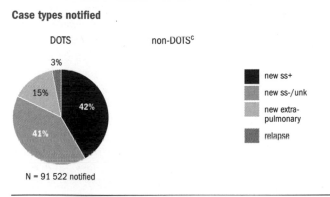

DOTS   non-DOTS[c]

new ss+
new ss-/unk
new extra-pulmonary
relapse

N = 91 522 notified

DOTS progress towards targets[d]

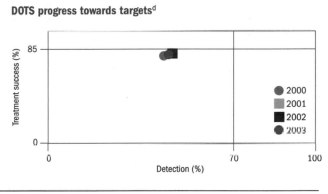

2000
2001
2002
2003

DOTS treatment outcomes (new ss+)

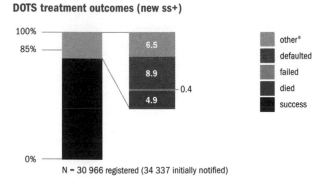

other[e]
defaulted
failed
died
success

N = 30 966 registered (34 337 initially notified)

Non-DOTS treatment outcomes (new ss+)

Notes

ss+ indicates smear-positive; ss-, smear-negative; pop, population; unk, unknown.

Absence of a graph indicates that the data were not available or applicable.

[a] See Methods for data sources. Prevalence and mortality estimates include patients with HIV.

[b] The sum of cases notified by age and sex is less than the number of new smear-positive cases notified for some countries.

[c] Non-DOTS is blank for countries which are 100% DOTS, or where no non-DOTS data were reported.

[d] DOTS case detection rate for given year, DOTS treatment success rate for cohort registered in previous year.

[e] "Other" includes transfer out and not evaluated, still on treatment, and other unknown.

impact of the DOTS programme will be hard to evaluate from routine surveillance data alone. A population-based survey of disease prevalence would give a better estimate of the current burden of TB in Kenya and provide a baseline against which to assess the future impact of control programmes.

Improving programme performance

The Government of Kenya is committed to providing anti-TB drugs for all new patients. The NTP also receives support for drugs from the GDF. The last official data from a drug resistance survey were reported in 1995. In December 2004, the GLC approved a DOTS-Plus pilot project, with funding from the GFATM.

A national TB control plan is being developed for 2005–2010. Tuberculin surveys were carried out in 1958–1959, 1986–1990 and 1990–1995. A fourth tuberculin survey has already started, in collaboration with KNCV, and should be completed in 2006.

An urban TB control project is planned, with a focus on expanding TB services to slum populations in cities; funds from the GFATM will allow several new activities to start. Diagnostic and treatment services are expanding, and NTP activities in collaboration with the national AIDS programme, private sector representatives (physicians and pharmacies), prison authorities and selected NGOs are continuing in several districts.

The COMBI communication plan was launched in April 2004, when materials developed by several agencies were presented. A system to monitor and evaluate the implementation, distribution and impact of these materials is being established.

Three other areas in which programme performance needs to be improved are diagnostic and laboratory services, TB/HIV coordination and links with other health-care providers and the community.

Diagnostic and laboratory services

Expansion of the diagnostic services continues, with the number of laboratories that perform smear microscopy increasing from 542 in 2003 to 619 in 2004. EQA for smear microscopy, in accordance with international guidelines, is being adopted for regional and district laboratories and its implementation started in May 2004 in some districts. Discussions on the establishment of a network of public and private laboratories and the inclusion of these laboratories in the existing EQA system are in progress. Major constraints for the laboratory services include inadequate human resources and an insufficient budget allocation for supervisory activities. Until 2003, the Central TB Reference Laboratory did not have a clear mandate to function as an NRL. At present, one of the main priorities for the NTP is to continue to improve the technical capacity of this laboratory. The NRL is currently equipped to carry out rapid liquid culture techniques and DST on all re-treatment cases from Nairobi as well as re-treatment and failure cases from other provinces. New laboratory guidelines for sputum examination by AFB microscopy have been developed and are to be published in 2005.

TB/HIV coordination

Kenya, like many other countries in sub-Saharan Africa, is severely affected by the HIV/AIDS epidemic. An estimated 29% of adult TB patients in Kenya are HIV-positive; a new survey of HIV in TB patients is planned for 2005. In 2003, a national TB/HIV coordinating body was set up, including representatives from the TB and HIV programmes, research institutions, technical agencies, donors and representatives of PLWHA. A national TB/HIV coordinator was appointed and is the secretary of the steering committee. TB/HIV activities have started in Nakuru District, and by the end of 2005, should have started in about 30 other districts.

Kenya is one of the pilot sites for the "3 by 5" initiative and is receiving funding from the President's Emergency Plan for AIDS Relief. In 2005, about 45 000 TB patients should be offered HIV testing and a package of prevention and care, including ART. It is estimated that about 35% of patients who are eligible for ART will be identified through the TB control services. A monitoring and evaluation system for TB/HIV activities is now being developed and tested in selected districts.

Links with other health-care providers

An initiative to encourage private physicians to provide DOTS services in Nairobi was started in 2001 and is now being implemented in several other towns and settings. This has led to an increase in case notification rates, and treatment results have been satisfactory. Guidelines for PPM-DOTS have been developed and staff trained. Collaboration between the NTP, NGOs and a variety of public sector health providers and related institutions, including general hospitals, medical colleges and health services in refugee camps, prisons, military and the police, is still in progress.

Links with the community

Community-based DOTS was successfully pilot tested in Machakos District between 1998 and 2000, and 11 other districts have recently started training community volunteers. District teams, comprising nurses, social workers, health educators and public health workers, train community volunteers in increasing awareness of TB, early referral of suspects and treatment support.

Partnerships

Financial support to the NTP in Kenya is mostly provided by CIDA, CDC and USAID. The NTP has a three-year agreement with the GDF for anti-TB drugs, which expired at the end of 2004. The World Bank supported the NTP through a loan for the purchase of anti-TB drugs. A GFATM grant agreement was signed in round 2 and will provide significant funding for DOTS expansion activities. KNCV and WHO are the main technical partners.

Budgets and expenditures

The NTP budget has increased steadily from US$ 5.2 million in 2002 to US$ 14 million in 2005; the budget per patient has increased from about US$ 67 per patient in 2002 (for about 60 000 patients) to US$ 142 per

(a) NTP budget by source of funding

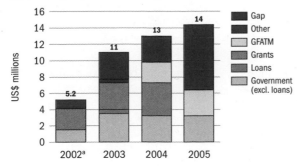

Legend:
- Gap
- Other
- GFATM
- Grants
- Loans
- Government (excl. loans)

(b) NTP budget by line item

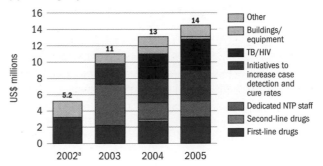

Legend:
- Other
- Buildings/equipment
- TB/HIV
- Initiatives to increase case detection and cure rates
- Dedicated NTP staff
- Second-line drugs
- First-line drugs

(c) Total TB control costs by line item[b]

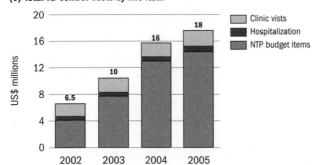

Legend:
- Clinic vists
- Hospitalization
- NTP budget items

(d) Per patient costs, budgets, available funding and expenditures

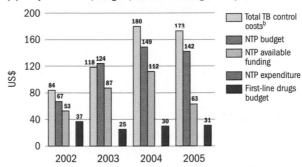

Legend:
- Total TB control costs[b]
- NTP budget
- NTP available funding
- NTP expenditure
- First-line drugs budget

[a] Does not include budget for buildings/equipment and dedicated NTP staff.

[b] Total TB control costs for 2002 and 2003 are based on available funding, whereas those for 2004 and 2005 are based on budgets. Estimates of the costs of clinic visits and hospitalization are WHO estimates based on data provided by the NTP and from other sources. See Methods for further details.

patient in 2005 (based on a projection by the NTP that about 100 000 patients will be treated in 2005). The government contribution to the NTP budget has been fairly constant at about US$ 3.5 million per year (although this is underestimated to some extent because funds budgeted for investment in buildings and equipment are not reflected in the NTP budget). All grants, except the GFATM grant, end in June 2005 and need to be renegotiated. This explains why a funding gap of US$ 8 million, equivalent to about 50% of the NTP budget, is reported for 2005. It is anticipated that external funding will be secured to reduce this gap.

The increased budgets in 2004 and 2005 are to allow increased spending on collaborative TB/HIV activities and initiatives aimed at improving case detection and cure rates. Implementation of these activities will depend on closing the funding gap. No expenditure data are available for the years 2002 or 2003.

If the NTP budget is fully funded and the money is spent, total TB control costs (which include visits to health clinics and expenditures related to hospitalization in addition to NTP budget items) will be about US$ 16–18 million in 2004 and 2005, or about US$ 180 per patient treated (compared with about US$ 120 in 2003). The increase in total costs per patient is almost entirely due to changes in costs included in the NTP budget.

Mozambique

Mozambique has a longstanding commitment to TB control, and the DOTS strategy was introduced in all districts by 2000. Nevertheless, the NTP still faces substantial difficulties in providing adequate TB services throughout the country. Efforts are being made to strengthen the country's health infrastructure, which has suffered in the past from inadequate resources as well as the destructive effects of civil unrest and natural disasters. Despite these difficulties, TB case detection and cure rates have improved in recent years. The award of a GFATM grant will greatly increase the amount of funds available for TB control in 2005 and make it possible to address problems related to staffing, training and medical supplies and equipment. With improvements in facilities for diagnosis and patient care, case detection and cure rates should continue to improve in the next few years. Progress will be gradual because it will take time to build up the necessary cadre of well-trained staff to carry out the full programme of DOTS activities. With the help of in-

ternational partners, Mozambique is beginning to tackle the special challenges associated with high rates of Tb and HIV coinfection. The extent of MDR-TB is being investigated in a new national survey.

System of TB control

The NTP was officially established in 1977 and consists of a central unit, 3 regional coordinators, 12 provincial coordinators and 149 health area district coordinators. There are 3 central hospitals (one in each region), 7 provincial hospitals, 27 rural hospitals and 162 health centres, all involved in DOTS implementation. There are also approximately 800 health posts, managed by rural health workers, which are not part of the DOTS programme.

The TB laboratory network has an NRL in Maputo City that performs culture and DST. There are 45 intermediate laboratories, 11 of which are located in the capital cities of the provinces, and 163 peripheral laboratories located mostly in health centres of the district capital cities. There are no

microscopy services in any of the health posts.

Surveillance and monitoring

The total number of TB cases notified, both smear-positive and all forms, continued to increase between 2002 and 2003. The proportion of new pulmonary cases diagnosed as smear-positive was 67% in 2003. This is towards the lower end of the expected range of 65–80%, as often seen in countries with high rates of HIV infection. For Mozambique, as for some other countries in southern Africa, the accuracy of the estimated case detection rate (45% in 2003) is uncertain. The treatment success rate was 78% for the 2002 cohort and has improved each year since 1995. In 2002, 11% of patients died and 10% defaulted or were lost to follow-up after transfer to other treatment centres. Both of the latter indicators were high for patients undergoing re-treatment following relapse, failure or default; the overall re-treatment success rate was 67%. Considering progress towards the MDGs, the priority for Mozambique is to bring treatment success and case detection rates closer to target levels.

Improving programme performance

Implementation of the NTP's five-year national strategic plan began in 2003. Financial constraints have hindered almost all aspects of programme performance in Mozambique, partly because of a change in financial transfer mechanisms at the central level. Future improvements in the programme rely heavily on the GFATM grant, which was signed in April 2004. Disbursement of funds started in September 2004 but has not yet reached the sub-recipients. However, it may prove difficult for the central unit to meet the staffing requirements needed to begin implementation of the overall GFATM plan. A number of key staff need to be recruited, including TB coordinators for the central, southern and northern regions as well as

---

PROGRESS IN TB CONTROL IN MOZAMBIQUE

Indicators

DOTS treatment success, 2002 cohort	78%
DOTS detection rate, 2003	45%
NTP budget available, 2004	44%
Government contribution to NTP budget, including loans, 2004	30%
Government contribution to total TB control costs, including loans, 2004	46%
Government health spending used for TB control, 2004	6%

Major achievements
— Implementation of a five-year strategic national plan for the NTP (2003–2008)
— Approval of GFATM funding for overall NTP strengthening, and GDF funding for FDC anti-TB drugs
— Development of a national TB/HIV collaborative project

Major planned activities
— Develop a drug management system to estimate the number of drugs and supplies needed at central and provincial level, and a plan to manage drug shortages
— Establish laboratory quality control in collaboration with provincial laboratory supervisors
— Commence collaborative TB/HIV activities in demonstration project sites, including surveillance of HIV in TB patients in 2005 and the introduction of isoniazid preventive therapy and co-trimoxazole preventive therapy

MOZAMBIQUE

LATEST ESTIMATES[a]		TRENDS	2000	2001	2002	2003
Population	**18 863 291**	DOTS coverage (%)	100	100	100	100
Global rank (by est. number of cases)	18	Notification rate (all cases/100 000 pop)	118	121	138	152
Incidence (all cases/100 000 pop/year)	457	Notification rate (new ss+/100 000 pop)	74	77	82	86
Incidence (new ss+/100 000 pop/year)	190	Detection of all cases (%)	30	29	32	33
Prevalence (all cases/100 000 pop)	636	Case detection rate (new ss+, %)	45	44	45	45
TB mortality (all cases/100 000 pop/year)	129	DOTS case detection rate (new ss+, %)	45	44	45	45
TB cases HIV+ (adults aged 15–49, %)	49	DOTS case detection rate (new ss+)/coverage (%)	45	44	45	45
New cases multidrug resistant (%)	3.5	DOTS treatment success (new ss+, %)	75	77	78	–

Notification rate (per 100 000 pop)

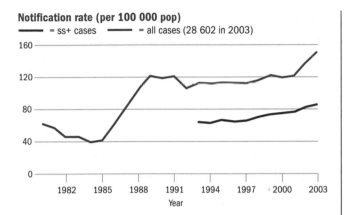

— = ss+ cases   — = all cases (28 602 in 2003)

Notification rate by age and sex (new ss+)[b]

Case types notified

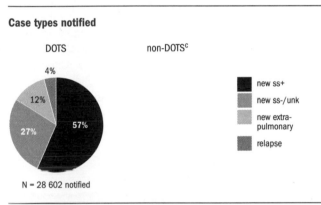

DOTS   non-DOTS[c]

4%
12%
27%
57%

new ss+
new ss-/unk
new extra-pulmonary
relapse

N = 28 602 notified

DOTS progress towards targets[d]

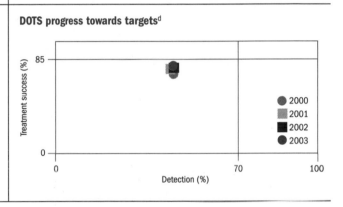

Treatment success (%)

Detection (%)

2000
2001
2002
2003

DOTS treatment outcomes (new ss+)

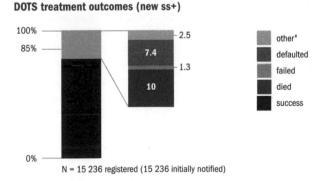

2.5
7.4
1.3
10

other[e]
defaulted
failed
died
success

N = 15 236 registered (15 236 initially notified)

Non-DOTS treatment outcomes (new ss+)

Notes

ss+ indicates smear-positive; ss-, smear-negative; pop, population; unk, unknown.

Absence of a graph indicates that the data were not available or applicable.

[a] See Methods for data sources. Prevalence and mortality estimates include patients with HIV.

[b] The sum of cases notified by age and sex is less than the number of new smear-positive cases notified for some countries.

[c] Non-DOTS is blank for countries which are 100% DOTS, or where no non-DOTS data were reported

[d] DOTS case detection rate for given year, DOTS treatment success rate for cohort registered in previous year.

[e] "Other" includes transfer out and not evaluated, still on treatment, and other unknown.

technical and administrative support staff and laboratory technicians. In preparation for the GFATM grant, six TB managers were trained at the WHO Collaborating Centre for TB and Lung Disease in Sondalo, Italy, in July 2003.

In 2003 and 2004, a serious shortage of anti-TB drugs occurred because of lack of funds. In May 2004, there were no stocks of ethambutol or pyrazinamide at the central level and a severe shortage of drugs was reported in some provinces. Fortunately, a three-year grant was approved by the GDF at the time of these shortages. FDC anti-TB drugs will be procured in place of loose formulations from 2004. A drug management system will be developed with GFATM funds; this will include a simple computer spreadsheet to estimate the amount of drugs and supplies needed at the central and provincial levels, a mandatory one-year national buffer stock of drugs and laboratory reagents to be maintained at the central level, and a mechanism for responding to unforeseen shortages by mobilizing additional support.

A new national drug resistance survey is planned. The protocol has been finalized and implementation should start in January 2005. DST is performed on isolates from patients failing re-treatment. However, no proper treatment is available for MDR-TB patients. A proposal will be submitted to the GLC in 2005.

Three other areas where programme performance needs to be improved are diagnostic and laboratory services, TB/HIV coordination and links with other health-care providers.

Diagnostic and laboratory services

The quality of DOTS implementation is limited by the poor laboratory network. Existing laboratories are inadequately distributed throughout the country, and more than half of the population is served by health centres that are 10 km or further from a diagnostic facility. The protocol for quality assurance of smear microscopy has been finalized but was not put into practice as scheduled in January 2004 because of lack of funds. Regular laboratory supervision has also stopped due to a lack of funds. There are plans to establish laboratory quality control (LQC) in collaboration with provincial laboratory supervisors and to identify and train staff in LQC. Pro-

vision of culture testing and quality control call for the upgrading of laboratories in Beira (central region) and Nampula (northern region), but infrastructure improvements have been postponed until GFATM funding becomes available. The NRL will be strengthened only if funds can be obtained from sources other than the GFATM. During 2003, a number of health facilities that had been out of service were rehabilitated and several health posts upgraded to health centres with smear microscopy services.

The lack of technicians throughout the laboratory services in Mozambique will be addressed through intensified training of existing technicians and, with forthcoming funding, re-hiring of qualified technicians.

TB/HIV coordination

A collaborative TB/HIV project (2004–2005) is being funded by WHO and USAID and implemented with support from KNCV. Good progress is being made at the central level. A TB/HIV coordinator has been recruited and a body to coordinate collaborative TB/HIV activities at all levels established. The team will oversee the develop-

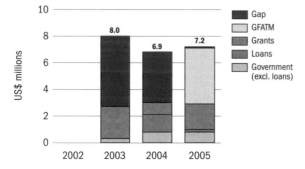

(a) NTP budget by source of funding

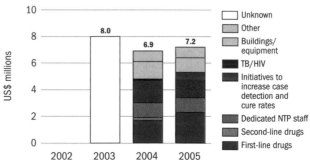

(b) NTP budget by line item

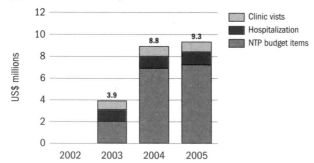

(c) Total TB control costs by line item[a]

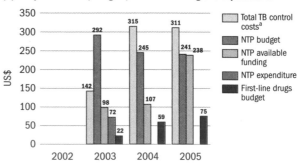

(d) Per patient costs, budgets, available funding and expenditures

[a] Total TB control costs for 2002 and 2003 are based on expenditures, whereas those for 2004 and 2005 are based on budgets. Estimates of the costs of clinic visits and hospitalization are WHO estimates based on data provided by the NTP and from other sources. See Methods for further details.

ment of a national policy for collaborative TB/HIV activities and its implementation, including planned demonstration projects. Planned project activities include surveillance of HIV in TB patients in 2005 and the introduction of isoniazid and cotrimoxazole preventive therapy. Training materials for TB/HIV are being developed and a workshop is planned. An important step has been the inclusion of the TB/HIV monitoring and evaluation indicators in the integrated health network system for HIV/AIDS; good progress is being made.

Links with other health-care providers
Private sector involvement is restricted to a few private hospitals that diagnose and treat TB under NTP guidance. The NTP is beginning to involve medical colleges, specialist TB clinics, and prison, army and police health facilities in DOTS activities.

Partnerships
External funding for TB control comes from the governments of Italy, Norway and the USA (USAID) and from the

GFATM. WHO and KNCV are the main technical partners; CARE International, CDC and MSF-Belgium/Luxembourg are additional partners in the TB/HIV project.

Budgets and expenditures
The NTP budget decreased from an estimated US$ 8.0 million in 2003 to US$ 6.9 million in 2004. However, available funding has increased from around US$ 3 million in 2003 to almost US$ 7 million in 2005. This means that the funding gap has fallen from 66% of the budget in 2003 to a projected 1% of the budget in 2005. This improved funding situation is mainly a result of an increase in loans and grants, including approval of a GFATM grant in round 2. The 2005 budget will be highly dependent on external financing, with around 85% of funds provided by grants, even though the government's contribution to the NTP budget has remained constant in absolute terms.

One of the largest budget line items is first-line anti-TB drugs. This budget has been increasing in recent years

to allow creation and consolidation of a buffer stock (this is why the budget per patient for first-line drugs has increased since 2003). There has also been a large increase in the budget for initiatives to increase case detection and cure rates between 2003 and 2005. These initiatives will be scaled up once GFATM funds become available. For the first time, there is a budget for collaborative TB/HIV activities in 2004 and 2005; however, this represents only around 1% of the NTP budget.

The total TB cost per patient based on budget data is about US$ 300 for the years 2004 and 2005. However, the total cost per patient based on actual expenditure was substantially lower in 2003 at US$ 142 because of the large funding gap. The total annual cost of TB control (including visits to health clinics and hospitalization as well as NTP budget items) is projected to increase from US$ 3.9 million in 2003 to US$ 9.3 million in 2005.

Myanmar

After a period of rapid DOTS expansion, Myanmar achieved nationwide DOTS coverage by the end of 2003. That year, more than 75 000 TB cases were reported, corresponding to a case detection rate of 73%; more than 80% of the 2002 cohort were treated successfully. With a strong national health infrastructure and government recognition of TB as a top priority, the country is now within sight of becoming the second of the current group of HBCs[1] to reach the global targets for DOTS implementation (after Viet Nam). Myanmar has made these commendable achievements with little external donor support. This situation will change radically with a massive increase in funding, mainly from the GFATM. When they become accessible, these funds will provide major opportunities for capital investment in infrastructure as well as important improvements in staffing at all levels and in the quality of laboratory services. They will also enable sustainability and strengthening of all aspects of the NTP including further boosting of treatment outcomes. Several NGOs now participate in the provision of TB control services, and the NTP is promoting the involvement of other health-care providers, particularly private physicians and clinicians from large hospitals. A national TB prevalence survey would provide a more accurate estimation of incidence and a baseline for assessing the impact of DOTS services on the TB epidemic.

System of TB control

The NTP functions through a central level office and 12 state or divisional TB centres. There is one central drug store and two subnational stores in upper and lower Myanmar. Township hospitals serve as the DOTS treatment units, and TB registers are maintained at this level for the population in each township.

The NRL was established in 2001, and there are two subnational laboratories. Since 2003, all state and divisional laboratories participate in a quality assurance network. Sputum smear microscopy is done in 309 of 324 townships. The NRL carries out drug susceptibility testing and, together with the subnational laboratory in Mandalay, also performs culture.

Surveillance and monitoring

The total number of reported TB cases increased from less than 15 000 in 1998 to more than 75 000 in 2003, with DOTS coverage reported to be 95% of the population during 2003 (rising to 100% towards the end of the year). During the same period, the smear-positive case detection rate increased from 29% to an estimated 73%, exceeding the 70% target. During this period of rapid DOTS expansion, the proportion of all new cases diagnosed as smear-positive fell from 68% (1998) to 36% (2003), which raises questions about the accuracy of the microscopic diagnosis. Treatment success has exceeded 80% since 1997, but moderately high default rates (9% in 2002) have limited the rate of success. As expected, the treatment success rates are somewhat lower for patients undergoing re-treatment (76% among relapses, 75% among all re-treatment cases combined). Nonetheless, on current evi-

---

PROGRESS IN TB CONTROL IN MYANMAR

Indicators

DOTS treatment success, 2002 cohort	81%
DOTS case detection rate, 2003	73%
NTP budget available, 2004	34%
Government contribution to NTP budget, including loans, 2004	6%
Government contribution to total TB control costs, including loans, 2004	18%
Government health spending used for TB control, 2004	0.4%

Major achievements

— DOTS expanded to all townships and case detection of new smear-positive patients above global target
— Operational guidelines on the involvement of private practitioners in DOTS published
— Treatment guidelines for HIV-infected TB patients published
— Nationwide introduction of FDC anti-TB drugs
— GFATM grant agreement signed in August 2004 and first funds distributed to principle recipient (UNDP)
— First nationwide drug resistance survey completed
— Technical Working Group on TB established by WHO to facilitate coordination and collaboration between agencies

Major planned activities

— Strengthen the national laboratory network by expanding the network of smear microscopy centres, improve quality control and upgrade the subnational laboratory in Mandalay
— Increase programme management capacity through GFATM funding (training, case management, supervision and monitoring, drug management, human resource development)
— Implement pilot project on ARV for HIV-infected TB patients in Mandalay
— Scale up PPM-DOTS projects
— Prepare 10-year plan for NTP (2006–2015), with emphasis on achievement of MDGs
— Apply to GDF for a second three-year grant
— Apply to ISAC for funding of technical assistance in GFATM project implementation

---

[1] Peru was excluded from the original group of HBCs, having met the targets and successfully reduced incidence.

LATEST ESTIMATES[a]		TRENDS	2000	2001	2002	2003
Population	**49 485 491**	DOTS coverage (%)	77	84	88	95
Global rank (by est. number of cases)	20	Notification rate (all cases/100 000 pop)	65	89	117	153
Incidence (all cases/100 000 pop/year)	171	Notification rate (new ss+/100 000 pop)	36	44	49	55
Incidence (new ss+/100 000 pop/year)	76	Detection of all cases (%)	38	52	68	90
Prevalence (all cases/100 000 pop)	187	Case detection rate (new ss+, %)	48	58	65	73
TB mortality (all cases/100 000 pop/year)	25	DOTS case detection rate (new ss+, %)	48	56	65	73
TB cases HIV+ (adults aged 15–49, %)	6.8	DOTS case detection rate (new ss+)/coverage (%)	62	67	74	77
New cases multidrug resistant (%)	4.0	DOTS treatment success (new ss+, %)	82	81	81	–

Notification rate (per 100 000 pop)

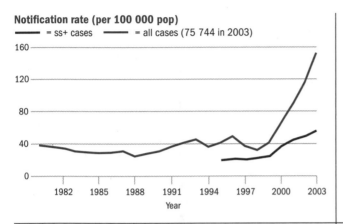

Notification rate by age and sex (new ss+)[b]

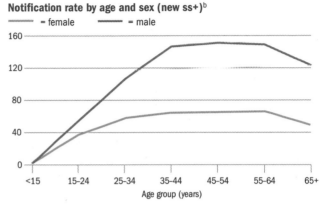

Case types notified

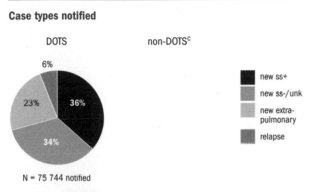

N = 75 744 notified

DOTS progress towards targets[d]

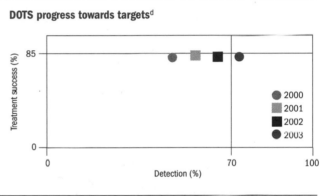

DOTS treatment outcomes (new ss+)

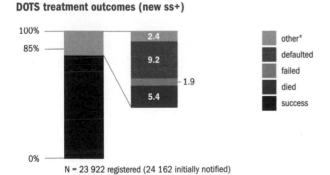

N = 23 922 registered (24 162 initially notified)

Non-DOTS treatment outcomes (new ss+)

Notes

ss+ indicates smear-positive; ss-, smear-negative; pop, population; unk, unknown.

Absence of a graph indicates that the data were not available or applicable.

[a] See Methods for data sources. Prevalence and mortality estimates include patients with HIV.

[b] The sum of cases notified by age and sex is less than the number of new smear-positive cases notified for some countries.

[c] Non-DOTS is blank for countries which are 100% DOTS, or where no non-DOTS data were reported.

[d] DOTS case detection rate for given year, DOTS treatment success rate for cohort registered in previous year.

[e] "Other" includes transfer out and not evaluated, still on treatment, and other unknown.

dence, Myanmar is close to reaching the targets for case detection and treatment success. One important caveat is that the denominator of the case detection rate – the estimated smear-positive incidence rate – is based on disease prevalence surveys carried out up to 1994. A decade later, a new national prevalence survey would provide a valuable reassessment of the burden of TB in Myanmar, give a baseline against which to evaluate DOTS impact and yield important information about the quality of diagnosis and treatment.

Improving programme performance

Development of human resource capacity has been strengthened, but many challenges still remain. An HR database is in place and shows that approximately a quarter of all sanctioned posts in the NTP are vacant. An HR development plan was prepared with WHO in 2003 and has already resulted in intensified training activities and the appointment of new staff. Future plans include cascade training of staff involved in TB control at all levels, including community volunteers, national NGOs and private physicians. The GFATM will support training activities and HR development; the NTP will apply for additional support through ISAC's second round of funding.

GFATM funding will also be used to increase monitoring, supervision and evaluation of programme activities and to strengthen DOTS by involving community and national NGOs and private providers, and by improving tracing of defaulters. The role of WHO will be to provide technical support to the principal recipient and subrecipients for planning, implementation and monitoring and evaluation of the TB component of the GFATM grant.

Myanmar currently receives anti-TB drugs through the GDF, which will provide a third year's supply of drugs for 2005, including a buffer stock. The GDF is considering a second term of three years beyond 2005. Following a successful pilot project to introduce FDC anti-TB drugs in the divisions of Mandalay and Yangon, all State/Divisional TB Officers were trained in FDC anti-TB drug management, and FDCs

have been introduced nationwide through cascade training of the Township Medical Officers. A nationwide drug resistance survey was completed in 2003, with the prevalence of MDR-TB among new cases estimated at 4.0%. There is no national policy on MDR-TB management; patients are treated on an individual basis.

Three other areas where programme performance needs to be improved are diagnostic and laboratory services, TB/HIV coordination and links with other health-care providers.

Diagnostic and laboratory services

Although the TB laboratory infrastructure is improving, strengthening of the national laboratory network is needed, especially the expansion of sputum smear microscopy centres, reinforcement of quality assurance at the township level and upgrading of the subnational laboratory in Mandalay. Another constraint is the shortage of qualified staff, especially junior laboratory technicians, which will be addressed as a priority for 2005. In addition, strengthening techniques for culture and drug susceptibility testing at the NRL in Yangon and the subnational laboratory in Mandalay are planned. It is also planned to introduce culture in four state/divisional laboratories in Bago, Mawlamyine, Pathein and Taunggyi.

TB/HIV coordination

The HIV prevalence among TB patients was estimated to be 4.5%, based on surveillance carried out in 20 sentinel sites from 1995–1997. This is lower than the current WHO estimate of 6.8%. No recent estimates from surveys are available, but a new HIV prevalence study among TB patients is planned once funding from the GFATM becomes accessible. Funding from GFATM will also support TB/HIV training for NTP staff at all levels. Political commitment has been demonstrated by the establishment by the MoH of a high-level coordinating body on TB/HIV. TB/HIV prevention and control activities were implemented in five pilot townships in 2000, including VCT for TB patients and provision of HIV education and prevention for HIV-infected TB patients. These activities were discontinued because of lack of

funding. Currently, there are limited collaborative TB/HIV activities in the country. Treatment guidelines for TB/HIV have been developed. VCT is available at a small number of VCT centres, at some drug treatment centres and at hospitals offering prevention of mother-to-child transmission programmes.

Although a supply of drugs for ART has arrived in Myanmar, ART is not yet available through the public sector. Some international NGOs such as MSF Holland and MSF Switzerland are providing ART to TB patients on a small scale. A WHO/National AIDS Programme/NTP/IUATLD/Total Exploration and Production Myanmar project will put 200 TB patients on ART in five townships in Mandalay Division in 2005. Partners within the government, and national and international NGOs have expressed interest in working with the NTP to strengthen existing TB/HIV activities and to actively engage in extending TB/HIV activities.

Links with other health-care providers

Involvement of general hospitals has increased rapidly during the past two years. In some areas, TB cases notified from general hospitals represent a substantial proportion of all cases registered under DOTS. However, a high proportion of the cases notified from hospitals are extrapulmonary or sputum smear-negative pulmonary TB, which raises some concern about the diagnostic quality in these hospitals. Involvement of army, police and prison health services has started but is still limited.

The Myanmar NTP has developed national guidelines for involvement of private practitioners in TB control. So far, two initiatives to involve private providers have been launched. In Mandalay Division, the NTP, together with the Department of Medical Research, started a project in 2002 to involve private physicians in diagnosis and treatment under the NTP. In Yangon, an international NGO (Population Services International) started implementing DOTS in 2004 as part of its existing franchising scheme, under which private physicians deliver diagnostic services at low cost and provide treatment with drugs free of charge from the NTP. Both initiatives have contributed substantially to increased case detection in targeted townships. Several additional initiatives are planned, including a training programme for private physicians, which will be coordinated by the Myanmar Medical Association, and a joint initiative by JICA and NTP to involve private practitioners in selected townships in Mandalay and Yangon Divisions.

Partnerships

Many national and a limited number of international NGOs work together on TB control in Myanmar. IUATLD supports operational research, TB/HIV activities including ART, and procurement of cars and laboratory equipment and supplies. WHO provides technical support and assists with HR development and procurement of drugs and laboratory supplies. JICA offers laboratory training, and anti-TB drugs are supplied by the GDF. The GFATM will soon be the main funding partner. The Country Coordination Mechanism has merged its working group with the Technical Working Group on TB hosted by WHO. The role of this working group is to support the United Nations Theme Group on Health (UNTGH) and the GFATM principal

recipient, the UNDP, by providing technical advice on all aspects of the implementation of the TB control programme funded by the GFATM and by other external sources, and by coordinating all operational and technical aspects between implementing agencies.

Budgets and expenditures

The NTP budget was around US$ 3 million in 2002, but a large funding gap meant that actual expenditures were only around US$ 1 million, primarily for staff and first-line drugs. The establishment of the GFATM has created new funding opportunities for the NTP, and following a successful GFATM application in 2003 the budget for 2004 was US$ 6.3 million. It was anticipated that the GFATM would provide about US$ 4 million of the required funds. However, because of delays in signing the initial two-year grant agreement, the first disbursement was only received by the GFATM principal recipient in September 2004, and thus a substantial funding gap remained. Provided that GFATM funds can be transferred to subrecipients and further disbursements are made according to the grant agreement, funding for the NTP will dramatically

improve in 2005, and the GFATM will be by far the most important source of financing. If this happens, funding per patient treated is likely to rise as well, from expenditures of US$ 20 per patient in 2002 to a budget of US$ 70 per patient in 2005. Since case detection is already high, increased funding will mainly provide for improvements in the quality of the existing infrastructure, which are needed to sustain the achievements that have already been made, and to support further improvements in case detection. Much of the increased budget in 2005 is for capital investments that will benefit patients for many years. Thus budgets for subsequent years will be lower (some of these investments were originally planned for 2004, but needed to be deferred to 2005 because of lack of funds; this explains why the budget developed for 2004 was higher than that for 2005). Costs beyond those reflected in the NTP budget are limited in Myanmar, at about US$ 1 million per year. If the NTP budget is fully funded in 2005, total TB control costs will rise from about US$ 2 million in 2002 and 2003 (about US$ 30 per patient treated) to US$ 6.1 million in 2005 (about US$ 80 per patient treated).

(a) NTP budget by source of funding

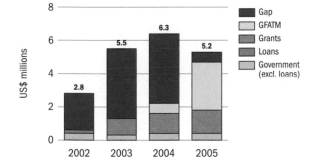

(b) NTP budget by line item

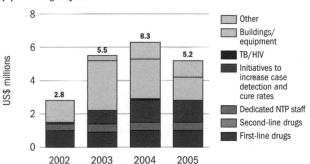

(c) Total TB control costs by line item[a]

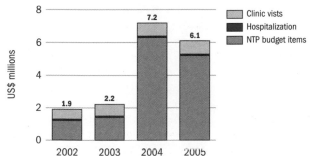

(d) Per patient costs, budgets, available funding and expenditures

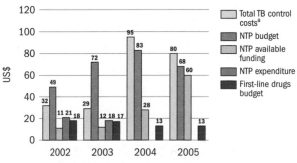

[a] Total TB control costs for 2002 and 2003 are based on expenditures, whereas those for 2004 and 2005 are based on budgets. Estimates of the costs of clinic visits and hospitalization are WHO estimates based on data provided by the NTP and from other sources. See Methods for further details.

Nigeria

Among African countries, Nigeria has the highest estimated number of new TB cases annually. Following the Abuja Declaration[1] in 2001, the DOTS strategy was adopted nationally and is now being applied in all states. There has been rapid progress in DOTS expansion in 2003, with relatively high treatment success. Unfortunately, political commitment has not yet been translated into strong support for the health system, and much of the approved government funding for health care has not been released for use in health programmes. This situation has discouraged a number of external donors, including the GFATM, who are reluctant to provide additional funds while government funding is very limited. Although Nigeria has an extensive national health infrastructure, it lacks the resources needed to function effectively. Nigeria is now decentralizing its health system and clarifying the responsibilities and services at each level, which should result in better management and

coordination. The spread of HIV infection is adding to the burden of TB; more than a quarter of adults with TB are coinfected with HIV. Notwithstanding the hesitation of some external donors, Nigeria now has an excellent opportunity to develop a programme of collaborative TB/HIV activities with the help of an award from the President's Emergency Plan for AIDS Relief.

System of TB control

Although the NTP was launched in 1991, the nationwide adoption and expansion of the DOTS strategy began only recently, following the Abuja Declaration to Stop TB in October 2001. Previously, only half of the states in Nigeria were supported by international NGOs (mainly dealing with leprosy) that were able to provide TB diagnosis and treatment; these did not include Lagos or the Federal Capital Territory (FCT), Abuja. All 37 states have at least one local government area (LGA) that is implementing DOTS.

The public health sector accounts for less than half of the health services provided in Nigeria, the rest being met by NGOs and the private sector, including hospitals, clinics and pharmacies. Health sector reform is under way in order to clearly establish the roles and responsibilities for health service provision at each level, and a Health Act will define the decentralization of functions. Tertiary care is provided and health regulations and technical guidelines developed at the federal level. States are responsible for secondary care and specialized services, while the LGAs are responsible for providing primary health care. The basic unit of health care is the ward. Each ward has 10 000–20 000 people and there are an average of 10 wards per LGA. Ward staff utilize community resources to help deliver the minimum package of care. Public health services will be decentralized from the LGA to the ward, and TB and leprosy control will be included in the minimum package of health services.

The NTP is organized at the federal, state and LGA levels. There is a central unit at the federal level led by a national coordinator. Each of the 37 state programmes is run by a state TB and leprosy control officer. The LGA is the main operational level of the programme, and most LGAs have a TB/leprosy control supervisor. The LGA TB/leprosy control supervisor is, in most cases, a community health officer or nurse who oversees activities in the health facilities.

The NRL in the National Institute for Medical Research in Lagos is responsible for overall supervision and quality assurance of the laboratory network. Six zonal reference laboratories supervise peripheral laboratories. The peripheral laboratories in PHC facilities, NGOs and private facilities all do direct smear microscopy.

PROGRESS IN TB CONTROL IN NIGERIA

Indicators

DOTS treatment success, 2002 cohort	79%
DOTS case detection rate, 2003	18%
NTP budget available, 2004	73%
Government contribution to NTP budget, including loans, 2004	37%
Government contribution to total TB control costs, including loans, 2004	66%
Government health spending used for TB control, 2004	4%

Major achievements

— Establishment of DOTS services in three more LGAs in each of 17 states, including training of general health workers and laboratory technicians, and purchase and distribution of laboratory materials

— Approval of a second year of funding from the GDF for anti-TB drugs and distribution of current anti-TB drugs to DOTS facilities throughout the country

— Appointment of a focal point for collaborative TB/HIV activities by the National AIDS and STD Control Programme

— Referral of TB patients with HIV/AIDS for HIV care and support, including ART in 25 pilot sites

Major planned activities

— Assess HR needs and strengthen capacity of general PHC and hospital staff in integrated TB control activities

— Establish at least one microscopy centre in each of the remaining LGAs, and strengthen collaboration between the microscopy centres and the NRL

— Establish a standardized quality assurance system for the entire country in 2005

[1] *Abuja declaration on HIV/AIDS, tuberculosis and other related infectious diseases*. Addis Ababa, The Economic Commission for Africa, 2001.

LATEST ESTIMATES[a]		TRENDS	2000	2001	2002	2003
Population	**124 009 171**	DOTS coverage (%)	47	55	55	60
Global rank (by est. number of cases)	4	Notification rate (all cases/100 000 pop)	23	39	32	36
Incidence (all cases/100 000 pop/year)	293	Notification rate (new ss+/100 000 pop)	15	20	18	23
Incidence (new ss+/100 000 pop/year)	126	Detection of all cases (%)	8.9	15	11	12
Prevalence (all cases/100 000 pop)	546	Case detection rate (new ss+, %)	14	17	15	18
TB mortality (all cases/100 000 pop/year)	85	DOTS case detection rate (new ss+, %)	14	14	13	18
TB cases HIV+ (adults aged 15–49, %)	27	DOTS case detection rate (new ss+)/coverage (%)	30	25	24	30
New cases multidrug resistant (%)	1.7	DOTS treatment success (new ss+, %)	79	79	79	–

Notification rate (per 100 000 pop)

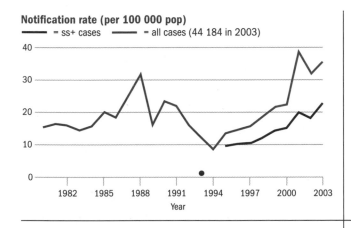

Notification rate by age and sex (new ss+)[b]

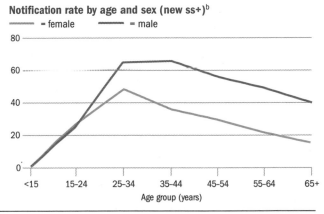

Case types notified

D

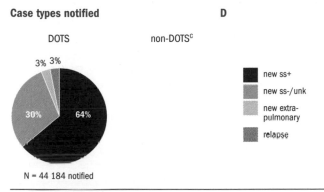

OTS progress towards targets[d]

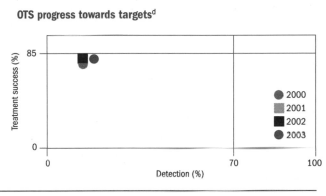

DOTS treatment outcomes (new ss+)

Non-DOTS treatment outcomes (new ss+)

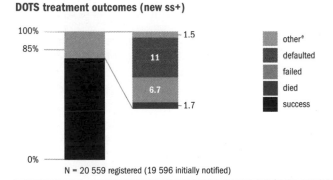

Notes

ss+ indicates smear-positive; ss-, smear-negative; pop, population; unk, unknown.

Absence of a graph indicates that the data were not available or applicable.

[a] See Methods for data sources. Prevalence and mortality estimates include patients with HIV.

[b] The sum of cases notified by age and sex is less than the number of new smear-positive cases notified for some countries.

[c] Non-DOTS is blank for countries which are 100% DOTS, or where no non-DOTS data were reported.

[d] DOTS case detection rate for given year, DOTS treatment success rate for cohort registered in previous year.

[e] "Other" includes transfer out and not evaluated, still on treatment, and other unknown.

Surveillance and monitoring

Among African countries, Nigeria has the highest estimated number of new TB cases each year. An estimated 6% of all adults, and 27% of adult TB patients, are infected with HIV. The increase in case notifications since 1994 is almost certainly due to a rise in TB incidence associated with the spread of HIV, rather than to improvements in case detection. DOTS coverage has changed little over the nine years for which data have been submitted to WHO (1995–2003), although there was a small increase between 2002 (55%) and 2003 (60%). The proportion of cases that were smear-positive fell between 1995 and 2003. While this could be due in part to increases in TB among HIV-infected people, the reasons for the observed trend need to be investigated further. Although the DOTS case detection rate has increased, the estimate for 2003 remains low at 18%. The treatment success rate was 79% in the 2002 DOTS cohort, with a high default rate (11%). Treatment success has increased only slightly since 1997. Nigeria has not yet taken steps to evaluate the impact of DOTS in reducing transmission, incidence, prevalence or deaths.

Improving programme performance

A major constraint for PHC and the TB control programme is the failure of the government to release funds that have been budgeted and allocated for health and TB control services at all levels. This reflects a low level of political commitment and results in reliance on external funding for TB control operations, mostly from CIDA, DFB, GLRA, NLR and USAID. CIDA funding from mid-2002 to the end of 2003 has made it possible to expand DOTS to the remaining 16 non-DOTS states and FCT Abuja (thus expanding DOTS to all the 36 states of the Federation, including FCT Abuja), to strengthen the central unit's infrastructure and coordination and to establish three zonal TB coordination and control offices. A TBCTA/USAID grant has provided funds for some TB control activities in 2004, including the expansion of the TB laboratory network, providing supervision and monitoring activities at the central and zonal levels, and training staff and developing human resources for collaborative TB/HIV activities.

Another challenge facing the NTP in Nigeria is the lack of professional health staff in the LGAs. The PHC facilities are staffed mainly by nurses and community health workers, and the physician to population ratio is between 1:160 000 and 1:400 000. Although the TB programme trains supervisors and other senior staff, very few general PHC and hospital staff have been trained in integrated TB control activities. HR needs are being assessed with a view to revising the HRD plan. Currently, states are responsible for training their own staff, while the federal government supports training programmes for TB control in collaboration with research institutions and universities. The National TB and Leprosy Training Centre in Zaria, established in 1991, is responsible for providing the necessary staff training at the LGA and health facility levels. The centre provides a three-month course for LGA TB control supervisors and a two-week course for laboratory technicians.

The supply of anti-TB drugs is adequate, and an application to the GDF for a second year of support has been approved. However, the country's drug policy dates from 1990 and is currently under revision. The federal government is responsible for legislation concerning drugs, while the management and procurement of drugs are decentralized to individual facilities. There is no system of drug control at national or provincial levels once drugs have been approved. There are no drug resistance data for the country.

Diagnostic and laboratory services

The number of TB laboratories is increasing, and smear microscopy is now available in 504 out of 774 LGAs. However, few of these laboratories are covered by a quality assurance system. Nigeria plans to establish a standardized quality assurance system for the whole country in 2005. Stocks of laboratory reagents are low because of the lack of government funding. Most laboratories receive reagents from the NTP (funded by WHO) or from NGOs, and some are charging patients. In 2005, the NTP plans to establish at least one microscopy centre in each of the remaining LGAs and to strengthen collaboration between the microscopy centres and the NRL.

TB/HIV coordination

The National AIDS and STD Control Programme has appointed a staff member to act as the focal point for collaborative TB/HIV activities. An NPO will be recruited to support these activities using funds provided by the Norwegian government. Many DOTS and ART centres are now starting collaborative TB/HIV activities. In 25 sites, TB patients with HIV/AIDS will have access to comprehensive HIV/AIDS care and support, including the provision of ART.

At the central level, a proposal to develop a strategy document for collaborative TB/HIV activities has been finalized and preparations for a high-level mission are being made in relation to the "3 by 5" initiative. Collaborative TB/HIV activities are constrained by the shortage and high cost of HIV test kits and the shortage of antiretrovirals and drugs for opportunistic infections at both HIV and TB treatment centres. Following a recent award from the President's Emergency Plan for AIDS Relief, collaborative TB/HIV activities will be expanded in 2005.

Links with other health-care providers

The NTP has successfully pilot tested the involvement of private clinics in the delivery of DOTS services; this initiative is being expanded to six states with financial support from FIDELIS. Several NGOs are already involved, with efforts being made to strengthen collaboration with general hospitals, specialist TB clinics, medical colleges and prison health services.

Partnerships

Major technical partners include DFB, DFID, GLRA, IUATLD, Netherlands Leprosy Relief and WHO. CIDA and USAID (TBCTA) are the main funding partners. The GDF provides anti-TB drugs and will start to provide laboratory test kits

(a) NTP budget by source of funding

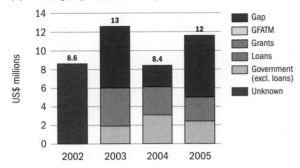

Gap
GFATM
Grants
Loans
Government (excl. loans)
Unknown

(b) NTP budget by line item

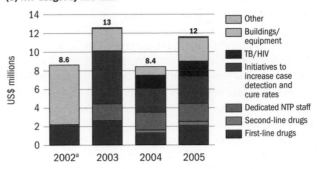

Other
Buildings/ equipment
TB/HIV
Initiatives to increase case detection and cure rates
Dedicated NTP staff
Second-line drugs
First-line drugs

(c) Total TB control costs by line item[b]

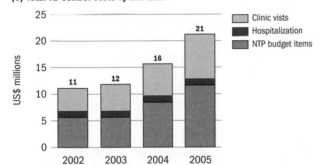

Clinic vists
Hospitalization
NTP budget items

(d) Per patient costs, budgets, available funding and expenditures

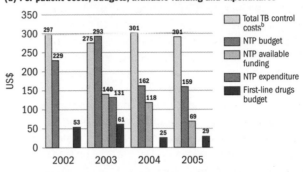

Total TB control costs[b]
NTP budget
NTP available funding
NTP expenditure
First-line drugs budget

[a] In the 2002 budget, the costs of dedicated staff and of building and equipment were not evaluated.
[b] Total TB control costs for 2002 and 2003 are based on expenditures, whereas those for 2004 and 2005 are based on budgets. Estimates of the costs of clinic visits and hospitalization are WHO estimates based on data provided by the NTP and from other sources. See Methods for further details.

in 2005. International leprosy organizations have provided technical assistance for TB control for more than a decade.

Budgets and expenditures

The NTP budget increased from US$ 8.6 million in 2002 to US$ 12 million in 2005. However, funding from both the government and donors has been declining since 2003, and in 2005 the funding gap is expected to be around US$ 7 million, equivalent to 57% of the budget. There are two main reasons for persistent funding gaps. One is that, while a GFATM grant was approved in January 2003, this

was subsequently revoked because of lack of counterpart funds from the government. In 2003, a second reason was that funding from the government was planned at US$ 3.9 million but reached only US$ 1.9 million. The largest budget line item each year between 2003 and 2005 is for expansion of DOTS to new LGAs (included in the line item "initiatives to increase case detection and cure rates"). Dedicated TB staff, first-line drugs and buildings and equipment are also relatively large budget items. The budget per patient treated has ranged from US$ 160 to US$ 300. Actual expenditures in 2003 were US$ 5.6 million

(equivalent to US$ 131 per patient treated), slightly lower than the available funding of US$ 6.0 million.

Total TB control costs, including visits to health clinics and spending on dedicated TB hospital beds as well as items covered by the NTP budget, are estimated at US$ 12 million in 2003 (about US$ 300 per patient treated). If the budget gap for 2005 is filled and the number of patients treated increased to nearly 73 000 as projected, then total TB control costs would reach about US$ 20 million in 2005 (also about US$ 300 per patient treated).

Pakistan

DOTS coverage has increased rapidly in Pakistan since 2000, reaching 63% in 2003. With plans to include the remaining districts, nationwide DOTS coverage should be achieved in 2005. Pakistan has been highly successful in mobilizing financial support for TB control from the international community, and this has given impetus to the programme. The NTP is well structured and has created a strong TB control network during the past five years, with an effective mechanism for coordinating a range of activities and partnerships. Both case detection and treatment outcomes are improving, but remain below the global targets at 17% and 77% respectively. Recent health sector reforms give increased responsibility to the districts for setting priorities for health programmes and to the NTP for ensuring that TB control is a priority at district level. As the programme advances towards nationwide DOTS coverage, the NTP will have to respond to the increasing demand for anti-TB drugs, equipment and reagents, and to ensure that the quality of the services continues to improve.

System of TB control

The NTP is responsible, under the MoH, for the overall coordination of TB control in the country. The specific responsibilities of the NTP include formulation of policy, strategic planning, technical support and supervision, monitoring and evaluation, coordination and communication with partners and research. The provincial and regional TB control managers are responsible for planning, implementing, monitoring and evaluating TB control activities in each province and region. However, districts serve as the main administrative units for the programme; the district authorities are primarily responsible for activities at that level. District hospitals and rural health centres provide diagnostic and treatment services; the basic health units and dispensaries provide treatment. In rural areas, "lady health workers" play an important role in referring TB suspects from communities and in providing DOT. In some big cities, treatment is not yet provided in all health centres.

Pakistan has one national, four provincial and two regional reference laboratories. The national laboratory and three of the provincial laboratories have facilities for culture and drug susceptibility testing. In the districts, 619 diagnostic centres do microscopy.

Surveillance and monitoring

No national survey of TB infection or disease has been carried out in Pakistan, and case notifications were erratic until the introduction of DOTS in the early 1990s. The incidence of TB and its trend are uncertain. DOTS coverage increased rapidly from 9% in 2000 to 63% by 2003. During the same period, the smear-positive case detection rate increased from 3% to 17%. While these two indicators have increased, their ratio has not changed, suggesting that the case detection rate within DOTS areas has stayed in the range 20–30% since 2000. A possible reason for the low rate of case detection is that only 30% of all notified TB cases were diagnosed as smear-positive in 2003. Since it is expected that about 45% of incident cases would be smear-positive, the low proportion of reported smear-positives suggests that some smear-positive cases may have been notified as smear-negative.

The treatment success rate in the 2002 cohort was 77%, similar to that in 2001; the default rate remained high at 14%. Furthermore, 13% of treated patients, who were counted as successfully treated, completed treatment without evidence of smear conversion. Information on treatment success outside the DOTS programme is not available. Among relapse cases treated under DOTS, the treatment success was high (81%), but the proportion of patients whose cure was not laboratory confirmed was even higher than among new patients (53%). Among patients who had defaulted on previous treatment, treatment success was only 58%, mostly as a result of patients defaulting again (22% of the cohort).

PROGRESS IN TB CONTROL IN PAKISTAN

Indicators

DOTS treatment success, 2002 cohort	77%
DOTS detection rate, 2003	17%
NTP budget available, 2004	27%
Government contribution to NTP budget, including loans, 2004	7%
Government contribution to total TB control costs, including loans, 2004	26%
Government health spending used for TB control, 2004	5%

Major achievements

— Rapid DOTS expansion to cover a total of 94 out of 121 districts
— Provincial and district capacity-building to improve monitoring and supervision
— Establishment of the National Pakistan Stop TB Partnership to increase TB awareness and political commitment of local authorities

Major planned activities

— Expand DOTS to cover all districts by 2005
— Develop an EQA system for smear microscopy
— Implement PPM-DOTS through FIDELIS and GFATM funding
— Launch communication strategies to improve TB awareness among health-care providers and the public

LATEST ESTIMATES[a]		TRENDS	2000	2001	2002	2003
Population	**153 577 848**	DOTS coverage (%)	9.0	24	45	63
Global rank (by est. number of cases)	6	Notification rate (all cases/100 000 pop)	7.7	23	35	48
Incidence (all cases/100 000 pop/year)	181	Notification rate (new ss+/100 000 pop)	2.3	7.5	11	14
Incidence (new ss+/100 000 pop/year)	82	Detection of all cases (%)	4.3	13	19	26
Prevalence (all cases/100 000 pop)	359	Case detection rate (new ss+, %)	2.8	9.2	13	17
TB mortality (all cases/100 000 pop/year)	43	DOTS case detection rate (new ss+, %)	2.8	5.2	13	17
TB cases HIV+ (adults aged 15–49, %)	0.6	DOTS case detection rate (new ss+)/coverage (%)	31	22	28	27
New cases multidrug resistant (%)	9.6	DOTS treatment success (new ss+, %)	74	77	77	–

Notification rate (per 100 000 pop)

— = ss+ cases　━ = all cases (73 100 in 2003)

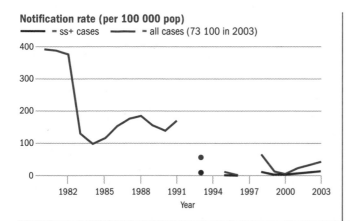

Notification rate by age and sex (new ss+)[b]

— = female　━ = male

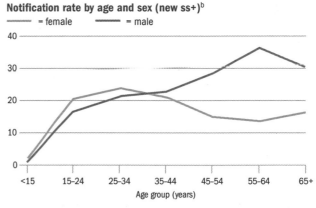

Case types notified

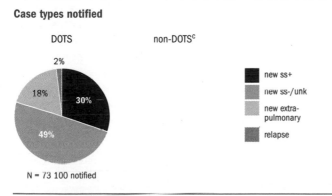

DOTS　　　non-DOTS[c]

- new ss+
- new ss-/unk
- new extra-pulmonary
- relapse

N = 73 100 notified

DOTS progress towards targets[d]

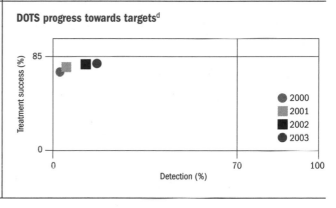

- 2000
- 2001
- 2002
- 2003

DOTS treatment outcomes (new ss+)

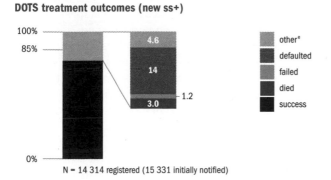

- other[e]
- defaulted
- failed
- died
- success

N = 14 314 registered (15 331 initially notified)

Non-DOTS treatment outcomes (new ss+)

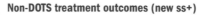

Notes

ss+ indicates smear-positive; ss-, smear-negative; pop, population; unk, unknown.

Absence of a graph indicates that the data were not available or applicable.

[a] See Methods for data sources. Prevalence and mortality estimates include patients with HIV.

[b] The sum of cases notified by age and sex is less than the number of new smear-positive cases notified for some countries.

[c] Non-DOTS is blank for countries which are 100% DOTS, or where no non-DOTS data were reported.

[d] DOTS case detection rate for given year, DOTS treatment success rate for cohort registered in previous year.

[e] "Other" includes transfer out and not evaluated, still on treatment, and other unknown.

Improving programme performance

Under the recent health reforms, district governments were authorized to prioritize their district health needs. The NTP needs to ensure that districts take ownership of their local TB control effort and make it a priority. The new National TB Control Programme Plan for 2006–2010 and Provincial TB Control Programme Strategic Plans for each of the four provinces for the same period have been drafted. These will be used to advocate for TB control at the national, provincial and district levels. The induction of national programme officers through USAID funding has helped to develop provincial and district capacity for monitoring and supervision.

The Government of Pakistan is committed to TB control under the DOTS strategy, and the programme is receiving adequate attention from policy-makers, as evidenced by the rapid expansion of DOTS since 2000. DOTS coverage will be expanded to the remaining 20 districts in 2005. With the rapid expansion of DOTS, the NTP faces constraints including inadequate public sector resources. As coverage is increased, the new national plan will progressively focus on the quality of care, enhanced case detection, monitoring and supervision and activities to de-stigmatize the disease. The Pakistan Stop TB Partnership is being launched and has appointed a Stop TB Ambassador. This is the first initiative in Pakistan to include non-traditional partners in TB control activities.

In 2002, the NTP received a two-year grant from the GDF, and this was extended to cover 2005. However, the current level of drug procurement will not be sufficient to meet the increasing needs arising from rapid DOTS expansion. As the use of FDCs is being advocated in the four provinces, the NTP has revised the treatment guidelines and has drafted training materials on their use. There are no drug resistance data available for Pakistan, although WHO estimates a prevalence of MDR in new TB patients of 10%. Patients in whom MDR-TB is diagnosed are not treated under the NTP.

The NTP has recognized the importance of behaviour change, communication and community mobilization in achieving countrywide implementation of DOTS, and support from various donors has been sought to develop effective strategies. Television spots, posters, leaflets, videos and other materials have been developed to raise public awareness. These strategies will be launched in 2005, with the aim of spreading public awareness among both health-care providers and the general public. Innovative approaches, coupled with operational research, are being explored to involve non-traditional partners such as politicians, industrialists, local district governments and religious leaders in TB control activities.

Three areas in which programme performance needs to be improved are diagnostic and laboratory services, TB/HIV coordination and links with other health-care providers.

Diagnostic and laboratory services

The NTP plans to establish an intermediate level laboratory network consisting of one reference laboratory in each district in 2004–2005 and to expand the number of hospitals and rural health centres that serve as diagnostic centres. The national and provincial reference laboratories have been strengthened with the procurement of laboratory equipment, materials and vehicles. Supervision and overall support for the provincial laboratories need further strengthening; guidelines need to be developed as well as tools for supervision, appropriate for the country setting. There are currently no systems in place for quality assurance of microscopy services at the district level, and this is a priority in the 2006–2010 national TB control plan. Other needs include training of laboratory staff and improvement in laboratory operating procedures.

TB/HIV coordination

The prevalence of HIV in the general population appears to be low, but the lack of adequate epidemiological data precludes an accurate assessment of the HIV situation in Pakistan. A TB/HIV plan and a national TB/HIV coordinating body are both being developed. TB/HIV awareness activities have been undertaken in conjunction with the South Asian Association for Regional Cooperation (SAARC) TB/HIV Awareness Year (2004).

Links with other health-care providers

Pakistan has developed a national strategy for PPM DOTS. Few initiatives have been launched so far, but there is a strong commitment to encourage the active involvement of more health-care providers, including governmental, semigovernmental and the private sector, in DOTS expansion. Funds from the GFATM are being used to expand PPM and BCC (behaviour change and communication) activities. Several FIDELIS projects linking the NTP to other health-care providers are planned, including improving TB case detection by encouraging intersectoral collaboration in three urban areas and strengthening DOTS implementation in four districts of Punjab. NGOs are involved in some districts of each province and territory of the country; these include the Abasseen Foundation, Aga Khan Foundation, Asia Foundation, Association for Social Development, Marie Adelaide Leprosy Center, Mercy Corps International, Pakistan Anti-TB Association and many other local NGOs.

Partnerships

Partnerships for TB control in Pakistan have been strengthened, and technical and financial support has increased significantly. The NTP has launched the National Pakistan Stop TB Partnership to increase TB awareness and the political commitment of local authorities. Major technical partners include GLRA, GTZ, IUATLD, JICA and WHO. DFID has offered assistance to develop PPM partnerships; USAID has provided support to strengthen the capacity for DOTS implementation in the districts. The governments of Canada, Germany and Japan are the main financial partners for TB control activities. Pakistan will receive ISAC initiative funding (through CIDA) for DOTS expansion and sustainability through the involvement of district governments.

(a) NTP budget by source of funding

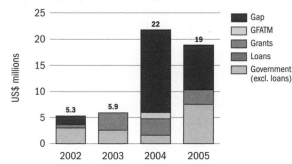

Legend:
- Gap
- GFATM
- Grants
- Loans
- Government (excl. loans)

(b) NTP budget by line item

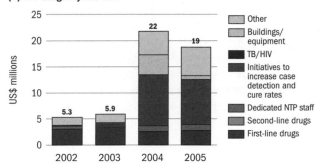

Legend:
- Other
- Buildings/ equipment
- TB/HIV
- Initiatives to increase case detection and cure rates
- Dedicated NTP staff
- Second-line drugs
- First-line drugs

(c) Total TB control costs by line item[a]

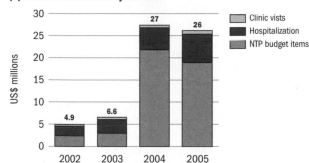

Legend:
- Clinic vists
- Hospitalization
- NTP budget items

(d) Per patient costs, budgets, available funding and expenditures

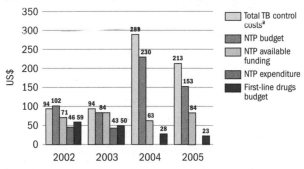

Legend:
- Total TB control costs[a]
- NTP budget
- NTP available funding
- NTP expenditure
- First-line drugs budget

[a] Total TB control costs for 2002 and 2003 are based on expenditures, whereas those for 2004 and 2005 are based on budgets. Estimates of the costs of clinic visits and hospitalization are WHO estimates based on data provided by the NTP and from other sources. See Methods for further details.

Budgets and expenditures

The budgets for both 2004 and 2005 are substantially higher than in previous years, at about US$ 20 million compared with US$ 5–6 million in 2002 and 2003 (US$ 153 per patient in 2005 compared with around US$ 100 in both 2002 and 2003). These budgetary increases reflect the development of more ambitious plans to accelerate DOTS expansion (to achieve 100% coverage by 2005) and to increase case detection and cure rates throughout the country, and the associated revision of existing national and provincial strategic plans and budgets in 2004 (most of the budgetary increase between 2003 and 2004 is in the category "initiatives to increase case detection and cure rates"). The revised plans include PPM-DOTS strategies and community mobilization activities.

While the funding available for 2004 and 2005 is similar to that in 2002 and 2003, the considerably increased budgets for 2004 and 2005 mean that large funding gaps currently exist: US$ 16 million in the fiscal year 2004 and US$ 8.6 million in 2005 (the fiscal year starts in July). The NTP is already engaged in efforts to mobilize funds to fill these gaps. For example, it is expected that PPM-DOTS strategies will be funded through the national health and population facility (this is supported by the Pakistani government and DFID), and a further application to the GFATM is planned. In addition, provinces are revising their budgetary allocations in the context of the revised strategic plans. Some positive results are already apparent: in December 2004, the Punjab government approved a revised three-year budget allocation of US$ 8.6 million

for TB control activities in the province, including US$ 2.4 million for the first year (of which US$ 1.3 million is for drugs).

If the revised NTP budget is fully funded, the total cost of TB control (including health clinic visits for observation of treatment and monitoring and limited hospitalization as well as NTP budget items) will increase from around US$ 5 million in 2002 to US$ 26 million in 2005 (and from around US$ 100 to US$ 213 per patient treated). It remains to be seen whether increased funding can be absorbed effectively and whether increased expenditures result in improved case detection and cure rates.

Philippines

The Philippines achieved full DOTS coverage in 2003, has met the global target for treatment success in each of the past four years and is coming close to the target for case detection. TB control has progressed thanks to strong government commitment and a relatively well-staffed programme, while innovative partnership arrangements are making important contributions to TB control activities and resource mobilization. The financial position is favourable, with the budget for TB control activities fully funded for 2004 and 2005. The use of barangay (small local district) health workers to treat and follow patients has been a very beneficial national policy that has helped to achieve high treatment success rates. Involving medical schools and private physicians in DOTS services is now a government priority because this will increase case detection and ensure that standard methods for diagnosis and treatment are used in the private sector. Surveillance for TB drug resistance is in progress. The Philippines is one of the few high-burden countries that has started to implement DOTS-Plus treatment for MDR-TB

cases. Providing TB control and other health services to population groups in remote mountainous areas and small islands, and accessing insecure areas, present continuing challenges.

System of TB control
The NTP has recently been reorganized as part of the national health sector reform process. Following restructuring and considerable decentralization of the Department of Health, the number of staff at central level was substantially reduced. Although additional staff have subsequently been employed at central level, there are still too few to carry out regular monitoring of programme activities in the regions. This means that regional coordinators are now responsible for most coordination and technical assistance, even though they may be responsible for more than one health programme and thus have limited time for TB control activities. Fortunately, the number of staff in the provinces and in rural health units is sufficient, and most staff have adequate training in all aspects of TB control. Each of the country's 16 regions has a centre for health devel-

opment that provides technical support to the provincial health offices. Provincial TB coordinators supervise staff in the rural health units, which are the main focus of TB control in the Philippines.

The TB laboratory network is structured as follows: the NRL is responsible for developing policy, management, training of microscopists, supervision of intermediate laboratories and DRS. Regional and provincial laboratories implement the policies developed by the NRL and provide EQA to the peripheral laboratories. The primary role of the peripheral laboratories at the rural and city health units is sputum smear microscopy. Culture and drug susceptibility testing are carried out by the NRL, one private laboratory and one NGO-affiliated laboratory. Seven regional laboratories have the capacity to perform culture.

Surveillance and monitoring
The TB case notification rate was decreasing before 2001 but has increased slightly since then. In 2003, as in previous years, the highest notification rates were among adults aged 45 years and older. These observations suggest that the TB incidence rate is probably in decline in the Philippines, with this reduction obscured since 2000 by DOTS expansion and the greater effort given to case-finding. The DOTS case detection rate increased rapidly to 48% in 2000 and then more slowly to 68% in 2003. Treatment success was reported as 88% in the 2000, 2001 and 2002 DOTS cohorts, and 91% of new smear-positive cases notified in 2002 were registered for treatment in that year.

With the public sector DOTS programme nearing full implementation, greater efforts are being made to diagnose and treat patients in collaboration with the private sector. The NTP must now also consider how to evaluate the epidemiological impact of the DOTS programme. Two prevalence surveys were done in the Philippines before the implementation of DOTS

PROGRESS IN TB CONTROL IN THE PHILIPPINES

Indicators

DOTS treatment success, 2002 cohort	88%
DOTS case detection rate, 2003	68%
NTP budget available, 2004	100%
Government contribution to NTP budget, including loans, 2004	36%
Government contribution to total TB control costs, including loans, 2004	82%
Government health spending used for TB control, 2004	3%

Major achievements
— Scaling up of PPM DOTS in two thirds of medical schools and more than 2000 private providers to increase the case detection rate
— Nationwide implementation of FDC anti-TB drugs, with increased health-worker capacity
— TB control in children was piloted in urban and rural areas, and TB control in high-risk populations started

Major planned activities
— Establish additional PPM-DOTS sites to cover the entire country
— Implement EQA for smear microscopy nationwide, including hospitals and private laboratories
— Strengthen the national reference laboratory function in laboratory networking

LATEST ESTIMATES[a]		TRENDS	2000	2001	2002	2003
Population	**79 999 016**	DOTS coverage (%)	90	95	98	100
Global rank (by est. number of cases)	9	Notification rate (all cases/100 000 pop)	158	139	151	168
Incidence (all cases/100 000 pop/year)	296	Notification rate (new ss+/100 000 pop)	89	77	83	91
Incidence (new ss+/100 000 pop/year)	133	Detection of all cases (%)	52	46	50	57
Prevalence (all cases/100 000 pop)	458	Case detection rate (new ss+, %)	65	57	62	68
TB mortality (all cases/100 000 pop/year)	49	DOTS case detection rate (new ss+, %)	48	57	62	68
TB cases HIV+ (adults aged 15–49, %)	0.1	DOTS case detection rate (new ss+)/coverage (%)	54	60	63	68
New cases multidrug resistant (%)	3.2	DOTS treatment success (new ss+, %)	88	88	88	–

Notification rate (per 100 000 pop)

— = ss+ cases   ▬ = all cases (134 375 in 2003)

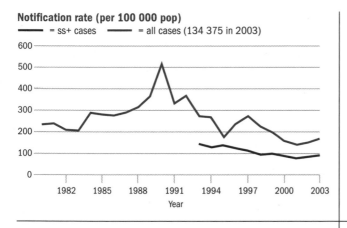

Notification rate by age and sex (new ss+)[b]

— = female   ▬ = male

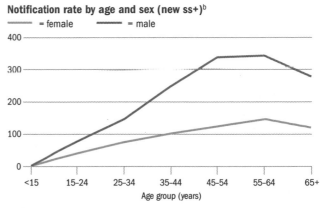

Case types notified

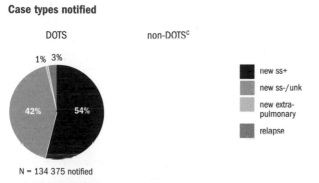

DOTS   non-DOTS[c]

- new ss+
- new ss-/unk
- new extra-pulmonary
- relapse

N = 134 375 notified

DOTS progress towards targets[d]

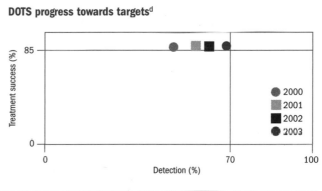

- 2000
- 2001
- 2002
- 2003

DOTS treatment outcomes (new ss+)

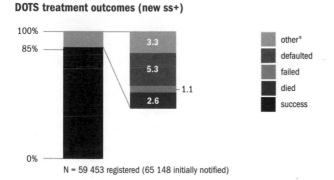

- other[e]
- defaulted
- failed
- died
- success

N = 59 453 registered (65 148 initially notified)

Non-DOTS treatment outcomes (new ss+)

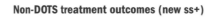

Notes

ss+ indicates smear-positive; ss-, smear-negative; pop, population; unk, unknown.

Absence of a graph indicates that the data were not available or applicable.

[a] See Methods for data sources. Prevalence and mortality estimates include patients with HIV.

[b] The sum of cases notified by age and sex is less than the number of new smear-positive cases notified for some countries.

[c] Non-DOTS is blank for countries which are 100% DOTS, or where no non-DOTS data were reported.

[d] DOTS case detection rate for given year, DOTS treatment success rate for cohort registered in previous year.

[e] "Other" includes transfer out and not evaluated, still on treatment, and other unknown.

that showed little reduction in culture-positive or smear-positive disease between 1981–1983 and 1997. A new national TB prevalence survey is scheduled for 2007. This will show whether or not the Philippines can meet, or has already met, the Millennium Development Goal of halving prevalence between 1990 and 2015.

Improving programme performance

The Philippines reached 100% DOTS coverage in 2003 as a result of strengthened DOTS expansion efforts, backed by government commitment and funding for TB control as a priority public health programme. As part of the health sector reform process, management capacity and programme infrastructure were upgraded, and TB control activities became the responsibility of the Infectious Diseases Office under the National Centre for Disease Control and Prevention. Following the reorganization of the Department of Health, the procedural manual for the NTP and the Comprehensive and Unified Policy for TB Control in the Philippines will be revised. This policy provides a framework for collaboration with other government agencies and with the private sector, which in turn will help to harmonize and unify TB control efforts in the Philippines.

Nationwide implementation of FDC anti-TB drugs started after successful training for health-care workers. To improve case detection, TB control initiatives focused on children were pilot tested in urban and rural areas, and TB control activities in high-risk populations begun. A TB outpatient benefit package, PhilHealth, was introduced to improve treatment success rates.

The first nationwide DRS survey started in June 2003. This will provide the first reliable estimate of the magnitude of MDR-TB in the country. In 2000, the GLC approved a DOTS-Plus project at Makati Medical Center in Manila (a private medical centre collaborating with the NTP), with an initial cohort of 200 patients. With support from the GFATM, this cohort has been expanded to 750 MDR-TB patients in 2004. As yet, no MDR-TB patients are treated in the public sector.

In addition to management of MDR-TB, diagnostic and laboratory services, TB/HIV coordination and links with other health-care providers could also be improved.

Diagnostic and laboratory services

The laboratory service at intermediate and peripheral levels is good and staff are well-trained; however, EQA for sputum smear microscopy is not in place in every laboratory and needs to be strengthened where it already exists. An updated national manual for EQA for direct sputum smear microscopy was developed and distributed in late 2004. A priority for 2005 is to establish models for EQA, to monitor and evaluate the model EQA implementation and to expand to other laboratories. Eventually, hospitals and private laboratory facilities will be included in EQA activities. Laboratory networking is to be developed at all levels of the health service; successful networking will require reinforcement of the NRL.

TB/HIV coordination

There are no existing data on TB/HIV coinfection in the Philippines. However, HIV prevalence in the general population, and among TB patients, remains low (<1%). Given the worsening HIV/AIDS epidemics in neighbouring countries, it is important to monitor HIV prevalence in the general population as well as among high-risk groups including TB patients.

Links with other health-care providers

With the aim of consolidating and scaling up initiatives to involve private health-care providers in DOTS, the Philippines issued guidelines on PPM DOTS in 2004, and a national committee for PPM DOTS has been established. Operational guidelines for PPM DOTS in the Philippines were published, endorsed by the Secretary of Health and distributed. PPM-DOTS units, whose role is to coordinate private sector involvement in provision of DOTS services, have been set up in over 50 sites nationwide. More than 2000 private providers have been trained, and six professional societies have introduced the DOTS strategy in

their training curricula. Two thirds of medical schools have become or are in the process of becoming involved in DOTS activities. The positive impact of these initiatives on case detection has been demonstrated in a few sites, but there is a need to incorporate a careful and more comprehensive strategy for monitoring and evaluation of the current scale-up of PPM DOTS in the Philippines.

Partnerships

The Philippines benefits from several partnerships that strengthen the programme and support DOTS expansion. Overall external technical collaboration is coordinated by WHO. Other external technical support is provided by CDC, JICA, KNCV, Medicos del Mundo (Spain), USAID and World Vision, which has helped to maintain technical quality during the expansion phase. An important innovation led by the Department of Health is the organization of the Philippines Coalition Against TB (PhilCAT). This includes a substantial group of NGO and private sector entities that collaborate to help private sector TB control activities and to mobilize local resources. The major funding partners are CIDA, GFATM, JICA and USAID.

Budgets and expenditures

The budget specifically for TB control activities has been similar in the four years 2002–2005, at about US$ 7–8 million. However, funding gaps existed in 2002 and 2003, whereas no funding gap has been reported for 2004 or 2005. This improved funding situation is linked to an increasing level of grant funding, much of which is related to initiatives to increase case detection – in particular, USAID funds for PPM DOTS. Funding from the government has fallen, related to austerity measures that affect public spending as a whole. In contrast to most other HBCs, there is also a budget for second-line drugs in 2004 and 2005, linked to implementation of DOTS-Plus in Manila. On a per patient basis, the overall NTP budget has fallen from US$ 66 in 2002 to US$ 48 in 2005. This is mainly explained by a reduction in the cost of first-line drugs, which has fallen from US$ 26 per pa-

(a) NTP budget by source of funding

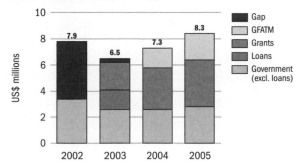

Legend: Gap, GFATM, Grants, Loans, Government (excl. loans)

(b) NTP budget by line item

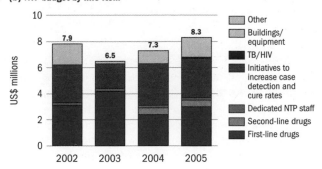

Legend: Other, Buildings/equipment, TB/HIV, Initiatives to increase case detection and cure rates, Dedicated NTP staff, Second-line drugs, First-line drugs

(c) Total TB control costs by line item[a]

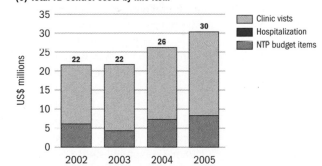

Legend: Clinic vists, Hospitalization, NTP budget items

(d) Per patient costs, budgets, available funding and expenditures

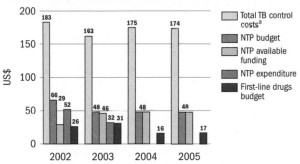

Legend: Total TB control costs[a], NTP budget, NTP available funding, NTP expenditure, First-line drugs budget

[a] Total TB control costs for 2002 and 2003 are based on expenditures, whereas those for 2004 and 2005 are based on budgets. Estimates of the costs of clinic visits and hospitalization are WHO estimates based on data provided by the NTP and from other sources. See Methods for further details.

tient treated in 2002 to US$ 17 per patient treated in 2005. When costs beyond those reflected in the budget specifically for TB control are also included, i.e. health clinic visits for DOT and monitoring during treatment, the cost per patient has been about US$ 160–180 for the past four years, and total TB control costs have been around US$ 22–30 million per year.

Russian Federation

Following a considerable rise in the TB burden in the Russian Federation during the 1990s, a peak was reached in 2000 when some 132 000 cases of TB were notified. Since then, a progressive reduction in the number of reported cases has occurred, mainly because of a decline in the number of cases registered in the prison sector. However, the number of cases in the general population has increased, particularly among children. The DOTS strategy is not widely used in the Russian Federation. In oblasts where it is being applied, both case detection and treatment outcomes are still low. However, government commitment to TB control is strong, and a recent World Bank loan will allow accelerated expansion of both TB and HIV/AIDS programmes. In addition, the Russian Federation made a successful application to the GFATM in 2004, opening up additional opportunities to extend and improve these programmes. The increasing public health importance of TB/HIV coinfection is being addressed through a national TB/HIV coordinating body, which has developed a national strategy for TB/HIV control. Also receiving special attention is the growing MDR-TB epidemic in the Russian Federation; links between the MDR-TB and TB/HIV epidemics are being investigated. A major challenge is to improve the laboratory network to meet international standards and provide reliable diagnostic services for the TB control programme.

System of TB control

The Russian Federal Target Programme "Prevention and Control of Social Diseases (2002–2006)", with the subprogramme "Urgent Measures of TB Control in Russia" was approved in 2001. The Programme aims to stabilize the epidemiological situation of social diseases through improvement of current organizations and newly established services. The plan covers strengthening the capacities of health facilities, research institutes and centres that carry out prevention, timely detection, diagnosis and treatment.

Several federal laws and regulations were developed to strengthen the foundation of the TB control programme. The national five-year plan, "Provision of guaranteed diagnostic and treatment procedures for TB patients and the development of TB services in Russia (2003–2006)", was developed as the main framework for activities and cooperation with international partners. Reduction of TB incidence, disability and mortality is currently one of the priorities of state policy in the Russian Federation.

Within the federal TB control programme, five research institutes are responsible for organizing and supervising research, training and implementation of TB control in a wide network of more than 500 TB control facilities in 88 regions of the Russian Federation. These are the Research Institute of Phthisiopulmonology of Sechenov Moscow Medical Academy (RIPP MMA), the Central TB Research Institute of the Russian Academy of Medical Sciences (CTRI RAMS), St Petersburg Institute of Phthisiopulmonology, Ural Research Institute of Phthisiopulmonology and the Novosibirsk TB Research Institute. The TB dispensaries in turn supervise and monitor regional TB hospitals, sanatoria and TB units at district polyclinics. Under the Ministry of Justice, 37 hospitals and 57 treatment facilities provide treatment for TB patients within the penitentiary system.

The five federal TB research institute laboratories and 377 TB dispensary laboratories perform culture and drug susceptibility testing. In the territories, 348 centres with hospitals and sanatoria perform culture, and more than 11 000 centres perform smear microscopy.

PROGRESS IN TB CONTROL IN THE RUSSIAN FEDERATION

Indicators

DOTS treatment success, 2002 cohort	67%
DOTS case detection rate, 2003	8.8%
NTP budget available, 2004	84%
Government contribution to NTP budget, including loans, 2004	83%
Government contribution to total TB control costs, including loans, 2004	87%
Government health spending used for TB control, 2004	4%

Major achievements

— Beginning of implementation of the AIDS and TB control project funded by a World Bank loan
— Approval by the MoH of the new recording and reporting system, including cohort analysis, introduced in 37 regions in 2004 and countrywide in 2005
— Successful application to the GFATM round 4 for TB control
— Development of a strategy on TB/HIV control and countrywide training of regional TB/HIV coordinators
— Training of trainers in the revised TB control strategy
— Substantial progress in the Thematic Working Group on MDR-TB control

Major planned activities

— Expand the revised TB control strategy through the World Bank loan project and prepare for GFATM project implementation
— Develop national guidelines and a framework for the management of MDR-TB
— Implement TB/HIV control strategy
— Strengthen laboratory system: capacity development for smear, culture and drug susceptibility testing; establish the national reference laboratories network and quality assurance system; implement drug resistance surveillance in 10 oblasts
— Improve anti-TB drug supply system

RUSSIAN FEDERATION

LATEST ESTIMATES[a]		TRENDS	2000	2001	2002	2003
Population	**143 246 223**	DOTS coverage (%)	12	16	25	25
Global rank (by est. number of cases)	12	Notification rate (all cases/100 000 pop)	97	91	89	87
Incidence (all cases/100 000 pop/year)	112	Notification rate (new ss+/100 000 pop)	19	18	19	20
Incidence (new ss+/100 000 pop/year)	50	Detection of all cases (%)	79	76	77	77
Prevalence (all cases/100 000 pop)	160	Case detection rate (new ss+, %)	35	34	37	40
TB mortality (all cases/100 000 pop/year)	20	DOTS case detection rate (new ss+, %)	4.6	5.2	6.9	8.8
TB cases HIV+ (adults aged 15–49, %)	6.2	DOTS case detection rate (new ss+)/coverage (%)	39	33	28	35
New cases multidrug resistant (%)	6.0	DOTS treatment success (new ss+, %)	68	67	67	–

Notification rate (per 100 000 pop)

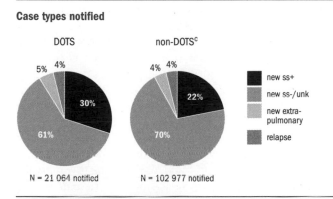

Notification rate by age and sex (new ss+)[b]

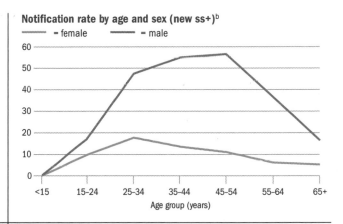

Case types notified

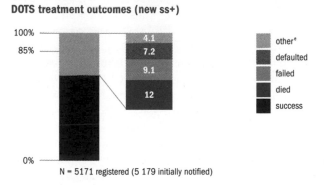

DOTS progress towards targets[d]

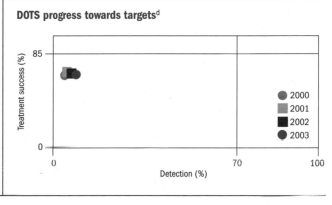

DOTS treatment outcomes (new ss+)

Non-DOTS treatment outcomes (new ss+)

Notes

ss+ indicates smear-positive; ss-, smear-negative; pop, population; unk, unknown.

Absence of a graph indicates that the data were not available or applicable.

[a] See Methods for data sources. Prevalence and mortality estimates include patients with HIV.

[b] The sum of cases notified by age and sex is less than the number of new smear-positive cases notified for some countries.

[c] Non-DOTS is blank for countries which are 100% DOTS, or where no non-DOTS data were reported.

[d] DOTS case detection rate for given year, DOTS treatment success rate for cohort registered in previous year.

[e] "Other" includes transfer out and not evaluated, still on treatment, and other unknown.

Surveillance and monitoring

The increase in the number of annual TB case notifications after 1990 reached a peak of around 141 000 cases in 2000, and the number of reported cases has fallen each successive year since then. Similar trends have also been observed in other countries of the former Soviet Union that have also reported fewer cases, or at least a slowing in the rate of increase in the number of patients. This stabilization in notification rates in the Russian Federation could be the result of improved TB control or of general improvements in peoples' health, but is most likely because of the decline in notified cases over the past few years observed in the prison sector. Since 2001, a decline of notified cases in the prison sector has occurred from more than 24 000 cases to around 16 000 in 2003. TB mortality rates remain increasingly high at around 20 per 100 000 population.

In 2003, DOTS coverage was low, with only 8.8% of cases detected under DOTS. It is therefore unlikely that the DOTS strategy had a major impact on incidence. In 2004, DOTS was implemented in 37 regions of the Russian Federation, with increased coverage to around 45% of the population; however, detection and treatment outcomes remain suboptimal. Moreover, treatment success in the 2002 cohort was low even in DOTS areas (67%) because many patients died (13%), failed treatment (9%) or were lost to follow-up (11%). The treatment outcomes for new smear-positive patients under DOTS have not improved in eight successive cohorts (1995–2002). Among the 962 DOTS relapse cases in 2002, fewer than half were successfully treated (46%), mainly because 26% failed re-treatment.

Treatment outcomes are not available for re-treatment after default or failure. Given the high prevalence of MDR-TB in the Russian Federation, it is important that these data be collated and analysed in future. Although sputum smear microscopy is increasingly used for diagnosis, the proportion of new pulmonary TB patients with a positive sputum smear was still only 33% in 2003 in DOTS regions and did not exceed 24% in non-DOTS regions,

with an overall average for the Russian Federation of 25.3%. Nevertheless, the Russian Federation is different from many other HBCs in having a fairly comprehensive system for recording and reporting the total numbers of TB cases and deaths. This system of routine surveillance (rather than population-based surveys) should, with some refinements, be adequate for monitoring epidemiological trends and the future impact of TB control.

Improving programme performance

The current state policy aims to stabilize and improve the epidemiological situation, which is evidenced by an increase in federal budget allocations for TB control. The commitment of the federal government to TB control continues to grow, with sustained activities of the high-level working group (HLWG), one of the mechanisms of international cooperation in the field of medicine. The HLWG comprises representatives of the Ministry of Health and Social Development of the Russian Federation, the Ministry of Justice, RIPP MMA, CTRI RAMS, WHO and the Council of Europe. The federal government has adopted a number of regulations for TB control including: the Executive Order No. 109 of 21 March 2003 "On Improvement of TB Control in the Russian Federation" that focuses on laboratory diagnosis, chemotherapy standards, organization of treatment, prevention of TB transmission, system of centralized control and management of main TB interventions at the level of TB facilities in regions of the Russian Federation, and the introduction of the new reporting and dispensary follow-up system; the Executive Order No. 50 of 13 February 2004 "On Implementation of Registration and Reporting Documentation for Tuberculosis Monitoring" that includes cohort analysis and assessment of detection and treatment effectiveness in line with international standards; a recording form "Individual Card of TB/HIV Patient"; and recommendations on decreasing TB burden among high HIV prevalence populations.

Registers for recording and report-

ing TB based on cohort analysis were introduced by the Russian MoH in February 2004. From April 2004, new reporting forms were being introduced in 37 territories in both the civil and penitentiary sectors, and will be used country-wide from January 2005.

The activities of the federal TB control programme and expansion of the revised strategy are constrained by the shortage of staff and age of the existing medical staff working in TB services, many of whom are retiring. A detailed assessment of HR needs is under way and several activities are in progress to address HR capacity, including a staff development plan, as part of the overall TB plan for 2003–2007, and further training of TB service personnel supported by the World Bank-funded TB/AIDS project. New national guidelines and recommendations have been developed, published and distributed on case detection, TB treatment, laboratory services and TB/HIV control.

MDR-TB is a major challenge for TB control in the Russian Federation. MDR-TB patients outside the DOTS-Plus projects are treated on an individual basis and according to the availability of second-line drugs. Data on the prevalence of drug resistance are reported routinely from Ivanovo, Orel and Tomsk oblasts where the prevalence of MDR-TB among new cases ranges from 2.6% in Orel to 13.7% in Tomsk. Data from a few additional oblasts will be available shortly, and a plan to survey oblasts systematically is being developed. GLC-approved DOTS-Plus projects are being implemented in Archangelsk, Ivanovo, Orel and Tomsk. The GLC has approved the treatment of 2830 MDR-TB patients. The project in Tomsk, which was the first of these projects to start, has been successful in treating MDR-TB patients and has recently been expanded with financial support from the GFATM.

Diagnostic and laboratory services

The physical infrastructure of many diagnostic facilities in the Russian Federation does not meet Russian and international standards for laboratory design and safety. In addition, in many instances, laboratory equipment is outdated. Updating infrastructure of existing facilities and ensuring availability of quality equipment and supplies is an enormous challenge facing the national TB control programme.

Quality assurance is being addressed by the introduction of a federal system of EQA for smear microscopy approved by the MoH. However, given the financial constraints, the system has not yet been introduced in all diagnostic centres, nor have internal quality control procedures. The TB laboratory network faces a serious shortage of staff; HR capacity building through training and development of a model for effective laboratory services at the central level should lead to improvements in laboratory diagnosis at all levels.

TB/HIV coordination
HIV/AIDS is becoming a significant public health problem in the Russian Federation. A thematic working group, "TB in HIV-infected people", has been established within the HLWG on TB and has developed recommendations on decreasing the TB burden among PLWHA. The group comprises leading national TB and HIV experts from re-

search institutes, health facilities, WHO and international partners. Its basic objective is to develop a framework for establishment of the national system of TB care among HIV-infected people. The first stage resulted in the preparation of the "Recommendations on decreasing TB burden in high HIV prevalence populations" based on national and international practices.

Regional TB/HIV coordinators have been appointed in many regions of the Russian Federation. A number of federal-level seminars were held in 2004 where these coordinators were trained in principles of the newly developed TB/HIV strategy.

Links with other health-care providers
Collaboration between all relevant public sector health-care providers and related institutions is being strengthened, including general hospitals, TB hospitals, medical colleges, prison health services and the health services of the armed forces and of the police. The Ministry of Railway Communication, the Federal Security Service and a number of other ministries and departments have their own TB control services, and links with them

need to be strengthened. The private sector plays a minor role in TB diagnosis and treatment.

Links with the community
Several community groups contribute to the provision of TB control activities in the Russian Federation, including an NGO of TB patients (NABAT), the Russian Red Cross, Russian TB Society and other regional foundations and societies. These groups participate in annual World TB Day campaigns and provide health education and social support for TB patients.

Partnerships
The HLWG, established in 1999, continues to play an important role in the development of TB control. It is responsible for coordinating TB activities between the national and international partners, and it works on recommendations for executive policy documents (prikaz) that regulate implementation of national TB control. Many national and International NGOs and technical agencies are partners in TB control within the 88 territories of the Russian Federation. Major donors include USAID, the Swedish

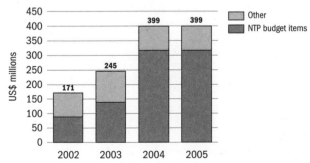

(a) NTP budget by source of funding

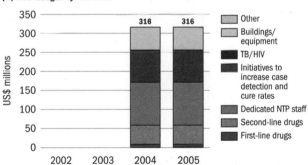

(b) NTP budget by line item

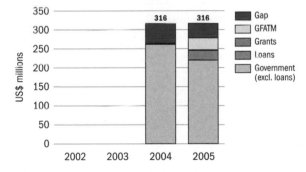

(c) Total TB control costs by line item[a]

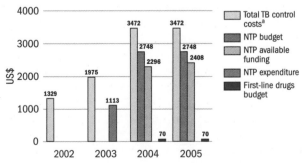

(d) Per patient costs, budgets, available funding and expenditures

[a] Total TB control costs for 2002 and 2003 are based on expenditures, whereas those for 2004 and 2005 are based on budgets. "Other" includes costs for hospitalization and fluorography not reflected in the budget estimates submitted to WHO.

International Development Agency, the EU, the Government of Finland and DFID. The Russian Federation successfully applied to the GFATM in round 4; funds for TB control activities should be available in 2005. A loan agreement between the Russian Federation and the World Bank to fund the project on "AIDS and TB Control" was signed in September 2003 and became effective in December 2003.

Budgets and expenditures

Financial data were prepared by WHO staff (Moscow office) using data available in the public domain, and are therefore estimates rather than official figures. Sources of data included the Ministry of Health and Social Development and the Federal Agency for Health Care and Social Development of the Russian Federation.

The total budget for TB control in both 2004 and 2005 is estimated at US$ 316 million (almost US$ 3000 per new TB patient). About US$ 250–260 million is available from the government in both 2004 and 2005 (including funds from a World Bank loan), a substantial increase compared with 2003. In 2005, the GFATM is expected to provide a further US$ 30 million, but grants from other sources are limited. While the available funding of about US$ 270 million in 2004 and 2005 is substantial by the standards of other HBCs, a funding gap of about US$ 40–50 million has been estimated for both years, primarily for the purchase of second-line drugs (US$ 18 million) and for investment in buildings and equipment (US$ 24 million). The Russian Federation accounts for almost one third of the total funding gap reported by the 22 HBCs.

The largest budget line items are for staff working exclusively on TB control (US$ 113 million in both years), initiatives to increase case detection and cure rates (US$ 84 million in both years), investment in buildings and equipment (US$ 60 million in both years) and second-line drugs (about US$ 45 million in both years). The budgets for staff, investment in buildings and equipment and second-line drugs are relatively large compared with those in other HBCs, and reflect the country's extensive network of dedicated TB control facilities and the large number of patients with MDR-TB. When costs beyond those reflected in the reported budgets are included (i.e. the operating costs of a network of 81 425 dedicated TB beds and the cost of mass screening using fluorography), the total cost of TB control is estimated to be about US$ 400 million in both 2004 and 2005 (about US$ 3500 per patient treated), up from an estimated US$ 245 million in 2003.

South Africa

In 1996, South Africa established an NTP and adopted DOTS as its TB control strategy. Despite government commitment to making TB control a priority, and the implementation of the DOTS strategy in all provinces and almost all districts, it is not known with confidence how much TB there is in the country. Inadequate case reporting systems, a shortage of trained staff at the provincial level and problems associated with the laboratory network hinder effective TB surveillance. Recognizing these shortcomings, the NTP has recently taken a number of steps to remedy the situation, and better data can be expected in the future. However, treatment success rates remain low and many patients are lost to follow-up. A concerted effort will be needed if South Africa is to reach the target cure rates. TB/HIV coinfection is a significant public health problem and is being addressed through a national programme of collaborative TB/HIV activities. MDR-TB prevalence is estimated to be about 2% in new TB patients and 7% in re-treatment cases. Second-line drug treatment is available in provincial MDR-TB units, though at high cost. A number of NGOs are involved in providing TB services and are also mobilizing support in the communities, but more needs to be done to encourage broader private sector participation.

System of TB control

South Africa's health system is decentralized. The National Department of Health provides general guidelines, but the implementation and delivery of services is the responsibility of the provincial authorities. The management structure and the implementation of TB control services vary considerably among provinces. The development of administrative districts, with health management structures in each province, is in progress and not yet complete. The basic unit for TB control and management is the individual primary care institution. Community health workers play an important role in patient care, but their involvement needs to be better organized and recorded.

The National Health Laboratory Service (NHLS) is the main provider of TB laboratory services in eight of the nine provinces in South Africa (all except KwaZulu-Natal) and is divided into central, coastal and northern regions. The laboratories of the NHLS are centralized, work under contract, and include primary health-care, regional, academic and referral laboratories. Communication between them is through a laboratory information system. Smear microscopy is performed in all laboratories; culture, identification and DST are performed in 11 referral laboratories throughout the country. In KwaZulu-Natal, 73 laboratories do smear microscopy, two have culture facilities and one referral laboratory carries out DST.

Surveillance and monitoring

The incidence of TB in South Africa is uncertain because of weaknesses in the reporting system. Furthermore, the rise in TB incidence caused by the spread of HIV cannot easily be distinguished from improvement in case detection. It is likely, however, that the actual incidence of TB is higher than the current WHO estimate because case detection in 2003 was reported to be 118%.[1]

The treatment success rate in the 2002 cohort was 68% and has been consistently low since recording began in 1996. In 2002–2003, 22% of new smear-positive patients were lost to follow-up, either through default or transfer, and 9% died. A further 14% completed treatment but without evidence of smear conversion. The outcome among re-treatment cases was substantially worse, with a treatment success rate of 53% and with 34% lost to follow-up. As noted in the 2004

PROGRESS IN TB CONTROL IN SOUTH AFRICA

Indicators

DOTS treatment success, 2002 cohort	68%
DOTS case detection rate, 2003	118%[1]
NTP budget available, 2004	NA
Government contribution to NTP budget, including loans, 2004	NA
Government contribution to total TB control costs, including loans, 2004	NA
Government health spending used for TB control, 2004	7%

Major achievements

— Implementation of the advocacy and social mobilization plan in five provinces (Eastern Cape, Western Cape, Gauteng, Limpopo and Free State)
— Implementation of a uniform, cohort-based reporting and recording system in all provinces
— Development of guidelines for care of HIV-infected TB patients, including access to ART

Major planned activities

— Strengthen DOT in the provinces and improve quality of data collected
— Implement and strengthen collaborative TB/HIV activities in subdistricts
— Shorten delays in diagnosis by sputum smear microscopy
— Improve laboratory infrastructure and coverage of services in remote areas

NA indicates not available.

---

[1] Note that the "case detection rate" can exceed 100% because this is calculated as the ratio of cases reported in a given year to the estimated incidence in that year. Because the numerator is derived from the pool of prevalent cases, a proportion of which has arisen in previous years, the ratio can exceed 100%.

LATEST ESTIMATES[a]		TRENDS	2000	2001	2002	2003
Population	45 026 470	DOTS coverage (%)	77	77	98	99.5
Global rank (by est. number of cases)	8	Notification rate (all cases/100 000 pop)	344	334	481	505
Incidence (all cases/100 000 pop/year)	536	Notification rate (new ss+/100 000 pop)	173	189	221	258
Incidence (new ss+/100 000 pop/year)	218	Detection of all cases (%)	74	68	94	94
Prevalence (all cases/100 000 pop)	458	Case detection rate (new ss+, %)	91	95	106	118
TB mortality (all cases/100 000 pop/year)	73	DOTS case detection rate (new ss+, %)	75	81	105	118
TB cases HIV+ (adults aged 15–49, %)	61	DOTS case detection rate (new ss+)/coverage (%)	97	105	107	119
New cases multidrug resistant (%)	1.6	DOTS treatment success (new ss+, %)	66	65	68	–

Notification rate (per 100 000 pop)

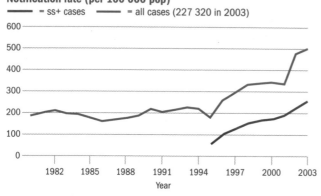

Notification rate by age and sex (new ss+)[b]

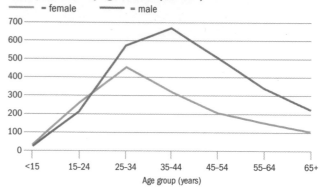

Case types notified

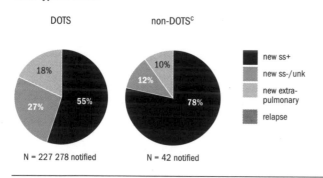

DOTS progress towards targets[d]

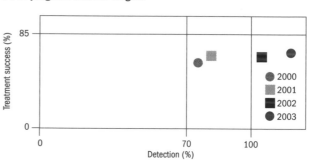

DOTS treatment outcomes (new ss+)

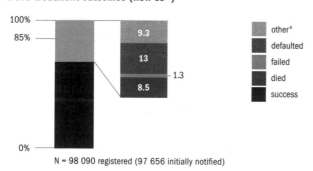

Non-DOTS treatment outcomes (new ss+)

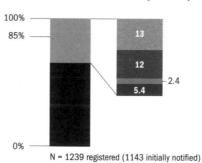

Notes

ss+ indicates smear-positive; ss-, smear-negative; pop, population; unk, unknown.

Absence of a graph indicates that the data were not available or applicable.

[a] See Methods for data sources. Prevalence and mortality estimates include patients with HIV.

[b] The sum of cases notified by age and sex is less than the number of new smear-positive cases notified for some countries.

[c] Non-DOTS is blank for countries which are 100% DOTS, or where no non-DOTS data were reported.

[d] DOTS case detection rate for given year, DOTS treatment success rate for cohort registered in previous year.

[e] "Other" includes transfer out and not evaluated, still on treatment, and other unknown.

WHO report, it remains unclear why so many patients are lost to follow-up, and efforts need to be made to promote better adherence and to achieve better treatment outcomes.

Because the surveillance and monitoring data are still weak, and the electronic TB register was introduced only at the end of 2003, it is difficult to assess the TB burden and trends and to evaluate the impact of the DOTS programme. A national disease prevalence survey would help to determine how much TB there is in South Africa and would provide a baseline against which to measure the future impact of DOTS and related control methods for HIV and AIDS.

Improving programme performance

The current TB control plan, the "Medium Term Development Plan" (2002–2005), was developed and endorsed by the national government and by eight of the country's nine provinces. A 10-year review of the programme is scheduled in 2005, and a new five-year plan will be developed in line with the strategies developed by the Department of Health.

South Africa has overcome some of the important constraints to achieving the global targets identified in the last report. A uniform, cohort-based recording and reporting system has been set up in all provinces, and the establishment of the electronic TB register will allow tracking of patients between health facilities. While staffing shortages still pose a problem at the provincial level, there has been an increase in staff at the national level. To address the lack of capacity, a training manual has been developed for medical practitioners and training workshops are being held in all provinces. The WHO training manual for trainers of facility health-care workers is being adapted and training of trainers will be conducted in all provinces. A database of trained staff has been established. A national TB manual is being developed.

A national advocacy and social mobilization plan entitled "Stop TB – because you can" is being used to improve community awareness about TB through sustained and highly visible campaigns. The plan has been used to advocate the need for more resources for TB control at all levels of the government and to bring together all partners involved in TB control. It is now implemented in five provinces (Eastern Cape, Western Cape, Gauteng, Limpopo and Free State).

New drug combinations, following the WHO-recommended treatment guidelines, were phased in during 2003 but this led to problems with drug supplies and to a shortage of first-line drugs. Furthermore, the sole supplier of streptomycin has stopped manufacturing the drug. While FDCs are now available in most districts, some districts have yet to train health staff in treatment regimens using FDCs.

Data collected from the most recent prevalence survey (2000–2002) estimated 7500 prevalent MDR-TB cases and about 450 new MDR-TB cases per year, corresponding to MDR-TB levels of 1.7% (new cases) and 6.6% (re-treatment cases). Treatment facilities for MDR-TB have been established in eight provinces. The Medical Research Council is currently developing a national policy on MDR-TB management. A standardized treatment regimen is provided to MDR-TB patients. The country is not planning to submit an application to the GLC as most second-line drugs are available in the country and many are locally produced.

Diagnostic and laboratory services

Nearly all laboratories participate in a quarterly EQA programme run by the NHLS, but the current programme does not yet completely satisfy international guidelines. The delays in sputum smear diagnosis are still too long and reporting mechanisms are inadequate in some laboratories. The NHLS plans to establish a national TB reference laboratory and to introduce a pilot EQA study for sputum smear microscopy that will comply with international guidelines. Other priorities for the NHLS are to improve the laboratory infrastructure and the coverage of services in remote rural areas, as well as training and monitoring.

TB/HIV coordination

South Africa had an estimated HIV prevalence of 22% among all adults at the end of 2003. A recent national survey estimated the HIV prevalence among TB patients to be 55% in 2002, close to the WHO estimate of 61% in 2003. There is a national TB/HIV coordinating body for collaborative activities, which have been implemented in 44 out of 174 subdistricts; it is planned to cover the entire country by 2007. TB/HIV provincial coordinators and national staff have been recruited and national guidelines for care of HIV-infected TB patients, including access to ART, have been developed. VCT is offered routinely to TB patients, but the acceptance rate remains low.

Links with other health-care providers and the community

A few public and private hospitals as well as prison health services implement DOTS. Several large private corporations, in particular in the mining industry, provide DOTS through their corporate health facilities and contribute about 20% of all reported cases. Several NGOs are involved in the delivery of TB control services and many have recruited community health workers and volunteers as DOTS providers. As noted in last year's report, a PPM-DOTS plan is still needed and more private sector participation should be encouraged.

Partnerships

South Africa has a country TB coordinating group that meets four times a year. Many partners and technical agencies support DOTS implementation and expansion, including CDC (surveillance and TB/HIV activities), DFID (district management and inpatient care of TB patients), IUATLD (laboratory support and programme management), KNCV (training and research) and WHO (training and TB/HIV activities). USAID is one of the main sources of funds and the GFATM has approved one grant to fund TB/HIV activities.

Budgets and expenditures

As in previous years, South Africa did not submit financial information to

WHO because the NTP does not have access to district and provincial financial data. South Africa was awarded one TB/HIV grant from the GFATM in round 2 for US$ 8.4 million over two years; to date no funds have been disbursed. The Government of Belgium is also funding TB/HIV activities to the amount of US$ 8.3 million over five years, of which US$ 1.2 million has been disbursed. Estimates made in previous WHO reports suggest that the total annual cost of TB control in South Africa is about US$ 300 million.

Thailand

Thailand has had nationwide DOTS coverage since 2002 and reached the global target for case detection in 2003. Recent data suggest that the incidence of TB is declining slowly in Thailand. Considerable efforts are being made to extend TB control services to marginalized and deprived population groups, and this has boosted the case detection rate. However, treatment success is still well below the DOTS target and too many patients die, fail to complete their treatment or are lost to follow-up. In contrast to most HBCs, diagnostic laboratories in Thailand are relatively well equipped and maintained, but the shortage of adequately trained staff is still a problem. The estimated prevalence of HIV in Thailand is higher than in any other country in the WHO South-East Asia Region. A national TB/HIV coordinating body has been set up and is planning joint TB/HIV activities. The recent reform and decentralization of the country's health sector is changing the responsibilities and funding arrangements for TB control; the full implications of this for TB control are still unclear.

System of TB control

The central office of the NTP has become a cluster within the Bureau of AIDS, TB and STIs, following the recent reorganization of the Department of Disease Control (DDC) of the MoPH. The TB cluster is responsible for the development of technical policies, planning and monitoring of TB control in the country. The procurement and distribution of anti-TB drugs have been decentralized to the provincial and district levels as part of the health-sector reform process. Twelve regional TB centres and the TB cluster in Bangkok are responsible for monitoring, training and supervising of provincial and district-level staff. Health inspectors monitor the provincial hospitals and health offices and have a strong influence on provincial and district health-care programmes. Certain programmes are now given priority and

efforts have been made to include TB control among these priority programmes.

Under the health-sector reform project, a number of managerial tasks for the TB control programme, including planning and budgeting for activities such as training and supervision, have been decentralized to the provincial and district levels. District TB Coordinators (DTCs) are responsible for coordinating TB control activities, and work in close collaboration with the TB clinics in the hospitals. One effect of the health-sector reform policies will be to weaken the role of provincial and district health offices, as planning and budgeting authority will now rest with the provincial and district hospitals. In many districts, clinic staff in TB hospitals have assumed some of the responsibilities of the DTCs.

Laboratory diagnostic services in Thailand are provided by one NRL, 167 provincial and 678 district laboratories. All laboratories do smear microscopy, about 85 do mycobacterial culture and eight have facilities for

DST. Regional and university laboratories perform culture on request for sputum smear-negative cases.

Surveillance and monitoring

Annual case notifications from 1980 to 1995 suggest that the underlying trend in incidence is downwards, masked since 1998 by improvements in case detection. Notification rates are highest in elderly men and women, which is consistent with a long-term downward trend in TB incidence. However, the recent impact of HIV on TB incidence cannot be determined from the nationally aggregated data. The prevalence of HIV among adult TB cases was estimated to be 8.7% in 2003, but HIV prevalence has been falling for several years, and TB incidence may also still be falling.

According to the most recent estimate, Thailand has exceeded the target for case detection, reaching 72% in 2003, following the rapid increase in DOTS population coverage between 1995 and 2002. In contrast, treatment success was well below target at 74% in the 2002 cohort, mainly

---

PROGRESS IN TB CONTROL IN THAILAND

Indicators

DOTS treatment success, 2002 cohort	74%
DOTS case detection rate, 2003	72%
NTP budget available, 2004	100%
Government contribution to NTP budget, including loans, 2004	NA
Government contribution to total TB control costs, including loans, 2004	NA
Government health spending used for TB control, 2004	0.5%

Major achievements
— A meeting of TB coordinators from the regions, Bangkok and the prison service that addressed the referral and transfer system and overall strengthening of the TB network
— Recent DOTS expansion to marginalized population groups including people in border areas, migrants, prisoners and the urban poor leading to increased case detection

Major planned activities
— Implement TB/HIV collaborative activities including routine VCT for all TB patients, according to national guidelines
— Develop a comprehensive human resource plan for all levels of the NTP
— Build capacity for mycobacterial culture in provincial hospitals and strengthening the existing culture facilities in regional TB reference laboratories

NA indicates not available.

LATEST ESTIMATES[a]		TRENDS	2000	2001	2002	2003
Population	62 833 330	DOTS coverage (%)	70	82	100	100
Global rank (by est. number of cases)	17	Notification rate (all cases/100 000 pop)	56	81	80	87
Incidence (all cases/100 000 pop/year)	142	Notification rate (new ss+/100 000 pop)	29	46	41	45
Incidence (new ss+/100 000 pop/year)	63	Detection of all cases (%)	39	57	56	61
Prevalence (all cases/100 000 pop)	208	Case detection rate (new ss+, %)	46	73	65	72
TB mortality (all cases/100 000 pop/year)	19	DOTS case detection rate (new ss+, %)	46	73	65	72
TB cases HIV+ (adults aged 15–49, %)	8.7	DOTS case detection rate (new ss+)/coverage (%)	66	89	65	72
New cases multidrug resistant (%)	0.9	DOTS treatment success (new ss+, %)	69	75	74	–

Notification rate (per 100 000 pop)

— = ss+ cases   — = all cases (54 504 in 2003)

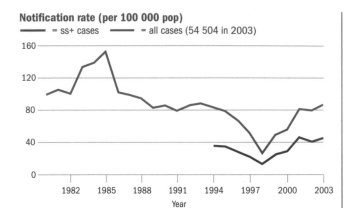

Notification rate by age and sex (new ss+)[b]

— = female   — = male

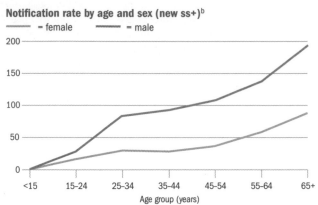

Case types notified

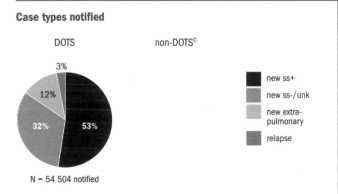

N = 54 504 notified

- new ss+
- new ss-/unk
- new extra-pulmonary
- relapse

DOTS progress towards targets[d]

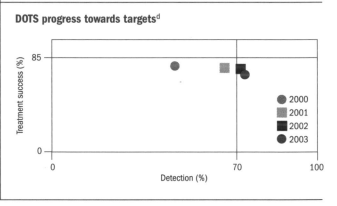

- 2000
- 2001
- 2002
- 2003

DOTS treatment outcomes (new ss+)

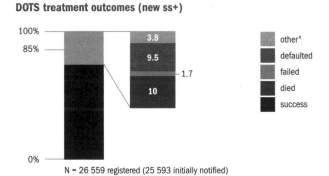

N = 26 559 registered (25 593 initially notified)

- other[e]
- defaulted
- failed
- died
- success

Non-DOTS treatment outcomes (new ss+)

Notes

ss+ indicates smear-positive; ss-, smear-negative; pop, population; unk, unknown.

Absence of a graph indicates that the data were not available or applicable.

[a] See Methods for data sources. Prevalence and mortality estimates include patients with HIV.

[b] The sum of cases notified by age and sex is less than the number of new smear-positive cases notified for some countries.

[c] Non-DOTS is blank for countries which are 100% DOTS, or where no non-DOTS data were reported.

[d] DOTS case detection rate for given year, DOTS treatment success rate for cohort registered in previous year.

[e] "Other" includes transfer out and not evaluated, still on treatment, and other unknown.

because 11% of patients died while on treatment and 13% defaulted or were transferred between treatment centres without subsequent follow-up of treatment outcome. Among patients registered for re-treatment, the success rate was only 62%; 17% of patients died while on treatment. There has been no systematic improvement in treatment success in Thailand since data were first submitted to WHO in 1995. Given the rapid recent increase in DOTS coverage, and the apparently high rate of case detection, Thailand should consider assessing the quality of treatment observation and ensure that reporting and recording are accurate. A recent programme review showed that parts of the database were incomplete and inconsistent.

Improving programme performance

In 2003, Thailand introduced a countrywide health insurance scheme for all clinical services known as the universal coverage (UC) scheme. The budget for this programme covers drugs and supplies for an "essential package of care" delivered at MoPH facilities and other health-care facilities under contract with the MoPH. Since 2002, following health-sector reforms, anti-TB drugs have been financed through the UC scheme. It is intended that training, supervision and monitoring activities for specific disease control programmes be financed through a non-UC budget available through the DDC at the MoPH. The TB cluster at the central level must use non-UC funds for the organization of national training courses, supervision in the regions and the organization of monitoring meetings for regional staff. During 2004, many training and monitoring activities required by NTP policy could not be carried out because of lack of funding at the peripheral level. Although funds are available for supervisory activities in 2004, the funding of training activities and monitoring meetings will require further negotiation with the DDC. The administrative process for the provision of non-UC funds at provincial and district levels is still being developed.

During the expansion of DOTS activities from 1996–2001, initial training was carried out for health-care workers at all levels. However, because of the high turnover of staff and the lack of systematic refresher courses, there is now a shortage of adequately trained TB control staff in Thailand. As noted last year, many of the regional TB offices have been weakened because staff posts have been cut and additional duties have been assigned to existing staff. A comprehensive HR development plan has been prepared; the immediate challenge is to ensure that sufficient funding is available to implement it.

Referral and transfer systems between treatment units and between prisons and MoPH facilities are weak. Timely information is often not communicated and there is no specific budget for communication between provinces. A TB network meeting was held in 2003 for the TB coordinators of the 12 regions, Bangkok and the prison service to address the referral and transfer system and overall strengthening of the TB network. Efforts are being made to improve data collection, and there are plans to introduce an electronic data management system.

The recent DOTS expansion to marginalized population groups including people living in border areas, migrants, prisoners and the urban poor have contributed to the high case detection rate in Thailand. NGOs and other organizations outside the MoPH system have been particularly active in expanding DOTS services to these groups.

Funding for anti-TB drugs has been adequate in the past but may be threatened if the purchase of drugs must be financed from fixed province and district budgets. Currently, most anti-TB drugs used by the NTP are manufactured in Thailand and are more costly than internationally procured drugs. Renegotiating prices with the government pharmaceutical organization or exploring additional procurement channels may help to release local funds for other TB-related activities such as training and supervision. The prevalence of MDR-TB among new cases decreased from 2.1% in 1997 to 0.9% in 2001. A nationwide drug resistance survey is planned for 2005. At present, the NTP does not diagnose and treat MDR-TB patients. However, policy guidelines on MDR-TB management are being developed.

Three areas where programme performance needs to be improved are diagnostic and laboratory services, TB/HIV coordination and links with other health-care providers.

Diagnostic and laboratory services

Compared with most other HBCs, Thailand has relatively well-equipped laboratories with few supply or maintenance problems. Thailand is planning to broaden the range of diagnostic services for TB by developing further capacity for doing TB culture in provincial hospitals and by strengthening the existing culture facilities of regional TB reference laboratories. The rapid detection of drug resistance is a priority for the NRL. EQA activities cover all TB laboratories in MoPH facilities, and efforts are to being made to include the private sector in the quality assurance scheme. Laboratory training activities are being expanded to include training for all TB control staff and targeted training for laboratory staff in technical areas where laboratory performance needs to be improved.

TB/HIV coordination

The estimated prevalence of HIV in Thailand (1.5% of adults aged 15–49 at the end of 2003) is the highest in the WHO South-East Asia Region. The prevalence of HIV among TB patients in sentinel surveys was between 10% and 15% in the country as a whole, but up to 30% in some regions (higher than the WHO estimate of 9% of adult TB patients). A national TB/HIV coordinating body was first established in 2001 and a national TB/HIV strategy has been in place since 2004. National TB/HIV guidelines were prepared in 2004 and will be implemented in January 2005.

VCT is offered to all TB patients in four pilot provinces: Chiang Rai, Ubon Ratchathani, Phuket and two districts in Bangkok. Data on specific indicators such as the proportion offered counselling, the proportion tested and the proportion found to be HIV positive will be collected and analysed. It is planned to train all TB clinic staff in the country in VCT by 2005.

Links with other health-care providers
The NTP has established a task force for PPM DOTS and has begun to collaborate with some private hospitals, private physicians and NGOs. There is a need to strengthen ties with all public sector providers and institutions involved in TB treatment and diagnosis, especially since the health-sector reform process has led to a more diversified network for delivering TB care. Public hospitals throughout the country are involved, but the participation of medical colleges and of prison and military health services remains limited.

Partnerships

CDC, RIT and WHO are the main technical partners in Thailand, assisting with DOTS expansion and TB/HIV activities. CDC (USAID) and GFATM are the major funding partners for surveillance, laboratory services, training and collaborative TB/HIV activities.

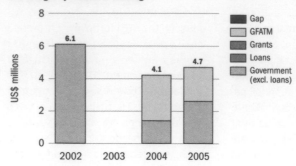

NTP budget by source of funding

Budgets and expenditures

Comprehensive data on NTP budgets and expenditures are not available for the period 2003–2005. This is because, under the new health insurance scheme introduced in 2003, provincial and district hospitals receive budgets (calculated on the basis of fixed per capita rates) to provide a package of clinical care. It is not clear how much funding for the TB control programme is provided from these budgets. Meanwhile, programme support functions such as training and supervision are covered through a separate budget. Budget figures reported to WHO for 2004 and 2005 therefore reflect only the budget managed by the TB cluster in Bangkok. As a result, the reported budget has fallen from US$ 6.1 million in 2002 to US$ 4.7 million in 2005, despite an increase in funding from the GFATM. The development of national budgets in future will depend on the NTP's ability to implement a comprehensive financial monitoring system that allows budgets and available funding to be reported by all provinces and districts. Estimates made in previous WHO reports indicate that the total cost of TB control is about US$ 10 million per year, and around US$ 170 per patient treated.

Uganda

Uganda is pursuing universal access to DOTS as its TB control strategy. All districts were implementing DOTS as far back as 1997, but the low coverage of general health services means that more than 50% of the population are still without access to TB services, although this proportion is decreasing. TB is a component of Uganda's minimum health-care package, and TB services are integrated in primary health care. However, many health facilities do not yet provide TB diagnosis and care. In 2000, Uganda adopted the community-based TB care model as the best strategy to control TB in the country. Community involvement is recognized as crucial for the success of TB control in Uganda. The NTP is committed to expanding community-based DOTS (CB-DOTS) to all 56 districts; 51 districts have already been covered. Although GFATM funds were approved for Uganda in round 2, a substantial funding gap still remains, meaning that some of the planned activities for 2005 may not be carried out. In December 2004, the Uganda Stop TB Partnership (USTP) was launched as a major initiative to raise awareness of TB as an important public health problem and to mobilize additional resources for TB control.

System of TB control

Uganda has a decentralized system of governance, with central ministries responsible for policies, standards, quality control, resource mobilization and training. Districts are responsible for management of services at peripheral level. Health service delivery, including TB control, is the responsibility of the health subdistricts (HSDs), which are the functional units for TB control. A total of 214 HSDs each serve about 100 000 people. TB service delivery is fully integrated in the primary health-care system.

TB control in Uganda is organized with a central unit at the MoH run by the NTP manager and one administrative officer. Hitherto, the NTP manager has been assisted by six zonal tuberculosis and leprosy supervisors (ZTLSs) based at the periphery, who oversee TB control in their zones. At district level, a district health team (DHT) oversees TB control. The District Tuberculosis and Leprosy Supervisor, a member of the DHT, is responsible for TB control including data collection, analysis and reporting. Below this level, general health workers handle TB control activities as part of their general duties.

The MoH has recently developed the second five-year "Health Sector Strategic Plan" (HSSP II) covering 2005/2006–2009/2010. HSSP II envisages continued implementation of the minimum health-care package of which TB is one component and foresees continued use of TB performance indicators for monitoring progress of HSSP II implementation. As part of continuing health sector reform, the NTP plans to recall the ZTLSs to the centre in order to form, under the guidance of the NTP manager, a strong central team with improved capacity in policy formulation and technical guidance to districts and partners on TB management. The ZTLSs will provide a strong technical link between government and partners, and support to the DHTs. Each district has three or more health facilities providing TB diagnostic and treatment services. Through CB-DOTS, treatment is provided at the community level. CB-DOTS is an important service delivery mechanism that is patient-centred and based on participation by civil society, providing accessible, cost-effective TB care; this mechanism is vital to the success of TB control in Uganda.

The NRL in Kampala is responsible for training, DST and EQA. The national coordinator of the laboratory network is responsible for the NRL. Ten regional laboratories based at regional hospitals also provide training and EQA, in addition to smear microscopy. The district laboratories' main responsibility is the supervision of peripheral laboratories, which serve as the main diagnostic units.

PROGRESS IN TB CONTROL IN UGANDA

Indicators

DOTS treatment success, 2002 cohort	60%
DOTS detection rate, 2003	44%
NTP budget available, 2004	83%
Government contribution to NTP budget, including loans, 2004	32%
Government contribution to total TB control costs, including loans, 2004	38%
Government health spending used for TB control, 2004	2%

Major achievements

— Expansion of community-based DOTS (CB DOTS) to an additional 11 districts, corresponding to an additional 20% of the country's population
— Formation and launch of the Uganda Stop TB Partnership (USTP) to better harness efforts of all partners on TB control
— Secured additional staff to build NTP capacity; secured additional resources through ISAC

Major planned activities

— Complete expansion and consolidation of CB DOTS, ensuring district-wide coverage and high quality of services
— Institute EQA of all laboratories in the country, and strengthen it where it exists
— Update NTP strategic TB control plan to include PPM DOTS as part of the DOTS expansion plan
— Operationalize the USTP

UGANDA

LATEST ESTIMATES[a]		TRENDS	2000	2001	2002	2003
Population	25 826 968	DOTS coverage (%)	100	100	100	100
Global rank (by est. number of cases)	16	Notification rate (all cases/100 000 pop)	129	152	163	162
Incidence (all cases/100 000 pop/year)	411	Notification rate (new ss+/100 000 pop)	73	71	76	79
Incidence (new ss+/100 000 pop/year)	179	Detection of all cases (%)	38	42	42	39
Prevalence (all cases/100 000 pop)	652	Case detection rate (new ss+, %)	50	46	46	44
TB mortality (all cases/100 000 pop/year)	96	DOTS case detection rate (new ss+, %)	50	46	46	44
TB cases HIV+ (adults aged 15–49, %)	21	DOTS case detection rate (new ss+)/coverage (%)	50	46	46	44
New cases multidrug resistant (%)	0.5	DOTS treatment success (new ss+, %)	63	56	60	–

Notification rate (per 100 000 pop)

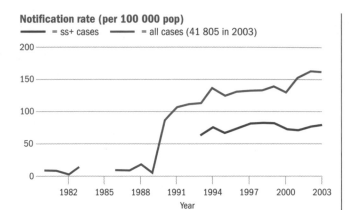

Notification rate by age and sex (new ss+)[b]

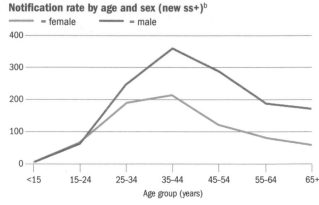

Case types notified

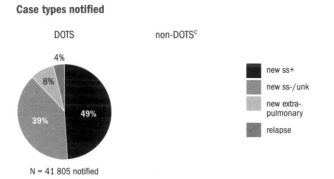

DOTS progress towards targets[d]

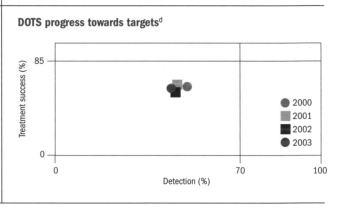

DOTS treatment outcomes (new ss+)

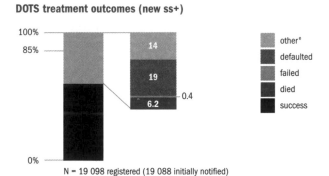

Non-DOTS treatment outcomes (new ss+)

Notes

ss+ indicates smear-positive; ss-, smear-negative; pop, population; unk, unknown.

Absence of a graph indicates that the data were not available or applicable.

[a] See Methods for data sources. Prevalence and mortality estimates include patients with HIV.

[b] The sum of cases notified by age and sex is less than the number of new smear-positive cases notified for some countries.

[c] Non-DOTS is blank for countries which are 100% DOTS, or where no non-DOTS data were reported.

[d] DOTS case detection rate for given year, DOTS treatment success rate for cohort registered in previous year.

[e] "Other" includes transfer out and not evaluated, still on treatment, and other unknown.

Surveillance and monitoring

While strong evidence exists that HIV prevalence has been falling in Uganda since the early 1990s, the notification rate of TB cases (all forms) has increased since 2000. The notification rate of new smear-positive cases has remained steady for the past decade. In order to estimate the case detection rate, it has been assumed that the increase in the notification rates of all forms of TB reflects an increase in incidence – and that the case detection rate of new smear-positive cases has fallen since 2000 from 50% to 44%. A plausible alternative explanation is that the case detection rate has improved as the coverage of CB DOTS has been extended throughout the country – and that TB incidence has stabilized or begun to fall. However, given the low access to health services (less than 50%), it is unlikely that the case detection rate is much higher than estimated here.

Notwithstanding the uncertainty surrounding the assessment of the case detection rate, it is clear that the NTP must work to improve treatment outcomes, which have been consistently low. Only 60% of new smear-positive patients were successfully treated in the 2002 cohort; 33% defaulted, were transferred without follow-up or were not evaluated. Cure was bacteriologically confirmed in only half the patients successfully treated; the final smear examination was not done for the other patients. The pattern is similar among patients registered for re-treatment.

A small disease prevalence survey was carried out in Kampala in 2001–2002,[1] finding a prevalence of smear-positive TB of 440 cases per 100 000 population in the periurban community sampled. However, a larger national survey is needed to assess the total burden of TB in Uganda and to set a baseline against which to measure the impact of DOTS. Alternatively, or in addition, a systematic evaluation of the process of diagnosis and reporting in Uganda would allow a reassessment of the case detection rate. The NTP acknowledges that progress has been hindered by non-prioritization of sputum smear examination (15% of new cases were put on treatment without sputum smear results), poor recording and the absence of strategies to recover interrupters and to capture the true treatment outcome of patients who transfer between treatment units. These factors are being addressed systematically.

Improving programme performance

Since early 2004, the NTP has benefited from the ISAC initiative, which greatly contributed to the increased capacity of the central team. An international WHO staff member supports the NTP central unit. The central unit has deployed three recently recruited professional officers at regional level to support the DHTs, with redistribution of regional supervisors to weak areas. However, major HR deficiencies still exist at the central level. CB DOTS is being expanded and, by the end of 2004, was being implemented in 51 out of 56 districts. The full impact of this expansion has not yet been seen.

CB DOTS is being implemented in a phased manner in the HSDs of some districts. Uganda has so far engaged two international NGOs (International Medical Corps and the Malaria Consortium) to implement CB DOTS in remote areas; the NTP plans to expand CB DOTS to the remaining districts early in 2005.

Supervision and monitoring activities have been expanded to all levels of TB control, including the community. A new DOTS expansion plan for the next five years is being developed by the NTP.

In 1996–1997, a DRS was conducted in areas of the country supported by GLRA, giving an estimate of 0.5% MDR in new pulmonary cases and 4.4% MDR in re-treatment cases. Resources are being sought to carry out a new DRS. Uganda plans to apply to the GLC in the context of the new DOTS expansion plan.

Three other areas in which programme performance needs to be improved are diagnostic and laboratory services, TB/HIV coordination and links with other health-care providers and the community.

Diagnostic and laboratory services

The two main challenges facing the diagnostic and laboratory services are the shortage of qualified laboratory personnel in the general health service and the lack of a countrywide EQA system for sputum smear microscopy. In 2003, only 12 out of 56 districts had implemented EQA for smear microscopy. In 2005, the NTP plans to establish routine EQA in the remaining districts and to strengthen it in those districts where it exists. The NTP will advocate for recruitment of qualified personnel in peripheral laboratories and will train existing personnel as microscopists in the interim.

TB/HIV coordination

An interim national TB/HIV coordinating body comprising the managers of the NTP and of the National AIDS Control Programme and partners (including the AIDS Information Centre, the AIDS Support Organization, GLRA, USAID-funded organizations and WHO) was formed in 2004 to formulate a policy as well as to prepare a proposal for collaborative TB/HIV activities. The committee will ensure phased implementation of collaborative TB/HIV activities in pilot districts and, based on the experiences gained, will frame the policy and strategy for rapid nationwide expansion.

In 2004, WHO appointed an NPO to coordinate TB/HIV activities and oversee the establishment of the committee; its first meeting was planned for mid-January 2005.

Links with other health-care providers

A situation analysis has shown that many patients in urban areas are treated in the private sector. The NTP has initiated a small-scale collaborative project with private hospitals, with plans to expand this initiative to involve individual private medical practitioners. NGOs play an important role in DOTS implementation, and the NTP has involved many general hospitals, a few medical colleges, and prison, army and police health facilities in TB control.

---

[1] Guwatudde D et al. Burden of tuberculosis in Kampala, Uganda. *Bulletin of the World Health Organization*, 2003, 81:799–805.

(a) NTP budget by source of funding

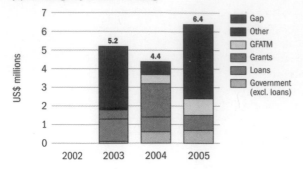

(b) NTP budget by line item

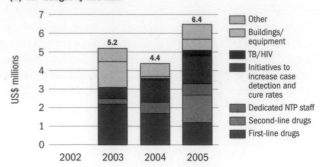

(c) Total TB control costs by line item[a]

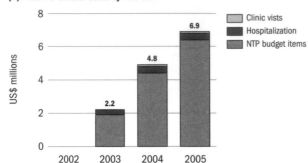

(d) Per patient costs, budgets, available funding and expenditures

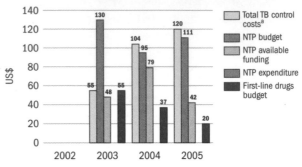

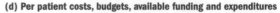

[a] Total TB control costs for 2003 are based on available funding, whereas those for 2004 and 2005 are based on budgets. Estimates of the costs of clinic visits and hospitalization are WHO estimates based on data provided by the NTP and from other sources. See Methods for further details.

Links with the community

The success and sustainability of CB DOTS is largely dependent on community involvement and ownership of the programme. In the CB-DOTS strategy, communities participate in selecting lay community members to support patients and ensure treatment compliance. The selected community members work on a voluntary basis, observing and recording the ingestion of each day's medication. In addition, they encourage patients to go for follow-up sputum smears and suspects to go for examination in health units. Community volunteers are responsible to the community and also to the formal health system through a public health worker who supervises and replenishes drug supplies.

Partnerships

The MoH is committed to attaining the targets for DOTS implementation, and has indicated an interest in forming a strong partnership to help the country accelerate towards the 2005 targets. The formation of the USTP was spearheaded by the MoH and supported by WHO and the Global Stop TB Partnership, as well as other part-

ners, in the context of the ISAC initiative. The USTP was launched in December 2004, with the aims of harnessing the contributions of all stakeholders to TB control and raising the profile of TB as a major public health problem. WHO Uganda has offered to host the USTP Secretariat; a Memorandum of Understanding is being prepared to guide their operations.

Budgets and expenditures

The NTP budget has been between US$ 4.4 million and US$ 6.4 million during the period 2003–2005 (equivalent to US$ 95–130 per patient). Despite the approval of a GFATM grant in round 2, Uganda suffers from a persistent funding gap, which is expected to reach US$ 4 million in 2005, representing 62% of the NTP budget.

The budget for first-line anti-TB drugs has decreased from US$ 2.2 million in 2003 to US$ 1.2 million in 2005, whereas the expected number of patients to be treated is rising. The drug budget per patient treated has thus been reduced from US$ 55 to US$ 20. This budget for first-line drugs is fully funded. In contrast, while the

budgets for initiatives to increase case detection and cure rates and for collaborative TB/HIV activities have been increasing between 2003 and 2005, implementation of all of the planned activities will depend on the availability of additional funds. A need for second-line drugs has also been identified; a budget of US$ 1.5 million has been included in 2005, which is for a stock sufficient to treat 1000 MDR-TB patients. However, funding has not yet been secured.

The total cost of TB control, including the costs of clinic visits and hospital stays as well as the NTP budget, will increase from an estimated US$ 2.2 million in 2003 to US$ 6.9 million in 2005 (US$ 55–120 per patient), provided the existing budget gap for 2005 is filled. If no additional funds are secured, total costs will reach only about US$ 3 million in 2005; the cost per patient will be US$ 51. The costs of clinic visits, at around US$ 0.1 million, is relatively low given the small number of visits required to health facilities following the nationwide introduction of CB DOTS.

United Republic of Tanzania

The United Republic of Tanzania was among the first countries to adopt the DOTS strategy. Nationwide DOTS coverage was attained in 2002, largely through the successful integration of TB control in the general health services. After reaching a peak in 2001, the number of reported TB cases has remained steady, which may perhaps indicate an end to the rise in TB incidence previously associated with the HIV epidemic. As the HIV prevalence has been constant in the country since 1996, the DOTS programme should be able to achieve a progressive reduction in TB incidence from now on. Improvements have been made in the treatment of patients, but a relatively high death rate is still an obstacle to reaching the global target for successful treatment. While progress has been made in control of both TB and HIV and in ART scale-up, the TB and HIV control programmes have not worked together in the past, and the particular needs arising from the epidemic of TB/HIV coinfection have not received special attention until recently. The government has now developed comprehensive plans for collaborative TB/HIV activities and, thanks to an award from the GFATM,

it should be possible to implement them all. Building on the well-managed TB control programme, the collaborative TB/HIV activities will give additional impetus to TB case-finding and treatment. The MoH is also preparing to establish DOTS-Plus within the regular DOTS programme. Further strengthening of human resources, particularly at central level, is essential to meet the needs of these rapidly expanding programme activities.

System of TB control

The NTP is well organized and managed. Under the direction of a small central unit, the regional and district TB coordinators supervise the activities of hospitals and other health centres and monitor programme performance, using formal quality assurance practices. The district health committees are responsible for developing district health plans that include both TB and HIV. Recognizing the importance of the dual epidemic of TB and HIV, the NTP has decided to implement the full package of collaborative TB/HIV activities as part of a comprehensive TB and HIV/AIDS control strategy.

The NRL oversees 2 zonal, 18 re-

gional and 701 district laboratories. Culture is done at the NRL and zonal laboratories, while DST is carried out only at the NRL.

Surveillance and monitoring

The total annual TB notification rate has increased three-fold between 1980 and 2001, and has fallen slightly since then. The notification rate of smear-positive cases has fallen slightly since 1998. Assuming that this is a consequence of the earlier levelling off of the HIV epidemic rather than a decline in case detection rates, the DOTS programme should now begin to reduce the incidence of TB, provided the programme performance is maintained or improved. The estimated rate of smear-positive case detection in 2003 (43%) was low, but the reliability of this estimate is not easily verified using the available tuberculin testing data because the usual methods of analysis based on the Stýblo ratio may not apply when the prevalence of HIV is high (see Methods). For this reason, a systematic and quantitative assessment of the completeness of surveillance data or a survey of the prevalence of disease would be very informative. Given the high rate of HIV infection in the country, the treatment success rates are good: 80% for new cases, 79% for relapse cases, 65% for re-treatment after failure and 71% for re-treatment after default. Treatment outcomes for new smear-positive patients have improved steadily since 1995, but the high death rates (11% for the 2002 cohort) are the main obstacle to reaching the 85% target for treatment success.

Improving programme performance

To improve case detection, the number of diagnostic centres has been increased in the districts, and a start has been made on integrating the delivery of TB control into the general health services and into the private sector. In 2003, 1250 general health-

---

PROGRESS IN TB CONTROL IN THE UNITED REPUBLIC OF TANZANIA

Indicators

DOTS treatment success, 2002 cohort	80%
DOTS case detection rate, 2003	43%
NTP budget available, 2004	76%
Government contribution to NTP budget, including loans, 2004	14%
Government contribution to total TB control costs, including loans, 2004	64%
Government health spending used for TB control, 2004	11%

Major achievements
— Increased number of diagnostic centres at district level
— Training of 1250 general health-care workers in case detection and treatment
— Maintained high treatment success despite high prevalence of HIV among TB patients
— Strengthening of MDR-TB services and infrastructure in preparation for application to the GLC

Major planned activities
— Expand DOTS by involving communities, the private sector, specialist TB clinics, medical colleges and prison health services
— Introduce DOTS Plus activities
— Expand collaborative TB/HIV activities to all districts by 2007

LATEST ESTIMATES[a]		TRENDS	2000	2001	2002	2003
Population	**36 976 622**	DOTS coverage (%)	100	100	100	100
Global rank (by est. number of cases)	14	Notification rate (all cases/100 000 pop)	156	173	166	167
Incidence (all cases/100 000 pop/year)	371	Notification rate (new ss+/100 000 pop)	69	69	67	67
Incidence (new ss+/100 000 pop/year)	157	Detection of all cases (%)	45	49	46	45
Prevalence (all cases/100 000 pop)	524	Case detection rate (new ss+, %)	47	46	43	43
TB mortality (all cases/100 000 pop/year)	86	DOTS case detection rate (new ss+, %)	47	46	43	43
TB cases HIV+ (adults aged 15–49, %)	36	DOTS case detection rate (new ss+)/coverage (%)	47	46	43	43
New cases multidrug resistant (%)	1.2	DOTS treatment success (new ss+, %)	78	81	80	—

Notification rate (per 100 000 pop)

— = ss+ cases   — = all cases (61 579 in 2003)

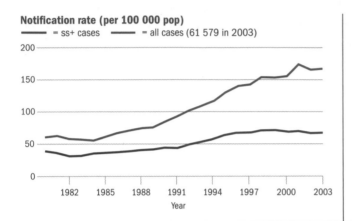

Notification rate by age and sex (new ss+)[b]

— = female   — = male

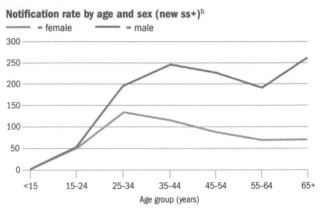

Case types notified

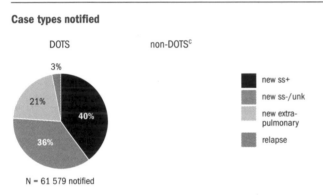

DOTS   non-DOTS[c]

- new ss+
- new ss-/unk
- new extra-pulmonary
- relapse

N = 61 579 notified

DOTS progress towards targets[d]

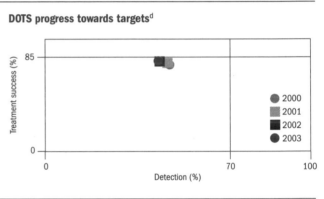

- 2000
- 2001
- 2002
- 2003

DOTS treatment outcomes (new ss+)

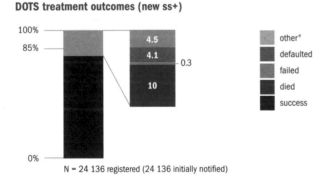

- other[e]
- defaulted
- failed
- died
- success

N = 24 136 registered (24 136 initially notified)

Non-DOTS treatment outcomes (new ss+)

Notes

ss+ indicates smear-positive; ss-, smear-negative; pop, population; unk, unknown.

Absence of a graph indicates that the data were not available or applicable.

[a] See Methods for data sources. Prevalence and mortality estimates include patients with HIV.

[b] The sum of cases notified by age and sex is less than the number of new smear-positive cases notified for some countries.

[c] Non-DOTS is blank for countries which are 100% DOTS, or where no non-DOTS data were reported.

[d] DOTS case detection rate for given year, DOTS treatment success rate for cohort registered in previous year.

[e] "Other" includes transfer out and not evaluated, still on treatment, and other unknown.

care workers were trained on case detection and treatment. The central unit has produced training guidelines and a facilitator module for clinical officers and will develop training guidelines for nurses.

To improve programme performance, it will be necessary to strengthen HR capacity at the central level. Currently, there are only four people to supervise and monitor the TB control programme, to expand DOTS services, to implement training at lower levels and to develop and implement collaborative TB/HIV activities. PATH, with funding from USAID, has recently developed a plan to strengthen HR capacity at central, regional and district level.

The MoH is planning to establish and integrate a DOTS-Plus component within the NTP. Following a WHO mission in spring 2004, plans have been made to: introduce DOTS-Plus, including developing a computerized TB notification system to monitor treatment outcomes among re-treatment cases; construct a new MDR-TB ward within the national TB hospital; set up a technical committee to oversee future implementation of MDR-TB activities; and provide training for medical personnel in management of MDR-TB. A drug resistance survey is scheduled to start in the middle of 2005.

Three areas where programme performance needs to be improved are diagnostic and laboratory services, TB/HIV coordination and links with other health-care providers.

Diagnostic and laboratory services

The quality of the central laboratory services has been significantly improved in preparation for an application to the GLC. New equipment has been installed, and internal quality control is now mandatory; the mycobacterial culture contamination rate has been reduced from 15% to 10% in less than a year. However, laboratories at all levels are still short of qualified staff and the implementation of EQA for smear microscopy is still not satisfactory. A further priority for the laboratory network is to improve the quality of supervision of the peripheral laboratories by the central unit.

TB/HIV coordination

A national TB/HIV strategic plan to cover all districts by 2007 has been developed and includes all the collaborative TB/HIV activities defined in the WHO interim policy. In 2003, the Tanzanian Government successfully applied to the GFATM (round 3) for resources to support collaborative TB/HIV activities in 45 of 120 districts. There is a gap in funding to scale up TB/HIV activities nationally, and there is a need to align TB/HIV activities with the national plan for scaling up access to ART to ensure that HIV-positive TB patients are able to access ART. Implementation of collaborative TB/HIV activities is slow; in order to accelerate their implementation, additional financial resources will be needed as well as increased HR capacity, particularly at central level.

Links with other health-care providers

Anti-TB drugs may only be prescribed and dispensed with the approval of the NTP and using drugs procured and distributed by the NTP. As a result, non-DOTS treatment of TB is very limited in both the private and the public sector, which facilitates the implementation of PPM-DOTS strategies. The NTP has involved NGOs and private hospitals in TB control by providing training, drugs and supervision, and is now expanding this effort to include private clinics. Links with specialist TB clinics, medical colleges and prison health services are also being strengthened.

Partnerships

A range of technical and financial partners are involved in TB control and they have formed an Interagency Coordination Committee that meets once a year. Development Cooperation Ireland, the Government of the Netherlands and the Swiss Agency for Development and Cooperation are the main sources of funds for TB control activities. GLRA, KNCV and WHO all support programme monitoring and offer other technical assistance.

Budgets and expenditures

The NTP budget has increased from about US$ 5 million in 2002–2003 to nearly US$ 9 million in 2004 (from about US$ 90 per patient in 2002–2003 to US$ 133 in 2004). Budget data are not yet available for 2005 since the fiscal year starts in July. The budget was increased in 2004 to pay for dedicated staff, for the implementation of collaborative TB/HIV activities and for investment in buildings and equipment. The available funding has also increased, from around US$ 5 million in 2002 and 2003 to US$ 6.7 million in 2004. Most NTP funding comes from grants, with the government contributing US$ 1.2 million (about 10% of the budget) in 2004. While a grant from the GFATM should make it possible to carry out the planned collaborative TB/HIV activities in selected pilot districts (provided that sufficient staff are available), a funding gap of US$ 0.8 million remains.

In 2003, the government contribution was only US$ 0.6 million rather than US$ 1.3 million as anticipated. However, total available funding was higher than expected, at US$ 5.6 million. Expenditures in 2003 were US$ 3.8 million, i.e. 62% of the funds received. As more funding becomes available through grants, the capacity of the programme to absorb this money may become an important issue.

The total cost of TB control, which includes the cost of dedicated TB beds, clinic visits during treatment and items included in the NTP budget, was between US$ 15 million and US$ 16 million in 2002 and 2003 (about US$ 250–275 per patient treated). If the 2004 budget is fully funded and the money is spent, this could increase to US$ 21 million in 2004 (US$ 320 per patient treated).

(a) NTP budget by source of funding

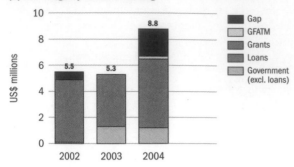

(b) NTP budget by line item

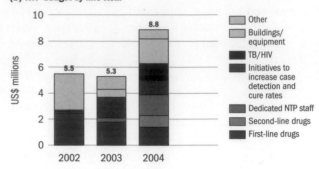

(c) Total TB control costs by line item[a,b]

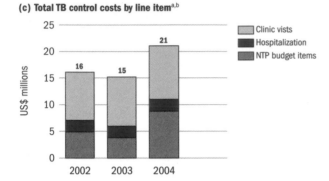

(d) Per patient costs, budgets, available funding and expenditures[a]

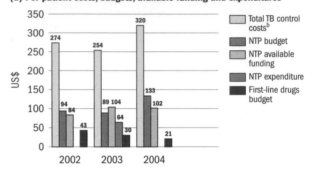

[a] No data available for 2005 – see text for explanation.

[b] Total TB control costs for 2002 are based on available funding, whereas those for 2003 are based on expenditures, and those for 2004 are based on budgets. Estimates of the costs of clinic visits and hospitalization are WHO estimates based on data provided by the NTP and from other sources. See Methods for further details.

Viet Nam

Viet Nam is the only member of the current group of HBCs[1] to have reached the targets for DOTS implementation, which were achieved before 2000 and exceeded subsequently. This outstanding success was made possible by the effective integration of political commitment, international technical assistance and funding, and efficient community mobilization. Viet Nam has continued to expand the programme so as to reach remote population groups who have not had access to TB services, and to strengthen the diagnostic laboratory network. An urgent priority is the development of a national plan for improved TB/HIV coordination. A planned national TB prevalence survey will be of critical importance for measuring the impact of DOTS on the TB epidemic. Because of its success in achieving the targets, Viet Nam does not need substantial budget increases in 2005.

System of TB control

The National Hospital of Tuberculosis and Respiratory Diseases, in Hanoi, is responsible for the activities for all of Viet Nam. Pham Ngoc Thach Hospital in Ho Chi Minh City is appointed to supervise the activities for the southern provinces. Each province has a provincial TB centre, under the direction of the provincial health service, which is responsible for the local implementation of the TB control programme. The district TB units, directed by the district health centres, coordinate the operation of peripheral TB activities. TB patients are referred to the district health centres from community health posts for sputum examination and initial treatment.

An effective national TB laboratory network operates under the supervision of the NTP. There are two reference laboratories (Hanoi and Ho Chi Minh City) that perform culture and drug susceptibility testing. Of the 64 provincial TB laboratories, nearly one quarter perform culture. Smear microscopy services are provided by more than 600 district TB laboratories.

Surveillance and monitoring

The best estimates of case detection for 2003 (86%) and treatment success for the 2002 cohort (92%) suggest, as in previous years, that Viet Nam has comfortably exceeded the targets for DOTS implementation. Given that DOTS coverage and case detection and cure rates have been very high since 1997, a fall in the incidence rate could be expected, which should be reflected in the trend in case notifications. It is unclear why no such decline is visible in the nationally aggregated data, but analysis by province could be more illuminating. Case-notification rates are highest among elderly men and women, suggesting that TB incidence has been higher in the past. It is possible that incidence is not falling perceptibly in Viet Nam because the case detection rate may be lower, and the incidence rate higher, than the WHO estimates. In this context, Viet Nam's long-planned prevalence survey would help to establish the true burden of TB in the country, as well as providing a baseline against which to evaluate the impact of the programme on the TB epidemic.

Improving programme performance

Although all provinces maintain 100% coverage by the DOTS strategy, there are populations living in remote and mountainous areas with limited access to DOTS services. The NTP is expanding DOTS to reach these areas while maintaining excellent services. Efforts to reach these remote populations and other vulnerable groups started in 2003 and continued in 2004. Maintaining a consistent supply of high-quality anti-TB drugs for the entire country, especially in newly covered areas, is another important challenge being addressed by the NTP. A regulatory framework and enforcement mechanism have been developed to ensure the high quality of

---

PROGRESS IN TB CONTROL IN VIET NAM

Indicators

DOTS treatment success, 2002 cohort	92%
DOTS case detection rate, 2003	86%
NTP budget available, 2004	98%
Government contribution to NTP budget, including loans, 2004	78%
Government contribution to total TB control costs, including loans, 2004	90%
Government health spending used for TB control, 2004	6%

Major achievements

— Expansion of the TB network to cover remote and mountainous areas and increased access to DOTS for vulnerable groups
— Establishment of nationwide EQA system for smear microscopy
— Development of a regulatory framework and enforcement mechanism to ensure the high quality of anti-TB drugs
— Pilot testing of isoniazid preventive therapy for PLWHA infected with *M. tuberculosis* and co-trimoxazole preventive therapy for TB patients coinfected with HIV in An Giang province
— Studies on FDCs for patients in remote areas and on PPM-DOTS

Major planned activities

— Develop five-year plan for NTP for 2006–2010
— Train staff in EQA and maintain system throughout the country
— Carry out third national drug resistance survey

---

[1] Peru was excluded from the original group of HBCs, having met the targets and successfully reduced incidence.

LATEST ESTIMATES[a]		TRENDS	2000	2001	2002	2003
Population	81 376 724	DOTS coverage (%)	99.8	99.8	100	100
Global rank (by est. number of cases)	13	Notification rate (all cases/100 000 pop)	115	115	118	114
Incidence (all cases/100 000 pop/year)	178	Notification rate (new ss+/100 000 pop)	68	68	71	69
Incidence (new ss+/100 000 pop/year)	80	Detection of all cases (%)	63	63	66	64
Prevalence (all cases/100 000 pop)	240	Case detection rate (new ss+, %)	83	84	88	86
TB mortality (all cases/100 000 pop/year)	23	DOTS case detection rate (new ss+, %)	83	84	88	86
TB cases HIV+ (adults aged 15–49, %)	2.8	DOTS case detection rate (new ss+)/coverage (%)	83	84	88	86
New cases multidrug resistant (%)	2.3	DOTS treatment success (new ss+, %)	92	93	92	–

Notification rate (per 100 000 pop)

— = ss+ cases   — = all cases (92 741 in 2003)

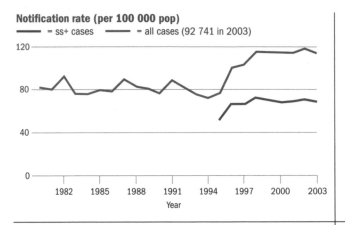

Notification rate by age and sex (new ss+)[b]

— = female   — = male

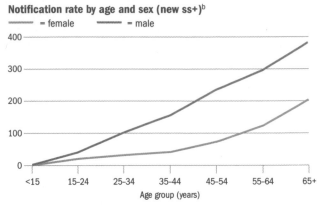

Case types notified

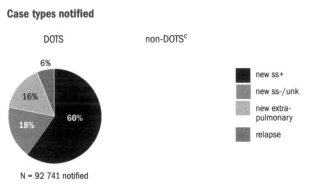

DOTS   non-DOTS[c]

- new ss+
- new ss-/unk
- new extra-pulmonary
- relapse

N = 92 741 notified

DOTS progress towards targets[d]

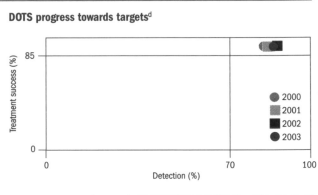

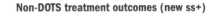

- 2000
- 2001
- 2002
- 2003

DOTS treatment outcomes (new ss+)

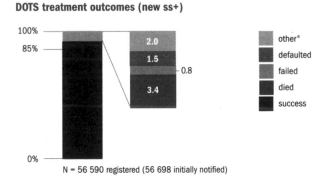

- other[e]
- defaulted
- failed
- died
- success

N = 56 590 registered (56 698 initially notified)

Non-DOTS treatment outcomes (new ss+)

Notes

ss+ indicates smear-positive; ss-, smear-negative; pop, population; unk, unknown.

Absence of a graph indicates that the data were not available or applicable.

[a] See Methods for data sources. Prevalence and mortality estimates include patients with HIV.

[b] The sum of cases notified by age and sex is less than the number of new smear-positive cases notified for some countries.

[c] Non-DOTS is blank for countries which are 100% DOTS, or where no non-DOTS data were reported.

[d] DOTS case detection rate for given year, DOTS treatment success rate for cohort registered in previous year.

[e] "Other" includes transfer out and not evaluated, still on treatment, and other unknown.

anti-TB drugs for TB services both within and outside the NTP. The feasibility of using FDCs for patients living in areas which are difficult to access is being explored. The last drug resistance survey was carried out in 1996 and estimated the prevalence of MDR-TB at 2.3% among new cases. A new survey is scheduled for 2005.

The NTP is developing the next five-year plan for TB control (2006–2010). Human resource capacity development will continue to be a priority, and the NTP will work with local authorities to recruit and maintain existing staff and to develop intensified training activities for staff at all levels.

Three other areas where programme performance needs to be improved are: diagnostic and laboratory services, TB/HIV coordination, and links with other health-care providers and the community.

Diagnostic and laboratory services

As DOTS services are expanded to remote and mountainous regions, diagnostic services also need to be provided to these areas. An EQA system for sputum microscopy based on new international guidelines is being established in laboratories at district level throughout Viet Nam. In 2004 and 2005, staff in 20 of 64 provinces will be trained on the EQA system, and methods will be developed to implement and maintain EQA throughout the country.

TB/HIV coordination

In 2002, the prevalence of HIV in new TB patients was estimated to be 3% based on HIV sentinel surveillance among TB patients. This is somewhat higher than the WHO national estimate of 1.8%. In 10 provinces HIV prevalence exceeded 3%, and in two provinces (Binh Duong and Haiphong) the prevalence was more than 10%. In An Giang Province a pilot project included the use of isoniazid preventive therapy for PLWHA infected with *M. tuberculosis*, and co-trimoxazole preventive therapy for TB patients with HIV coinfection. ART for HIV-infected TB patients is not yet available. There is an urgent need for a well-defined national plan for TB/HIV coordination, including strategies for TB prevention and control for PLWHA, HIV/AIDS prevention, and health promotion and treatment for TB patients.

Links with other health-care providers

Private providers treat a considerable proportion of patients in metropolitan Ho Chi Minh City, but the situation is uncertain in other parts of the country. A project aimed at involving private providers in TB control in Ho Chi Minh was implemented from 2001 to 2004 with mixed results. Case notification increased, but the treatment success rate was poor in the private clinics involved, probably because anti-TB drugs were not provided free of charge. No other private sector initiatives have been undertaken.

Links with the community

The community (i.e. villages, Women's Union, Farmer's Union) is involved in a successful IEC campaign for TB control activities, and there are plans to scale up these activities.

Partnerships

Effective international partnerships are a major feature of Viet Nam's TB control programme. Viet Nam's longstanding relationship with the Medical Committee Netherlands Viet Nam and, more recently, technical and funding partnerships with KNCV and

(a) NTP budget by source of funding

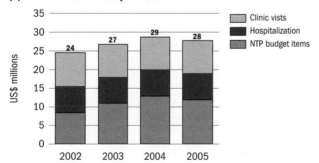

(b) NTP budget by line item

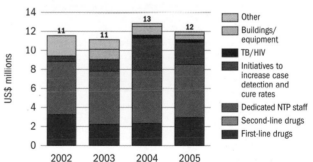

(c) Total TB control costs by line item[a]

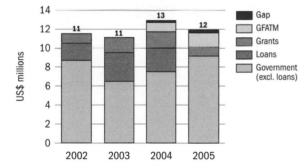

(d) Per patient costs, budgets, available funding and expenditures

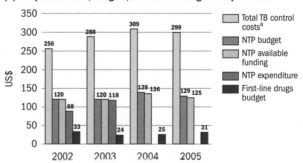

[a] Total TB control costs for 2002 and 2003 are based on expenditures, whereas those for 2004 and 2005 are based on budgets. Estimates of the costs of clinic visits and hospitalization are WHO estimates based on data provided by the NTP and from other sources. See Methods for further details.

the Dutch Government, have created nationwide TB services of high quality. A grant from the GFATM (signed in late 2003) is being used to reach TB patients among high-risk groups, remote populations and PLWHA. WHO and CDC provide technical and financial support for TB control activities, and CDC operates a Global AIDS Programme office in Viet Nam. A World Bank loan assists with purchase of anti-TB drugs.

Budgets and expenditures

The NTP budget has consistently been about US$ 11–13 million per year between 2002 and 2005. Unlike most other HBCs, there has been no need for large increases in the budget during the period 2002–2005 because case detection and treatment success rates were already at target levels in 2002. Nevertheless, some budget increases have been planned, for example to allow better access to DOTS in remote areas and for a national prevalence survey.

Most funding is provided by the government (including loans), but grants also make an important contribution, and GFATM funding accounts for about 13% of the budget in 2005. Actual expenditures in 2003 were very similar to the planned budget. The NTP budget is consistently about US$ 120–140 per patient treated, while the total cost of TB control (including a network of dedicated hospital beds for TB patients and visits to clinics for DOT and monitoring during treatment) is consistently about US$ 250–300 per patient treated. The total estimated cost of TB control has remained stable at US$ 24–30 million per year.

Zimbabwe

Zimbabwe adopted the DOTS strategy in 1992 and has been reporting nationwide coverage since 2000. TB treatment is provided free of charge to all patients and an adequate supply of anti-TB drugs is assured until 2006. Nevertheless, Zimbabwe still has some way to go to reach the global targets for case detection and treatment success. Many difficulties face TB control efforts, including insufficient funding, severe staff shortages and the impact of the HIV/AIDS epidemic. WHO estimates that, in 2003, 69% of TB patients were HIV-positive. Efforts to address the needs arising from widespread TB/HIV coinfection are still in the developmental stage.

System of TB control

Zimbabwe's NTP was established in the 1960s. In 1983, the government introduced a policy of integrating all TB control activities into the general health services. The DOTS strategy was officially adopted by the NTP in 1997. The NTP operates at three levels: central, provincial/local authority and district. At the central level, the NTP is part of the HIV/AIDS/STI and TB unit and is responsible for planning, coordination, monitoring, training and evaluation of programme performance. At the provincial level, training of staff and collection and analysis of TB data are the responsibility of the provincial epidemiology and disease control officer. Four local authorities (Bulawayo, Gweru, Harare and Mutare) run their own TB control programmes, but follow national guidelines and report to the NTP. Mission hospitals, health services of the uniformed forces and some large private organizations also provide TB control services according to national guidelines. The district is the basic management unit for TB control and is responsible for diagnosis, treatment and follow-up of patients, as well as supervision and monitoring of treatment, registration and compilation of quarterly and annual reports. There are rural health centres or municipal clinics in most urban localities that function as primary health-care facilities. These centres and clinics assist in the identification and referral of TB suspects, supervision and observation of treatment and follow-up of contacts and defaulters.

The laboratory network consists of an NRL, 10 intermediate (province/city) laboratories and 96 peripheral laboratories. All intermediate and peripheral laboratories do smear microscopy and refer re-treatment and failure cases for culture and drug susceptibility testing to the NRL. In addition, the NRL is responsible for providing overall assistance and EQA to all laboratories in the network. There are more than 30 private laboratories that do smear microscopy for private and public providers and that participate in the NTP laboratory network, but they are not involved in the NRL EQA.

Surveillance and monitoring

The total number of TB cases reported in Zimbabwe rose from 6000 in 1988 to 60 000 in 2002. However, the rate of increase has been slowing since 1997, and the number of reported cases fell between 2002 and 2003. The smear-positive case notification rate has been fairly stable since 1997, so the proportion of cases diagnosed as smear-positive has fallen. This proportion was only 27% in 2003, indicating poor diagnostic technique. In 2003, Zimbabwe experienced nationwide industrial action in the public health sector for three months, which adversely affected diagnosis and treatment of TB. It is not clear whether these trends reflect the underlying trends in incidence or variations in the quality of reporting, but the pattern is similar in some other eastern and southern African countries with high rates of HIV infection. Case detection under DOTS was in the range 40–50% between 2000 and 2003, but further investigation is needed to verify this estimate.

The treatment success rate was 67% for patients registered in 2002 and has remained at this level since 1998. In the 2002 cohort, 11% of patients died and 22% either defaulted or were transferred between

PROGRESS IN TB CONTROL IN ZIMBABWE

Indicators

DOTS treatment success, 2002 cohort	67%
DOTS case detection rate, 2003	42%
NTP budget available, 2004	58%
Government contribution to NTP budget, including loans, 2004	27%
Government contribution to total TB control costs, including loans, 2004	59%
Government health spending used for TB control, 2004	4%

Major achievements

— Training of all laboratory staff and strengthening of laboratory supervision
— Training of prison health workers on DOTS
— Joint MoH/WHO review of the NTP in November 2003

Major planned activities

— Strengthen the EQA system in both public and private laboratories
— Improve the recording and reporting system that links the national reference laboratory and public and private laboratories
— Introduce DOTS to prison services and train prison health-care workers
— Introduce community-based DOTS in one pilot district
— Introduce FDCs
— Revise national TB manual
— Train TB microscopists

LATEST ESTIMATES[a]		TRENDS	2000	2001	2002	2003
Population	12 891 242	DOTS coverage (%)	100	100	100	100
Global rank (by est. number of cases)	19	Notification rate (all cases/100 000 pop)	402	441	461	413
Incidence (all cases/100 000 pop/year)	659	Notification rate (new ss+/100 000 pop)	114	120	124	112
Incidence (new ss+/100 000 pop/year)	265	Detection of all cases (%)	65	68	70	63
Prevalence (all cases/100 000 pop)	660	Case detection rate (new ss+, %)	46	46	47	42
TB mortality (all cases/100 000 pop/year)	153	DOTS case detection rate (new ss+, %)	46	46	47	42
TB cases HIV+ (adults aged 15–49, %)	69	DOTS case detection rate (new ss+)/coverage (%)	46	46	47	42
New cases multidrug resistant (%)	1.9	DOTS treatment success (new ss+, %)	69	71	67	–

Notification rate (per 100 000 pop)

— = ss+ cases   — = all cases (53 183 in 2003)

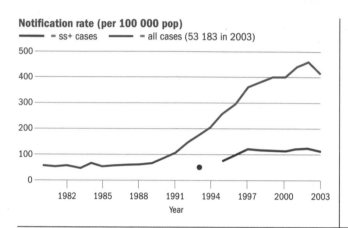

Notification rate by age and sex (new ss+)[b]

— = female   — = male

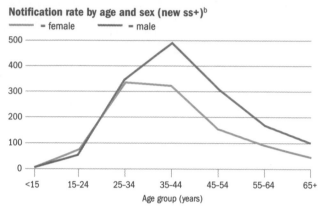

Case types notified

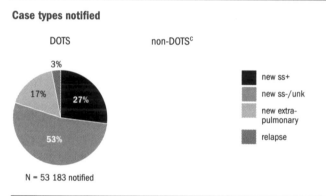

N = 53 183 notified

- new ss+
- new ss-/unk
- new extra-pulmonary
- relapse

DOTS progress towards targets[d]

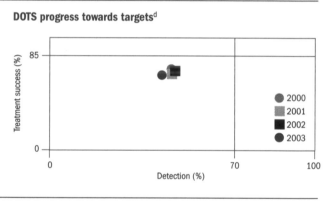

- 2000
- 2001
- 2002
- 2003

DOTS treatment outcomes (new ss+)

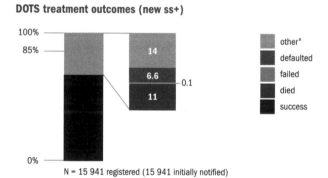

N = 15 941 registered (15 941 initially notified)

- other[e]
- defaulted
- failed
- died
- success

Non-DOTS treatment outcomes (new ss+)

Notes

ss+ indicates smear-positive; ss-, smear-negative; pop, population; unk, unknown.

Absence of a graph indicates that the data were not available or applicable.

[a] See Methods for data sources. Prevalence and mortality estimates include patients with HIV.

[b] The sum of cases notified by age and sex is less than the number of new smear-positive cases notified for some countries.

[c] Non-DOTS is blank for countries which are 100% DOTS, or where no non-DOTS data were reported.

[d] DOTS case detection rate for given year, DOTS treatment success rate for cohort registered in previous year.

[e] "Other" includes transfer out and not evaluated, still on treatment, and other unknown.

treatment centres without follow-up. Among patients registered for re-treatment, 20% were reported to have died, 16% defaulted or transferred without follow-up.

While it would be valuable to assess the impact of DOTS on the burden of TB in Zimbabwe, the immediate priority is to evaluate more accurately the progress made in programme implementation (case detection, treatment success) against the background of changing TB incidence, prevalence and death rates.

Improving programme performance

The high rates of HIV infection together with unfavourable socioeconomic conditions have had an impact on general health services in Zimbabwe in the past year, and will also affect TB control activities. A national review of the NTP by MoH/WHO carried out in November 2003 included a review of activities at the central level, in all eight provinces and the three major cities (Bulawayo, Chitungwiza and Harare). Recommendations were made on strengthening existing TB control and collaborative TB/HIV activities in order to reverse the downward trends in case detection and treatment success. Senior ministry officials are committed to improving TB control and a national TB policy, strategic plan and manual have been developed. However, the strategic plan for DOTS expansion has not been adopted nationally and there are serious financial and infrastructural deficiencies at all levels.

There is a severe shortage of human resources at all levels, especially at the central level. The NTP continues to be adversely affected by the departure of experienced staff from the public to the private sectors and to other countries. Five of the eight provincial TB coordinators were appointed in the past year and many districts have no TB coordinators. The NTP is planning to identify districts without coordinators, appoint new staff and ensure that all district hospitals have a staff member responsible for TB. Staffing at the central level has been strengthened by the appoint-

ment of a national TB coordinator to assist the NTP manager and by NTP advisers and officers that have been seconded by IUATLD and CDC. Training for staff has been intensified and efforts have been made to train prison health workers on the DOTS strategy.

IEC material is generally available at most facilities; however, it is produced centrally, which reduces its impact in areas where other languages are spoken. No national advocacy plan has been developed.

The supply of high quality anti-TB drugs is guaranteed until the end of 2006, with funding from the European Union, but FDCs and paediatric formulations are not available. The NTP intends to introduce FDCs in early 2005. The last national DRS was done in 1994–1995, when the prevalence of MDR-TB in previously untreated patients was 1.4%. No recent data on the prevalence of MDR-TB are available, but another DRS is planned for 2005. The draft policy document on MDR-TB management is awaiting finalization. Consequently, no second-line drugs are currently being used.

Other areas where programme performance needs to be improved include diagnostic laboratory services, TB/HIV coordination and links with other health-care providers.

Diagnostic and laboratory services

Training of laboratory staff and strengthening of laboratory supervision were undertaken in 2003–2004, but many facilities still have untrained staff. Similarly, while EQA systems were strengthened, financial and staffing constraints mean that some quality assurance activities were not routinely performed or have been suspended at national and provincial levels. A major problem for the laboratory services in Zimbabwe is the shortage of staff associated with the elimination of many posts for microscopists, and the movement of trained staff to the private sector or to other countries. The country is planning to train basic-level TB microscopists in 2005 to help to rectify this problem.

TB/HIV coordination

The number of AIDS cases and AIDS-related deaths continues to increase in Zimbabwe. There is no routine HIV surveillance among TB patients, but WHO estimates that 69% of adult TB patients are infected with HIV. The government has set up units to manage opportunistic infections, including provision of co-trimoxazole and fluconazole to PLWHA, and plans to begin delivery of ART in Harare and Mpilo hospitals in the near future. The government has also signed a policy on the use of co-trimoxazole among HIV-positive TB patients, though not yet on the use of isoniazid preventive therapy in PLWHA.

A TB/HIV working group has been set up and collaborative TB/HIV activities have been planned. To date, few of these activities have started. WHO is funding a community TB/HIV care initiative in one district and HIV surveillance among TB patients is planned for 2005.

Links with other health-care providers

Private laboratories have been included in the NTP laboratory network. A small-scale PPM-DOTS project involving private practitioners and hospitals is being piloted in Harare. The NTP is involving medical colleges, specialist TB hospitals, prison health services, mission hospitals and health services operated by the police and the armed forces in DOTS implementation. A few large agricultural and mining companies also provide TB control services to their employees and dependants according to national guidelines.

Partnerships

Technical assistance is provided by IUATLD and WHO. The CDC provides laboratory support (reagents and other consumables) and the EU provides funding for anti-TB drugs. There is a national TB expert committee that guides policy development and implementation, but there is currently no interagency body coordinating TB control. However, a country coordination committee meets monthly and functions as the national TB/HIV coordinating body.

(a) NTP budget by source of funding

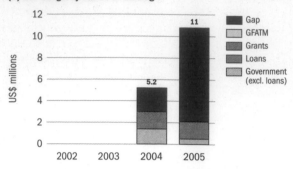

Legend: Gap, GFATM, Grants, Loans, Government (excl. loans)

(b) NTP budget by line item

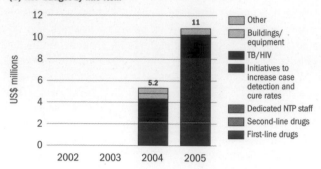

Legend: Other, Buildings/equipment, TB/HIV, Initiatives to increase case detection and cure rates, Dedicated NTP staff, Second-line drugs, First-line drugs

(c) Total TB control costs by line item[a]

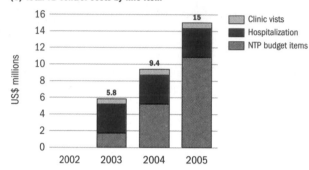

Legend: Clinic vists, Hospitalization, NTP budget items

(d) Per patient costs, budgets, available funding and expenditures

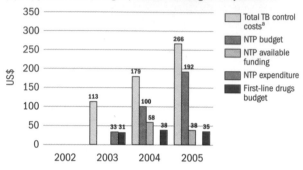

Legend: Total TB control costs[a], NTP budget, NTP available funding, NTP expenditure, First-line drugs budget

[a] Total TB control costs for 2003 are based on expenditures, whereas those for 2004 and 2005 are based on budgets. Estimates of the costs of clinic visits and hospitalization are WHO estimates based on data provided by the NTP and from other sources. See Methods for further details.

Budgets and expenditures

The NTP budget for 2005 is US$ 11 million, compared with US$ 5 million in 2004 (about US$ 200 per patient vs US$ 100 per patient). The increased budget reflects plans to increase spending on various initiatives, including collaborative TB/HIV activities, training, monitoring and evaluation, and community TB care. However, available funding is limited, at only around US$ 2 million in 2005. This is down from available funding of US$ 3 million in 2004, but a slight increase compared with expenditures of US$ 1.7 million in 2003. The government's contribution to funding is likely to be higher than reported, as finan-cial support for buildings and equip-ment is not reflected in disease con-trol programme budgets. Most of the grant funding for first-line drugs is pro-vided by the EU through the essential drugs programme and has remained constant between 2003 and 2005 at around US$ 1.6 million each year (equivalent to about US$ 35 per pa-tient treated). At around US$ 9 mil-lion, the funding gap in 2005 is equivalent to 80% of the budget. Zim-babwe is likely to apply to the GFATM in round 5 to address this gap.

The total cost of TB control, which includes the cost of dedicated TB beds and clinic visits during treatment as well as items included in the NTP budget, was about US$ 6 million in 2003 (just over US$ 100 per patient treated). If the 2005 NTP budget is fully funded and spent, this will in-crease to about US$ 15 million in 2005 (about US$ 270 per patient treated). The estimated cost of dedi-cated TB hospital beds, at US$ 3.5 million, is based on an estimate of 1660 dedicated TB beds, including those in mission hospitals. However, since occupancy in district hospitals is decreasing (for example because of a new admission policy introduced in the late 1990s) and beds are be-ing reallocated to other diseases, this may be an overestimate.

Explanatory notes

Country-specific data grouped by WHO region. For each country we present:

■ Estimated burden of TB in 1990 (baseline year for MDG) and 2003 (the latest year covered by this report). Estimates of TB include incidence, prevalence and death rates.

■ Population, TB notifications (numbers and rates), detection rates (countrywide and under DOTS), DOTS coverage and percentage of pulmonary cases that were smear-positive (DOTS and non-DOTS) in 2003.

■ Treatment outcomes for cases registered in 2002 – the new smear-positive cohort for both DOTS and (where available) non-DOTS programmes, and all re-treatment cases (taken together, where available) from DOTS programmes.

■ Treatment outcomes for specific re-treatment cohorts from DOTS programmes in 2002 – relapse, after-failure and after-default cohorts.

■ Trends in DOTS treatment success (1994–2002) and DOTS case detection (1995–2003).

■ Age and sex distribution (numbers) of new smear-positive notifications from DOTS and non-DOTS programmes.

■ Age and sex rates of new smear-positive notifications countrywide.

■ Notifications (numbers and rates) of TB (all forms) since 1980.

■ Notifications (numbers and rates) of new smear-positive cases since 1993.

■ Country notes: remarks from respondents that may help to explain data in selected countries' reports.

Notation for 1st table
Country data ... estimated burden of TB
See Methods section for information on how estimates are derived.

"Incl. HIV+" means including HIV+ TB cases; "Excl. HIV+" means excluding HIV+ TB cases.

Rate: the number per 100 000 population. (For incidence and death rates, the number represents events occurring annually.)

Notation for 2nd table
Country data ... notification, detection and DOTS coverage, 2003
Pop thousands: the population of the country or territory, expressed in thousands, from the United Nations Population Division, World Population Prospects, 2002 revision.

All cases, country, number [a]: the total number of TB cases according to the country's count.

All cases, WHO, number [b]: the total number of TB cases notified to WHO (WHO definition of a TB case notification, which includes new and relapse cases and, for the WHO European region only, cases with previous history unknown).

All cases, rate: cases notified to WHO per 100 000 population.

New cases, smear-positive, rate: per 100 000 population.

New cases, pulm confirmed: new pulmonary laboratory-confirmed cases.

Re-treatment cases: see definitions in Methods section. "Other" re-treatment includes cases that were classified as re-treatment but were not specified as relapse, after-failure or after-default.

Other, number: TB cases that were not classified as new or re-treatment. These cases plus re-treatment cases other than relapse cases make up the gap (if any) between the country's count of TB cases and WHO notifications.

Detection rate, all cases: the proportion of all estimated cases (all forms) that were notified.

Detection rate, new ss+: the proportion of estimated new smear-positive cases that were notified.

DOTS % of pop: the percentage of the population living in geographical areas nominally serviced by health facilities implementing DOTS.

DOTS, DDR: the new smear-positive detection rate of DOTS programmes.

DOTS, % of pulm. cases ss+: the percentage of new pulmonary cases in DOTS programmes that are smear-positive.

Notation for 3rd table
Country data ... treatment outcomes for cases registered in 2002
Number of cases notified: the number of new smear-positive cases notified in 2002 and representing, in theory, a cohort of cases for which treatment outcomes should be monitored.

Number of cases registered: the number of new smear-positive cases ultimately reported as constituting the cohort for treatment outcome monitoring which, ideally, should be close the number of cases initially notified (see Methods section).

% of notif registered: the percentage of notified cases that was ultimately represented by the number of cases registered

% not eval: the difference between the number registered and the sum of the six mutually exclusive outcomes (cured, completed, died, failed, defaulted, transferred-out, see definitions in the Methods section).

Africa

AFR

	STATUS[a]	MANUAL[b]	MICROSCOPY[c]	SCC[d]	DOT[e]	MONITORING OUTCOME[f]
ALGERIA	DOTS	YES				
ANGOLA	DOTS	YES				
BENIN	DOTS	YES				
BOTSWANA	DOTS	YES				
BURKINA FASO	DOTS	YES				
BURUNDI	DOTS	YES				
CAMEROON	DOTS	YES				
CAPE VERDE	NON-DOTS	YES				
CENTRAL AFRICAN REPUBLIC	DOTS	YES				
CHAD	DOTS	YES				
COMOROS	DOTS	YES				
CONGO	DOTS	YES				
CÔTE D'IVOIRE	DOTS	YES				
DR CONGO	DOTS	YES				
EQUATORIAL GUINEA						
ERITREA	DOTS	YES				
ETHIOPIA	DOTS	YES				
GABON	DOTS					
GAMBIA	DOTS	YES				
GHANA	DOTS	YES				
GUINEA	DOTS					
GUINEA-BISSAU	DOTS	YES				
KENYA	DOTS	YES				
LESOTHO	DOTS	NO				
LIBERIA						
MADAGASCAR	DOTS	YES				
MALAWI	DOTS	YES				
MALI	DOTS	YES				
MAURITANIA						
MAURITIUS	DOTS	NO				
MOZAMBIQUE	DOTS	YES				
NAMIBIA	DOTS	YES				
NIGER	DOTS					
NIGERIA	DOTS	YES				
RWANDA	DOTS	YES				
SAO TOME AND PRINCIPE						
SENEGAL	DOTS	YES				
SEYCHELLES	DOTS					
SIERRA LEONE	DOTS	YES				
SOUTH AFRICA	DOTS	YES				
SWAZILAND	DOTS	NO				
TOGO	DOTS	YES				
UGANDA	DOTS	YES				
UR TANZANIA	DOTS	YES				
ZAMBIA	DOTS	YES				
ZIMBABWE	DOTS	YES				

Implemented in all units/areas

Implemented in some units/areas

Not implemented

Unknown

a Status: DOTS status (bold indicates DOTS introduced in 2003. Blank indicates no report received)
b Manual: national TB control manual (recommended)
c Microscopy: use of smear microscopy for diagnosis (core component of DOTS)
d SCC: short course chemotherapy (core component of DOTS)
e DOT: directly observed treatment (core component of DOTS)
f Outcome monitoring: monitoring of treatment outcomes by cohort analysis (core component of DOTS)

Country data for Africa: estimated burden of TB

	Incidence, 1990				Prevalence, 1990				Death, 1990				Incidence, 2003				Prevalence, 2003				Death, 2003			
	All cases incl. HIV+		New ss+ incl. HIV+		All cases incl. HIV+		All cases excl. HIV+		All cases incl. HIV+		All cases excl. HIV+		All cases incl. HIV+		New ss+ incl. HIV+		All cases incl. HIV+		All cases excl. HIV+		All cases incl. HIV+		All cases excl. HIV+	
	number	rate	number	rate	number	rate	number	rate	number	rate	number	rate	number	rate	number	rate	number	rate	number	rate	number	rate	number	rate
Algeria	9 094	36	4 091	16	20 647	83	20 647	83	2 383	10	2 383	10	16 790	53	7 552	24	16 774	53	16 757	53	609	2	607	2
Angola	19 729	211	8 636	92	42 306	453	41 603	445	5 520	59	4 802	51	35 236	259	15 424	113	36 997	272	34 835	256	3 446	25	2 699	20
Benin	3 576	77	1 584	34	7 972	171	7 931	171	958	21	915	20	5 869	87	2 600	39	9 713	144	9 506	141	994	15	822	12
Botswana	3 266	241	1 291	95	6 711	496	6 500	480	934	69	704	52	11 307	633	4 469	250	9 202	515	6 105	342	1 530	86	610	34
Burkina Faso	13 142	147	5 718	64	25 420	285	24 172	271	4 066	46	2 790	31	21 174	163	9 213	71	40 946	315	39 370	303	5 912	45	4 342	33
Burundi	6 727	120	2 876	51	13 120	234	12 488	223	2 041	36	1 353	24	23 585	346	10 083	148	38 090	558	35 441	519	6 308	92	4 011	59
Cameroon	7 304	63	3 127	27	16 141	138	15 984	137	1 901	16	1 731	15	28 911	180	12 379	77	38 598	241	35 443	221	5 606	35	3 441	21
Cape Verde	563	161	252	72	1 277	366	1 277	366	147	42	147	42	778	168	349	75	1 526	329	1 519	328	186	40	180	39
Central African Republic	3 318	113	1 379	47	6 622	225	6 352	216	982	33	688	23	12 558	325	5 219	135	21 197	548	19 039	493	4 360	113	2 100	54
Chad	10 722	184	4 666	80	23 085	397	22 731	390	2 986	51	2 624	45	19 385	225	8 437	98	39 188	456	37 752	439	5 645	66	4 151	48
Comoros	449	85	202	38	1 019	193	1 019	193	118	22	118	22	382	50	172	22	795	103	794	103	60	8	59	8
Congo	3 285	132	1 423	57	6 310	253	5 974	240	1 013	41	647	26	14 134	380	6 124	164	19 382	521	18 202	489	2 937	79	2 132	57
Côte d'Ivoire	17 182	137	7 369	59	34 571	276	33 251	266	5 038	40	3 602	29	65 849	396	28 239	170	109 675	659	102 713	618	17 678	106	11 323	68
DR Congo	47 828	128	20 806	56	98 411	263	95 349	255	13 661	37	10 328	28	194 627	369	84 667	160	297 861	564	283 284	537	42 996	81	31 314	59
Equatorial Guinea	558	158	238	67	1 207	341	1 191	337	154	44	137	39	954	193	407	82	1 846	374	1 733	351	312	63	191	39
Eritrea	6 874	222	3 027	98	15 294	493	15 206	490	1 845	59	1 755	57	11 233	271	4 946	119	18 405	444	17 861	431	2 556	62	2 162	52
Ethiopia	60 373	124	26 255	54	131 545	269	129 730	266	16 028	33	14 052	29	251 685	356	109 452	155	377 030	533	358 001	507	56 146	79	42 508	60
Gabon	1 300	136	556	58	2 843	298	2 807	295	343	36	304	32	3 102	233	1 326	100	3 566	268	3 218	242	502	38	302	23
Gambia	1 783	190	796	85	4 042	432	4 040	432	468	50	466	50	3 325	233	1 485	104	4 865	341	4 808	337	591	41	552	39
Ghana	33 599	220	14 771	97	73 925	484	73 260	480	9 136	60	8 456	55	43 881	210	19 292	92	79 466	380	77 193	369	10 572	51	8 513	41
Guinea	7 224	118	3 173	52	16 135	264	16 060	262	1 931	32	1 854	30	19 999	236	8 784	104	34 528	407	33 451	394	4 611	54	3 668	43
Guinea-Bissau	1 647	162	721	71	3 702	364	3 692	363	437	43	426	42	2 962	198	1 296	87	4 659	312	4 476	300	648	43	503	34
Kenya	26 329	112	11 306	48	54 904	233	53 422	227	7 399	31	5 787	25	195 207	610	83 822	262	282 816	884	262 708	821	42 660	133	28 527	89
Lesotho	2 918	186	1 155	74	6 539	416	6 503	414	744	47	704	45	13 203	733	5 228	290	10 598	588	7 030	390	1 972	109	823	46
Liberia	4 363	204	1 882	88	9 172	430	8 965	420	1 246	58	1 035	48	8 422	250	3 633	108	17 073	507	16 287	484	2 639	78	1 797	53
Madagascar	22 936	192	10 184	85	51 917	434	51 873	434	6 032	50	5 987	50	37 605	216	16 697	96	57 622	331	56 494	325	7 059	41	6 201	36
Malawi	24 845	263	10 259	108	49 478	523	47 428	502	7 369	78	5 137	54	53 503	442	22 093	183	66 672	551	56 754	469	13 008	107	6 337	52
Mali	26 883	297	11 889	131	59 223	655	58 711	649	7 299	81	6 777	75	37 470	288	16 571	127	77 191	593	75 738	582	9 799	75	8 346	64
Mauritania	4 755	234	2 128	105	10 781	531	10 778	531	1 248	61	1 244	61	8 295	287	3 712	128	19 324	668	19 220	664	2 232	77	2 120	73
Mauritius	716	68	322	30	1 624	154	1 624	154	188	18	188	18	783	64	352	29	1 666	136	1 664	136	139	11	138	11
Mozambique	21 336	158	8 865	66	44 646	332	43 489	323	5 970	44	4 711	35	86 130	457	35 787	190	120 004	636	105 146	557	24 420	129	11 708	62
Namibia	3 530	251	1 434	102	7 923	562	7 881	559	899	64	854	61	14 351	722	5 829	293	12 630	635	9 486	477	2 422	122	1 029	52
Niger	9 833	129	4 381	57	22 222	290	22 193	290	2 591	34	2 562	33	18 840	157	8 393	70	32 998	276	32 571	272	3 962	33	3 603	30
Nigeria	87 333	102	37 636	44	190 477	221	187 905	218	23 154	27	20 354	24	362 819	293	156 358	126	676 879	546	642 327	518	105 311	85	70 864	57
Rwanda	8 789	130	3 783	56	17 010	251	16 146	238	2 689	40	1 749	26	31 353	374	13 497	161	55 701	664	52 643	628	8 732	104	5 811	69
Sao Tome & Principe	158	136	71	61	358	309	358	309	41	36	41	36	173	108	78	48	410	256	410	256	4	5	4	5
Senegal	14 703	200	6 570	89	33 230	452	33 187	452	3 874	53	3 831	52	24 742	245	11 055	110	43 652	432	43 259	429	5 061	50	4 727	47
Seychelles	31	44	14	20	70	99	70	99	8	11	8	11	28	35	13	16	53	65	53	65	4	5	4	5
Sierra Leone	8 950	221	3 966	98	20 160	497	20 115	496	2 368	58	2 322	57	21 220	427	9 404	189	40 210	809	39 485	794	5 047	102	4 386	88
South Africa	68 593	186	27 890	76	152 637	414	151 465	411	17 682	48	16 407	45	241 537	536	98 208	218	206 110	458	153 694	341	32 794	73	12 459	28
Swaziland	2 259	267	888	105	4 724	558	4 601	543	633	75	498	59	11 666	1 083	4 585	426	10 687	992	7 361	683	2 553	237	893	83
Togo	12 276	355	5 359	155	27 605	799	27 530	797	3 254	94	3 178	92	17 221	351	7 518	153	34 188	696	33 029	673	4 807	98	3 633	74
Uganda	27 641	159	12 018	69	46 922	270	42 367	244	9 547	55	4 589	26	106 201	411	46 176	179	168 387	652	160 315	621	24 692	96	18 233	71
UR Tanzania	47 831	183	20 294	78	96 732	371	93 199	358	13 942	53	10 095	39	137 260	371	58 235	157	193 610	524	175 953	476	31 745	86	19 101	52
Zambia	24 333	297	9 987	122	40 326	492	36 042	440	8 567	104	3 904	48	70 975	656	29 130	269	68 996	638	54 954	508	13 152	122	6 584	61
Zimbabwe	13 719	131	5 507	53	24 035	230	21 984	210	4 614	44	2 381	23	85 015	659	34 126	265	85 129	660	64 474	500	19 749	153	7 869	61
Region	724 602	146	310 745	63	1 525 020	307	1 489 099	300	203 451	41	164 627	33	2 371 745	345	1 012 416	147	3 486 914	507	3 212 558	467	538 212	78	351 432	51

See Explanatory notes, page 151.

Country data for Africa: notification, detection and DOTS coverage, 2003

Country	Pop thousands	All cases Country number	All cases WHO number	All cases rate	New cases Smear-positive number	Smear-positive rate	Pulm confirmed number	Smear-negative or unknown number	Extra-pulmonary number	Re-treatment Relapse number	After failure number	After default number	Other number	Other number	Detection rate All cases %	New ss+ %	DOTS % of pop	DOTS Notif All cases number	rate	New ss+ number	rate	DDR %	% of pulm cases ss+	non-DOTS All cases number	New ss+ number	% of pulm ss+
Algeria	31 800	19 730	19 730	62	8 549	27	8 924	1 812	8 861	508	38	86			118	113	100	19 730	62	8 549	27	113	83	1 987	807	44
Angola	13 625	37 053	36 079	265	18 971	139	0	12 790	2 921	1 397	433	541			102	123	65	34 032	250	18 164	133	118	61			
Benin	6 736	3 172	2 932	44	2 438	36	2 506	68	317	109	63	177			50	94	100	2 547	38	2 438	36	94	100	385		0
Botswana	1 785	10 030	9 862	552	3 050	171	3 050	5 021	1 183	608	55	113			87	68	100	9 852	552	3 050	171	68	38			
Burkina Faso	13 002	2 765	2 620	20	1 703	13	1 703	266	535	116	85	60			12	18	100	2 620	20	1 703	13	18	86			
Burundi	6 825	6 846	6 822	100	3 017	44	3 017	1 467	2 242	96	6	18			29	30	100	6 822	100	3 017	44	30	67			
Cameroon	16 018	16 509	15 964	100	10 692	67	10 692	2 951	1 649	672	82			463	55	86	100	15 964	100	10 692	67	86	78			
Cape Verde	463	323	316	68	165		165	111	21	111	2	5			41	47	0							316	165	60
Central African Republic	3 865	2 817	3 932	102	2 818	73	2 817	752	362	19					31	54	68	507	13	320	8	6	72	3 425	2 498	80
Chad	8 598	4 499	4 679	54	3 599	42	3 599	700	200	160	72	260			24	43	25	1 149	13	899	10	11	84	3 530	2 700	84
Comoros	768	91	89	12	63	8	63	3	20	3	0	2			23	37	100	89	12	63	8	37	95			
Congo	3 724	9 053	7 782	209	3 477	93		2 080	2 075	150	15	67			55	57	80	7 782	209	3 477	93	57	63			
Côte d'Ivoire	16 631	18 213	17 782	107	11 411	69		2 250	3 564	557	274	157			27	40	74	16 998	102	10 915	66	39	83	784	496	85
DR Congo	52 771	86 715	84 687	160	53 578	102	53 578	9 352	18 357	3 400	676	965		387	44	63	75	84 687	160	53 578	102	63	85			
Equatorial Guinea	494																									
Eritrea	4 141	4 708	4 708	114	887	21	887	2 363	1 308	101	15	31		3	42	18	60	4 708	114	887	21	18	27			
Ethiopia	70 678	118 276	117 600	166	39 698	56	39 698	35 141	40 883	1 873	242	434			47	36	95	117 600	166	39 698	56	36	53			
Gabon	1 329	2 174	2 174	164	1 233	93		683	149	109	27	55			70	93	22	2 174	164	1 233	93	93	64			
Gambia	1 426	1 985	1 945	136	1 040	73	1 040	786	95	24	3	37			58	70	100	1 945	136	1 040	73	70	57			
Ghana	20 922	11 891	11 891	57	7 714	37		2 860	759	553					27	40	100	11 891	57	7 714	37	40	73			
Guinea	8 480	6 570	6 570	77	4 495	53		486	1 376	213	43			213	33	51	100	6 570	77	4 495	53	51	90			
Guinea-Bissau	1 493	1 647	1 647	110	963	65	963	450	59	123		47			56	74	40	1 327	89	715	48	55	64	320	248	83
Kenya	31 987	95 310	91 522	286	38 158	119		37 135	13 403	2 826	104	1 023		2 661	47	46	100	91 522	286	38 158	119	46	51			
Lesotho	1 802	13 341	12 007	666	3 652	203	3 652	5 404	2 402	549	67	371		887	91	70	100	12 007	666	3 652	203	70	40			
Liberia	3 367																									
Madagascar	17 404	19 799	19 309	111	12 881	74	12 881	1 910	3 580	938	134	356			51	77	100	19 309	111	12 881	74	77	87			
Malawi	12 105	28 234	25 841	213	7 716	64	8 766	11 246	5 829	1 050				2 393	48	35	100	25 841	213	7 716	64	35	41			
Mali	13 007	4 545	4 496	35	3 015	23	3 015	501	652	228	18	31			12	18	100	4 496	35	3 015	23	18	83			
Mauritania	2 893																									
Mauritius	1 221	137	137	11	99	8	99	17	17	17	1	1			18	28	100	137	11	99	8	28	85			
Mozambique	18 863	29 107	28 602	152	16 138	86	16 138	7 847	3 441	1 176	182	323			33	45	100	28 602	152	16 138	86	45	67			
Namibia	1 987	12 931	11 776	593	5 004	252		4 642	1 365	765				1 155	82	86	100	11 776	593	5 004	252	86	52			
Niger	11 972	7 423	7 078	59	4 505	38		1 070	1 106	397	156	189			38	54	50	7 073	59	4 505	38	54	81			
Nigeria	124 009	46 596	44 184	36	28 173	23		13 276	1 525	1 210	888	1 263		261	12	18	60	44 184	36	28 173	23	18	68			
Rwanda	8 387	6 046	5 895	70	3 710	44	3 710	652	1 194	335	45	34		72	19	27	100	5 895	70	3 710	44	27	85			
Sao Tome & Principe	161																									
Senegal	10 095	9 796	9 380	93	6 587	65		1 421	951	421	49	367			38	59	100	9 380	93	6 587	65	59	82			
Seychelles	81	10	10	12	5	6		4	4	0	0	0			36	40	100	10	12	5	6	40	56			
Sierra Leone	4 971	5 421	5 289	106	3 113	63		1 695	388	93	33	99			25	33	100	5 289	106	3 113	63	33	65			
South Africa	45 026	255 422	227 320	505	116 364	258	116 364	56 540	37 686	16 730	1 603	3 317	23 182		94	118	100	227 278	505	116 331	258	118	67	42	33	87
Swaziland	1 077	7 869	7 749	719	1 585	147		4 582	1 012	570	37	83			66	35	100	7 749	719	1 585	147	35	26			
Togo	4 909	1 766	1 766	36	1 257	26		125	283	101	26				10	17	100	1 766	36	1 257	26	17	91			
Uganda	25 827	42 901	41 805	162	20 320	79	20 320	16 612	3 249	1 624	128			1 096	39	44	100	41 805	162	20 320	79	44	55			
UR Tanzania	36 977	64 665	61 579	167	24 899	67	46 810	21 511	12 959	1 810		250		2 708	45	43	100	61 579	167	24 899	67	43	53			
Zambia	10 812	58 032	53 932	499	18 934	175	18 934	24 900	7 930	2 168	431			3 669	76	65	100	53 932	499	18 934	175	65	43			
Zimbabwe	12 891	57 117	53 183	413	14 488	112	32 702	28 246	8 916	1 533				3 934	63	42	100	53 183	413	14 488	112	42	34			
Region	**687 405**	**1 129 361**	**1 072 671**	**156**	**510 164**	**74**	**405 410**	**322 228**	**194 825**	**45 358**	**6 007**	**10 762**	**23 182**	**19 902**	**45**	**50**	**85**	**1 061 882**	**154**	**503 217**	**73**	**50**	**61**	**10 789**	**6 947**	**73**

See Explanatory notes, page 151.

Country data for Africa: treatment outcomes for cases registered in 2002

New smear-positive cases – DOTS

	Number of cases notified	Number of cases regist'd	% of notif regist'd	% cured	% compl-eted	% died	% failed	% default	% trans-ferred	% not eval	% success
Algeria	8 246	9 200	112	72	17	2	0	4	4		89
Angola	17 345	17 345	100	65	9	3	1	20	2		74
Benin	2 415	2 420	100	55	25	6	2	11	1		80
Botswana	3 334	3 458	104	35	36	9	1	8	12		71
Burkina Faso	1 544	1 518	98	58	7	12	3	13	6		64
Burundi	2 791	3 138	112	37	42	4	0	16	1		79
Cameroon	7 365	7 365	100	61	8	6	2	20	1	2	70
Cape Verde	2 657										
Central African Republic											
Chad	3 417	791	23	22	50	5	1	11	11		72
Comoros		72		94	1	3		1			96
Congo	5 019	5 019	100	56	14	3	1	22	4		71
Côte d'Ivoire	10 255	10 236	100	54	13	7	2	16	8		67
DR Congo	44 518	45 013	101	71	8	7	1	8	5	2	78
Equatorial Guinea											
Eritrea	646	853	132	73	9	6	2	6	4		82
Ethiopia	36 541	36 541	100	59	17	7	1	5	10	2	76
Gabon	1 033	1 033	100	47		5	1	40	2	5	47
Gambia	1 035	1 035	100	67	7	5	3	11	7		74
Ghana	7 732	7 732	100	55	5	8	0	15	6	10	60
Guinea	4 300	4 246	99	61	10	9	1	10	9		72
Guinea-Bissau	532	532	100	33	14	3	0	19	30		48
Kenya	34 337	30 966	90	65	14	5	0	9	7		79
Lesotho	3 167	3 167	100	29	23	11	1	5	5	27	52
Liberia											
Madagascar	11 387	11 145	98	65	9	2	6	15	3		74
Malawi	7 703	7 703	100	70	3	19	1	4	3	0	72
Mali	2 757	2 757	100	33	18	5	2	19	5	19	50
Mauritania											
Mauritius	86	86	100	88	3	2	2	3	2	0	92
Mozambique	15 236	15 236	100	77	1	11	1	7	2	0	78
Namibia	4 690	4 649	99	42	19	8	2	13	7	9	62
Niger											
Nigeria	19 596	20 559	105	69	10	2	7	11	1		79
Rwanda	3 956	3 975	100	48	10	7	1	4	21	9	58
Sao Tome & Principe											
Senegal	5 796	5 796	100	59	8	4	1	17	7	5	66
Seychelles	9	11	122	45		27			27		45
Sierra Leone	2 938	2 915	99	60	21	1	5	13	0		81
South Africa	97 656	98 090	100	54	14	9	1	13	9		68
Swaziland	1 410	1 412	100	16	31	9	0	14	30		47
Togo	421	990	235	67	1	13	2	15	2		68
Uganda	19 088	19 098	100	30	31	6	0	19	7	7	60
UR Tanzania	24 136	24 136	100	76	4	11	0	4	4	0	80
Zambia	11 694	11 694	100	67	16	10	0	3	1		83
Zimbabwe	15 941	15 941	100	62	6	11	0	7	15		67
Region	**442 729**	**437 873**	**99**	**60**	**13**	**7**	**1**	**11**	**7**	**1**	**73**

New smear-positive cases – non-DOTS

	Number of cases notified	Number of cases regist'd	% of notif regist'd	% cured	% compl-eted	% died	% failed	% default	% trans-ferred	% not eval	% success
Algeria	742										
Cameroon	556										
Cape Verde	111	34	31	53		9		18	21		53
Central African Republic	101										
Chad	102	2 630	2 578	14	40	8	18	5	15		54
Côte d'Ivoire	771	336	336	9	7	3	2	64	15		16
Guinea-Bissau	367	367	100	38	30	13	1	14	5		68
Madagascar		69		57	10	7		23	3		67
Nigeria	2 340										
Rwanda	42										
South Africa	1 143	1 239	108	59	6	5	2	13	8	6	65
Togo	782										
Zambia	4 657	4 657	100	55	16	13	8	7	5		71
Region	**11 714**	**9 332**	**80**	**42**	**22**	**10**	**8**	**10**	**8**	**1**	**63**

Smear-positive re-treatment cases – DOTS

	Number regist'd	% cured	% compl-eted	% died	% failed	% default	% trans-ferred	% not eval	% success
Algeria	644	65	13	4	1	13	3	1	78
Angola	2 320	40	11			20		29	51
Benin	338	49	26	5	6	13	1		75
Botswana	294	30	35	15	1	11	9		65
Burkina Faso	185	51	8	11	8	13	10		58
Burundi	51	41	22	12		24	2		63
Cameroon	185	59	9	10	6	14	1		69
Cape Verde	12	67				8	25		67
Chad	89	42	47	3	1	2	4	1	89
Congo	132	61	17	6		15	1		78
Côte d'Ivoire	486	38	12	7	11	26	6		50
DR Congo	4 618	61	6	9	4	10	7	3	67
Eritrea	119	79	8	3	4	3	2	1	87
Ethiopia	1 716	52	9	7	3	5	2	22	60
Gambia	149	41				3	35		41
Guinea	340	50	11	12	5	12	9		61
Guinea-Bissau	103	38	28	2		16	17		66
Kenya	2 476	65	12	10	0	7	6		77
Madagascar	975	61	8	4	6	15	6		69
Malawi	862	66	4	24	1	4	1		71
Mali	207	34	13	6	1	29	8	8	47
Mauritius	4	50			50				50
Mozambique	1 721	65	1	12	2	9	4	6	67
Namibia	849	42	24	12	4	12	6	1	66
Nigeria	2 373	63	11	5	8	11	1	2	73
Rwanda	376	40	4	10	4	4	22	17	44
Senegal	924	43	6	5	2	20	7	17	49
Sierra Leone	170	52	11	6	8	21	3		62
South Africa	28 755	43	10	11	2	17	10	7	53
Swaziland	367	2	27	8	1	14	49		29
Togo	150	35	3	3	6	10		47	35
Uganda	2 555	28	27	10	1	16	5	13	55
UR Tanzania	2 081	71	6	13	1	13	4	1	77
Zambia	1 577	63	13	3	2	3	4		76
Zimbabwe	1 371	58	5	20	1	8	9		63
Region	**59 574**	**49**	**11**	**10**	**2**	**14**	**8**	**7**	**59**

See Explanatory notes, page 151.

Country data for Africa: re-treatment outcomes for cases registered in 2002

Country	Relapse – DOTS number regist'd	% cured	% compl-eted	% died	% failed	% default	% trans-ferred	% not eval	% success	After failure – DOTS number regist'd	% cured	% compl-eted	% died	% failed	% default	% trans-ferred	% not eval	% success	After default – DOTS number regist'd	% cured	% compl-eted	% died	% failed	% default	% trans-ferred	% not eval	% success
Algeria	510	70	13	3	1	9	4		83	46	41	11	7	7	20	6	15	52	88	45	17	6		30	1	1	63
Angola																											
Benin																											
Botswana																											
Burkina Faso	93	54	3	12	10	9	13		57	54	52	9	7	11	15	6		61	38	42	16	13		21	8		58
Burundi																											
Camercon																											
Cape Verde																											
Central African Republic																											
Chad	24	79	13	4	4	4			92	5	80	20						100	60	23	63	3		3	7		87
Comoros																											
Congo	132	61	17	6		15	1		78																		
Côte d'Ivoire	3 124	64	5	9	2	7	8	4	70	581	49	5	13	12	12	8	1	54	913	56	8	9	2	17	5	2	64
DR Congo																											
Equatorial Guinea																											
Eritrea	82	83	7	1	4	4	1		90	12	67	8	8	8			8	75	25	72	12	4	4	4	4		84
Ethiopie																											
Gabon																											
Gambia	34	50		26		6	18		50	3	67		33					67	112	38		18	1	3	41		38
Ghana																											
Guinea																											
Guinea-Bissau	67	42	31	3		9	15		73	1	100							100									
Kenya	2 476	65	12	10	0	7	6		77										35	29	23			29	20		51
Lesotho																											
Liberia																											
Madagascar																											
Malawi	862	66	4	24	1	4	1		71																		
Mali	207	34	13	6	1	29	8	8	47																		
Mauritania																											
Mauritius	2	50			50				50	1				100					1	100							100
Mozambique	1 148	68	1	13	2	8	5	3	59	202	52		8	7	11	5	6	62	371	60	2	11	2	12		13	62
Namibie	849	42	24	12	4	12	6	1	66																		
Niger																											
Nigeria																											
Rwanda																											
Sao Tome & Principe																											
Senegal																											
Seychelles																											
Sierra Leone	72	69	10	4	6	11			79	22	41	5	18	9	27	14	15	45	76	38	13	4	9	29	7		51
South Africa	12 562	44	13	10	1	12	9	12	56	1 010	33	11	12	2	13	7	15	44	3 075	34	12	9	2	24	8	12	46
Swaziland																										100	
Togo	43							100		11							100		16								
Uganda	1 771	29	25	9	1	14	4	19	54																		
UR Tanzania	1 703	76	3	13	0	4	3	0	79	140	60	5	17	4	5	7	2	65	238	42	30	11	1	11	6		71
Zambia	1 577	63	13	14	2	3	5		76																		
Zimbabwe	1 371	58	5	20	1	8	9		63																		
Region	**28 709**	**53**	**11**	**11**	**1**	**10**	**7**	**7**	**64**	**2 088**	**43**	**8**	**12**	**6**	**12**	**10**	**9**	**51**	**5 048**	**41**	**12**	**9**	**2**	**20**	**8**	**9**	**52**

AFR

See Explanatory notes for previous table, page 151.

Country data for Africa: trends in DOTS treatment success and detection rates, 1994–2003

	DOTS new smear-positive treatment success (%)									DOTS new smear-positive case detection rate (%)								
	1994	1995	1996	1997	1998	1999	2000	2001	2002	1995	1996	1997	1998	1999	2000	2001	2002	2003
Algeria			86			87	87	84	89			134			126	115	114	113
Angola		73	72	15	68	77	68	66	74		92	69	44	58		85	118	118
Benin	76		70	73	77	77	79	79	80		92	92	91	97	98		96	94
Botswana	72	67	70	70	47	71	77	78	71	94	87	87	88	72	76	71	76	68
Burkina Faso		25	29	61	59	61	60	65	64	11	19	15	17	18	19	18	17	18
Burundi	44	45		67	74	75	80	80	79	20	25	31	19	39		35	30	30
Cameroon				80	75		77	62	70		5		11		35	43	63	86
Cape Verde																42	54	
Central African Republic		37						61			64					9		6
Chad	63	47			64		57		72	34	14		54	42			42	11
Comoros	94	90				93	93	92	96	54	57		49		49	52		37
Congo	69					61	69	66	71	66					86	81	88	57
Côte d'Ivoire	17	68	56	61	62	63		73	67	54	53	49	49	46	36	10	39	39
DR Congo	71	80	48	64	70	69	78	77	78	43	49	46	57	56	53	58	57	63
Equatorial Guinea	89	89	77	82						75	69	71	86					
Eritrea				83	73	44	76	80	82			3	4	13	14	16	14	18
Ethiopia	74	61	73	72	74	76	80	76	76	16	21	23	25	26	35	35	36	36
Gabon		79						49	47								83	93
Gambia	74	76	80	70		55	70	71	74	76	69	72	76				73	70
Ghana		54	51	48	59	55	50	56	60	16	14	32	33	31	39	41	41	40
Guinea	78	78	75	74	73	74	68	74	72	46	53	52	54	53	55	53	52	51
Guinea-Bissau						35		51	48						46		43	55
Kenya	73	75	77	65		78	80	80	79	53	54	50	54	52	44		46	46
Lesotho	56	47		63	77	69		71	52	62	72	83	75		74	47	66	70
Liberia				75							31		46					
Madagascar	51	55		64			70	69	74	52	66		70			72	71	77
Malawi	22	71	68	71		71	73	70	72	38	40	42	46	41	40	40	36	35
Mali	68	59	65	62	69	68		50	50	14	16	18	17		15		17	18
Mauritania					70									16	15			
Mauritius	96				91	87	93	93		34			32	35		24	25	28
Mozambique	67	39	54	67	69	71	75	77	78	56	50	48	48		45	44	45	45
Namibia			66	64		68	64	68	62	23	85	86	87	84	81	85	85	86
Niger			57	66		60	66					21	17		37			54
Nigeria	65	49	32	73	73	75	79	79	79	12	12	12	12	14	14	14	13	18
Rwanda			61	68	72	67	61		58	35	35	41	54	45	34	27	31	27
Sao Tome & Principe																		
Senegal	35	39	41	52	48		52	53	66	67	71	61	60	53		60	54	59
Seychelles		89	100	100		90	82	67	45		82	98	69		85	94	71	40
Sierra Leone	75	69	74	79	74	75	77	80	81	28	41	40	37		34	34	34	33
South Africa			69	73		60	66	65	68			6	22		75	81	105	118
Swaziland					74			36	47								34	35
Togo	45	60	65	73	69	76	63	55	68	15	15		14	13	14		6	17
Uganda			33	40	62	61	78	56	60			58	58	58	50	46	46	44
UR Tanzania	80	73	76	77	76	78		81	80	55	54	51	52	50	47	46	43	43
Zambia								75	83								41	65
Zimbabwe					70	73	69	71	67				51	49	46	46	47	42
Region	**59**	**62**	**57**	**63**	**70**	**69**	**72**	**71**	**73**	**24**	**26**	**29**	**35**	**36**	**37**	**40**	**47**	**50**

Country data for Africa: age and sex distribution of smear-positive cases in DOTS areas, 2003 (absolute numbers)

	MALE							FEMALE							ALL						
	0-14	15-24	25-34	35-44	45-54	55-64	65+	0-14	15-24	25-34	35-44	45-54	55-64	65+	0-14	15-24	25-34	35-44	45-54	55-64	65+
Algeria	40	1 316	1 633	706	429	231	328	74	1 017	702	326	242	241	356	114	2 333	2 335	1 032	671	472	684
Angola	380	2 282	2 484	1 841	1 018	483	344	551	2 983	2 525	1 660	1 111	374	128	931	5 265	5 009	3 501	2 129	857	472
Benin	20	266	504	370	188	117	92	32	226	304	150	93	47	25	52	492	808	520	281	164	117
Botswana	22	203	552	446	244	136	78	32	338	524	276	104	52	43	54	541	1 076	722	348	188	121
Burkina Faso	14	148	313	321	162	129	80	19	102	131	132	70	46	36	33	250	444	453	232	175	116
Burundi	32	348	572	488	260	106	35	75	308	361	276	119	27	10	107	656	933	764	379	133	45
Cameroon	100	1 176	2 274	1 516	788	330	160	136	1 273	1 542	745	363	217	72	236	2 449	3 816	2 261	1 151	547	232
Cape Verde																					
Central African Republic																					
Chad	39	64	105	137	76	48	19	28	52	91	124	65	38	13	67	116	196	261	141	86	32
Comoros	1	7	12	5	1	3	3	0	5	7	1	1	1	1	1	12	19	6	2	4	4
Congo																					
Côte d'Ivoire	205	1 200	2 009	1 473	799	402	362	141	1 152	1 546	845	425	213	143	346	2 352	3 555	2 318	1 224	615	505
DR Congo	854	5 885	8 427	6 193	3 776	1 836	1 047	1 233	6 630	7 711	4 826	2 866	1 457	592	2 087	12 515	16 138	11 019	6 642	3 293	1 639
Equatorial Guinea																					
Eritrea	17	90	85	55	46	44	36	27	120	149	100	60	36	22	44	210	234	155	106	80	58
Ethiopia	1 110	6 923	6 648	3 737	2 022	976	483	1 387	5 936	5 908	2 780	1 239	412	137	2 497	12 859	12 556	6 517	3 261	1 388	620
Gabon	14	165	225	149	103	48	22	16	138	144	107	51	33	18	30	303	369	256	154	81	40
Gambia	3	162	236	149	83	52	31	8	81	85	52	39	27	17	11	243	321	211	122	79	48
Ghana	79	579	1 265	1 234	924	509	441	83	487	744	586	380	200	203	162	1 066	2 009	1 820	1 304	709	644
Guinea	34	617	1 052	671	368	172	134	53	353	451	307	137	106	40	87	970	1 503	978	505	278	174
Guinea-Bissau	5	81	116	94	73	44	17	6	76	63	58	36	28	18	11	157	179	152	109	72	35
Kenya	341	4 918	8 515	4 560	2 167	928	567	487	5 003	5 023	2 618	1 171	551	309	828	9 921	14 538	7 178	3 338	1 479	876
Lesotho	10	219	614	592	466	219	83	32	328	567	313	219	59	33	42	547	1 181	905	685	278	116
Liberia																					
Madagascar	123	1 249	1 830	1 839	1 413	723	438	216	1 164	1 578	1 240	743	326	191	339	2 413	3 408	3 079	2 156	1 049	629
Malawi	43	596	1 374	936	489	209	128	76	963	1 531	790	374	155	52	119	1 559	2 905	1 726	863	364	180
Mali	32	348	619	438	330	201	115	29	172	278	212	123	73	45	61	520	897	650	453	274	160
Mauritania																					
Mauritius	0	9	12	10	17	11	9	1	6	8	4	4	3	5	1	15	20	14	21	14	14
Mozambique																					
Namibia	24	344	1 033	770	383	168	68	41	413	862	494	202	83	92	65	757	1 895	1 264	585	251	160
Niger	41	485	1 051	779	512	299	169	30	201	356	279	177	83	42	71	686	1 407	1 058	689	382	211
Nigeria	267	3 263	5 388	3 590	2 106	1 139	719	356	3 394	3 956	1 973	1 159	536	327	623	6 657	9 344	5 563	3 265	1 675	1 046
Rwanda	32	364	517	424	270	83	48	36	312	340	161	79	41	17	68	676	857	585	349	124	65
Sao Tome & Principe																					
Senegal	50	1 005	1 438	896	531	293	250	77	629	600	398	212	122	86	127	1 634	2 038	1 294	743	415	336
Seychelles	0	1	0	0	1	2	0	0							0	1	0	0	1	2	0
Sierra Leone	19	351	564	481	264	149	77	26	308	394	249	122	77	32	45	659	958	730	386	226	109
South Africa	1 767	10 105	20 389	17 858	9 535	3 600	1 491	2 341	12 599	16 863	9 204	4 080	1 972	1 171	4 108	22 704	37 252	27 062	13 615	5 572	2 662
Swaziland	15	120	298	171	96	48	19	14	242	325	145	60	20	8	29	362	623	316	156	68	27
Togo	10	126	229	192	120	66	57	15	102	149	80	55	26	28	25	228	378	272	175	92	85
Uganda	261	1 643	4 142	3 011	1 578	719	501	377	1 770	3 176	1 815	749	356	214	638	3 413	7 318	4 826	2 327	1 075	715
UR Tanzania	181	2 172	4 964	3 728	2 166	1 237	1 025	244	2 063	3 504	1 833	929	509	344	425	4 235	8 468	5 561	3 095	1 746	1 369
Zambia	302	1 733	4 182	2 390	995	386	308	292	2 061	3 439	1 626	680	297	243	594	3 794	7 621	4 016	1 675	683	551
Zimbabwe	133	874	3 048	2 228	981	367	205	180	1 232	2 856	1 480	565	225	114	313	2 106	5 904	3 708	1 546	592	319
Region	6 620	51 437	88 719	64 478	35 780	16 513	9 989	8 771	54 239	69 793	38 275	19 104	9 069	5 227	15 391	105 676	158 512	102 753	54 884	25 582	15 216

Note: the sum of cases notified by age is less than the number of new smear-positive cases notified for some countries.

Country data for Africa: age and sex distribution of smear-positive cases in non-DOTS areas, 2003 (absolute numbers)

	MALE							FEMALE							ALL						
	0-14	15-24	25-34	35-44	45-54	55-64	65+	0-14	15-24	25-34	35-44	45-54	55-64	65+	0-14	15-24	25-34	35-44	45-54	55-64	65+
Algeria																					
Angola	29	73	114	67	72	29	17	40	95	116	87	46	21	1	69	168	230	154	118	50	18
Benin																					
Botswana																					
Burkina Faso																					
Burundi																					
Cameroon																					
Cape Verde	3	12	32	32	9	7	8	1	6	7	13	7	4	11	4	18	39	45	16	11	19
Central African Republic																					
Chad	116	192	323	412	227	143	59	84	154	272	373	194	113	38	200	346	595	785	421	256	97
Comoros																					
Congo																					
Côte d'Ivoire	7	49	94	65	32	21	14	9	39	68	44	26	15	13	16	88	162	109	58	36	27
DR Congo																					
Equatorial Guinea																					
Eritrea																					
Ethiopia																					
Gabon																					
Gambia																					
Ghana																					
Guinea																					
Guinea-Bissau	4	20	37	24	35	19	10	1	21	19	20	22	10	6	5	41	56	44	57	29	16
Kenya																					
Lesotho																					
Liberia																					
Madagascar																					
Malawi																					
Mali																					
Mauritania																					
Mauritius																					
Mozambique																					
Namibia																					
Niger																					
Nigeria																					
Rwanda																					
Sao Tome & Principe																					
Senegal																					
Seychelles																					
Sierra Leone																					
South Africa	2	2	3	4	5	4	4	0	1	4	3	0	0	1	2	3	7	7	5	4	5
Swaziland																					
Togo																					
Uganda																					
UR Tanzania																					
Zambia																					
Zimbabwe																					
Region	161	348	603	604	380	223	112	135	316	486	540	295	163	70	296	664	1 089	1 144	675	386	182

Note: the sum of cases notified by age is less than the number of new smear-positive cases notified for some countries.

Country data for Africa: smear-positive notification rates (per 100 000 population) by age and sex, 2003

	MALE							FEMALE							ALL						
	0-14	15-24	25-34	35-44	45-54	55-64	65+	0-14	15-24	25-34	35-44	45-54	55-64	65+	0-14	15-24	25-34	35-44	45-54	55-64	65+
Algeria	1	37	60	36	34	36	54	1	30	27	16	20	35	47	1	34	44	26	27	35	51
Angola	13	181	305	345	293	214	222	18	234	302	301	285	146	63	15	207	304	323	289	178	134
Benin	1	38	122	130	102	108	107	2	32	71	45	44	40	27	2	35	96	84	71	73	65
Botswana	6	99	423	544	450	491	386	9	166	396	312	165	127	140	8	133	409	424	297	274	238
Burkina Faso	0	11	37	71	71	81	63	1	8	15	26	23	20	17	1	9	26	47	43	45	34
Burundi	2	46	141	194	149	118	48	5	40	84	104	58	21	8	3	43	112	148	99	60	23
Cameroon	3	70	208	216	165	100	60	4	76	140	101	70	59	22	3	73	174	157	116	79	39
Cape Verde	3	23	101	133	94	143	105	1	11	21	49	43	45	82	2	17	60	89	62	80	90
Central African Republic																					
Chad	8	31	77	156	127	124	66	6	25	64	136	101	87	35	7	28	71	146	113	105	49
Comoros	1	8	21	13	4	22	34	0	6	13	3	4	7	9	0	7	17	8	4	14	20
Congo																					
Côte d'Ivoire	6	67	184	204	142	108	134	4	64	147	133	89	68	59	5	65	166	170	117	90	98
DR Congo	7	110	240	292	282	212	178	10	124	218	227	199	142	74	8	117	229	259	239	174	118
Equatorial Guinea																					
Eritrea	2	21	30	29	39	64	105	3	28	53	52	48	46	42	2	25	41	41	44	54	67
Ethiopia	7	99	144	124	99	73	52	9	85	126	89	57	28	12	8	92	135	106	77	50	30
Gabon	5	123	243	232	228	177	85	6	102	149	167	113	122	56	6	113	195	200	171	150	69
Gambia	1	121	240	202	164	152	130	3	60	84	80	73	73	61	2	91	161	140	117	111	93
Ghana	2	25	82	124	139	120	136	2	22	48	57	54	43	53	2	23	65	90	95	80	91
Guinea	2	72	181	168	136	110	120	2	42	79	78	50	63	30	2	57	131	123	93	85	72
Guinea-Bissau	3	73	160	194	262	232	130	2	69	83	122	130	126	94	2	71	121	157	193	176	110
Kenya	5	129	373	350	252	198	131	7	131	259	185	121	104	62	6	130	316	264	182	148	94
Lesotho	3	104	643	1170	1026	615	217	9	148	430	358	310	114	70	6	126	520	656	590	319	136
Liberia																					
Madagascar	3	75	156	224	256	232	183	6	70	133	149	132	95	67	4	72	144	186	194	160	120
Malawi	2	51	179	200	154	91	64	3	81	192	153	103	63	23	2	66	186	175	127	77	43
Mali	1	26	76	93	119	114	87	1	13	33	41	37	33	25	1	20	55	66	75	68	51
Mauritania																					
Mauritius	0	9	12	10	22	29	28	1	6	8	4	5	7	11	0	7	10	7	14	17	18
Mozambique																					
Namibia	6	177	762	868	713	472	208	10	212	618	496	306	178	215	8	194	689	671	489	306	212
Niger	1	41	137	161	170	186	154	1	18	48	58	58	46	32	1	30	93	110	113	113	88
Nigeria	1	25	65	66	56	49	40	1	27	49	36	30	22	16	1	26	57	51	43	35	27
Rwanda	2	44	102	130	128	60	52	2	32	54	43	32	26	14	2	38	75	84	76	42	31
Sao Tome & Principe																					
Senegal	2	96	204	190	171	164	249	4	60	84	82	64	60	61	3	78	144	135	116	108	139
Seychelles																					
Sierra Leone	2	74	169	214	173	154	123	2	64	114	105	73	69	40	2	69	141	158	120	109	76
South Africa	24	214	574	671	510	336	220	32	266	460	325	206	151	105	28	240	516	493	354	234	148
Swaziland	6	98	479	522	369	238	118	6	193	433	297	164	87	39	6	146	454	388	250	158	74
Togo	1	25	69	90	82	72	82	1	23	44	36	35	26	33	1	23	56	62	58	48	55
Uganda	4	63	248	359	288	190	171	6	63	190	214	122	82	60	5	66	219	266	200	132	110
UR Tanzania	2	55	196	248	226	193	262	3	53	134	116	88	71	71	3	54	164	180	154	128	156
Zambia	12	149	569	671	389	208	213	12	177	479	455	236	137	133	12	163	525	563	308	170	168
Zimbabwe	5	56	349	494	310	168	99	7	73	337	321	157	91	46	6	67	343	407	228	127	70
Region	4	72	190	216	180	134	108	6	77	148	124	90	66	45	5	75	169	170	133	98	73

Note: rates are missing where data for smear-positive cases are missing, or where age- and sex-specific population data are not available.

Country data for Africa: number of TB cases notified, 1980–2003

	1980	1981	1982	1983	1984	1985	1986	1987	1988	1989	1990	1991	1992	1993	1994	1995	1996	1997	1998	1999	2000	2001	2002	2003
Algeria	2 702		13 916	13 681	13 133	13 832	12 917	11 212	11 325	11 039	11 607	11 332	11 428	13 345	13 345	13 507	15 329	16 522	15 324	16 647	18 572	18 250	18 934	19 730
Angola	10 117	7 501	7 911	6 625	10 153	8 653	9 363	8 510	8 184	9 587	10 271	11 134	11 272	8 269	7 157	5 143	15 424	15 066	14 296	14 235	16 062	21 713	29 996	36 079
Benin	1 835	1 862	1 793	1 804	1 913	2 041	2 162	1 901	2 027	1 941	2 084	2 162	2 420	2 340	2 119	2 332	2 284	2 255	2 316	2 552	2 706	2 830	2 830	2 932
Botswana	2 662	2 605	2 705	2 883	3 101	2 706	2 627	3 173	2 740	2 532	2 938	3 274	4 179	4 654	4 756	5 665	6 636	7 287	7 960	8 647	9 292	9 618	10 204	9 862
Burkina Faso	2 577	2 391	2 265	3 061	877	4 547	1 018	1 407	949	1 616	1 497	1 488		1 443	861	2 572	1 814	1 643	2 074	2 310	2 310	2 406	2 376	2 620
Burundi	789	643	951	1 053	1 904	2 317	2 569	2 739	3 745	4 608	4 575	4 883	4 464	4 677	3 840	3 326	3 796	5 335	6 546	6 365		6 478	6 371	6 822
Cameroon	2 434	2 236	3 765	3 445	3 338	3 393	2 138	3 878	4 982	5 521	5 892	6 814	6 803	7 064	7 312	3 292	3 049	3 952	5 022	7 660	5 251	11 307	11 057	15 964
Cape Verde	516	344	393	230	285	259		285	276	210	221					303	179	196	205			291	195	316
Central African Republic	651	758	1 475	1 686	468	520	779	499	814	64	2 124	2 045				3 339	3 623	4 459	4 875	5 003		2 550	4 837	3 932
Chad	220	286	127	1 977	1 430	1 486	1 285	1 086	2 977	2 572	2 591	2 912	2 684	2 871	3 303	3 186	1 936	2 180	2 784	4 710			5 077	4 679
Comoros									212	139	140	119	108	129	115	123	138	134	132	153	120	138		89
Congo	742	1 214	3 716	4 156	2 776	2 648	3 120	3 473	3 878	4 363	591	618	1 179	1 976	2 992	3 615	4 469	3 417	3 863	5 023		9 735	9 888	7 782
Côte d'Ivoire	4 197	4 418	5 000	6 000	6 062	5 729	6 072	6 422	6 556	6 982	7 841	8 021	9 093	9 563	14 000	11 988	13 104	13 802	14 841	15 056	9 239		16 071	17 782
DR Congo	5 122	3 051	9 905	13 021	20 415	26 082	27 665	27 096	30 272	31 321	21 131	33 782	37 660	36 647	38 477	42 819	45 999	44 783	58 917	59 531	60 627	66 748	70 625	84 687
Equatorial Guinea				181		17	1	11	20	157	260	331	262	309	356	306	319	366	416					
Eritrea											3 699			11 664	15 505	21 453	5 220	8 321	7 789	6 037	6 652	2 743	2 805	4 708
Ethiopia	40 096	42 423	52 403	56 824	65 045	71 731	80 846	85 867	95 521	80 795	88 634	60 006	60 006		99 329	26 034	41 889	59 105	69 472	72 095	91 101	94 957	110 289	117 600
Gabon	865	796	761	752	654	855	769	864	721	912	917	906	926	972	1 034	1 115	951	1 434	1 380	1 598			2 034	2 174
Gambia	239	58														1 023	1 242	1 357	1 558	1 514			1 859	1 945
Ghana	5 207	4 041	4 345	2 651	1 935	3 235	3 925	5 877	5 297	6 017	6 407	7 136	7 044	8 569	17 004	8 636	10 449	10 749	11 352	10 386	10 933	11 923	11 723	11 891
Guinea		1 884	1 469	832	1 203	1 317	1 128	1 214	1 740	1 869	1 988	2 267	2 941	3 167	3 300	3 523	4 357	4 439	4 768	5 171	5 440	5 874	6 199	6 570
Guinea-Bissau	645	465	205	376	368	530	1 310	752	778	1 362	1 163	1 246	1 059	1 558	1 647	1 613	1 678	1 445	846	1 164	1 273		1 566	1 647
Kenya	11 049	10 027		11 966		10 460	10 022	10 515	10 957	12 592	11 788	12 320	14 599	20 451	22 930	28 142	34 980	39 738	48 936	57 266	64 159	73 017	80 183	91 522
Lesotho	4 082	3 830	4 932	3 443	2 923	2 927		225	2 346	2 463	2 525	2 994	3 327	3 384	4 334	5 181	5 598	6 447	7 806	8 552	9 746		10 111	12 007
Liberia	774	1 002	835	885		425	232	384	894				1 948	1 766	1 764	1 393	840		1 753					
Madagascar	9 082	7 464	3 573	3 588	8 673	3 220	3 717	4 007	4 393	5 417	6 261	6 015	8 126	9 855	10 671	21 616	12 718	20 676	14 661	24 396	23 604	16 447	16 718	19 309
Malawi	4 758	5 033	4 411	4 404	4 404	5 335	6 260	7 581	8 359	9 431	12 395	14 743	14 237	17 105	19 496	19 155	20 630	22 674	22 674			26 094	24 595	25 841
Mali	839	933	187	532	1 872	1 621	1 851	2 534	2 578	1 626	2 933	2 631	3 113	3 204	3 075	3 849	3 655	5 022	6 112	4 466	4 216		4 457	4 496
Mauritania	7 576	9 427	2 327	2 333	3 977	4 406	2 257	3 722	3 928	4 040	5 284	3 064	4 316	3 996			3 837	3 788	3 617	3 649	3 067			
Mauritius	132	157	121	152	118	111	119	117	114	129	119	134	130	159	149	131	116	121	120	154	160	123	139	137
Mozambique	7 457	6 984	5 787	5 937	5 204	5 645	8 263	10 996	13 863	15 958	15 899	16 609	15 085	16 588	17 158	17 882	18 443	18 842	19 672	21 329	21 158	22 094	25 544	28 602
Namibia						4 840	4 427	3 640	2 815	3 703	2 671	2 500	1 756	5 500	3 784	1 540	9 625	9 950	11 142	10 026	10 653	12 935	13 283	11 776
Niger	717	2 871	754	673	665	698	570	556	631	608	5 200			626		1 980		3 311	3 419	4 054	4 292			7 078
Nigeria	9 877	10 838	10 949	10 212	11 439	14 937	14 071	19 723	25 700	13 342	20 122	19 626	14 802	11 601	8 449	13 423	15 020	16 660	20 249	24 157	25 821	45 842	38 628	44 184
Rwanda	1 495	1 386		1 364	1 419	1 327	2 460	3 287	4 145	4 741	6 387	3 200				3 054	3 535	4 710	6 112	6 483	6 093	5 473	6 011	5 895
Sao Tome & Principe	131	37	40	59	49	40	8	55	13		17	120		97	41				106	96	97	97	94	
Senegal	2 014	2 573	1 612	2 417		1 065	927	6 145	5 611	5 965	4 977	6 781	7 408	6 841	6 913	7 561	8 525	8 232	8 245	7 282	8 924	8 554	8 366	9 380
Seychelles	16	0	16	16	10	10	24	14	10	6	41			5		8	15	18	11	21	20	19	29	10
Sierra Leone	750	847	889	293	816	865	358	130	120		632	1 466	1 665	2 691	2 564	1 955	3 241	3 160	3 270		3 760	4 673	4 793	5 289
South Africa	55 310	59 943	64 115	62 556	62 717	59 349	55 013	57 406	61 486	68 075	80 400	77 652	82 539	89 786	90 292	73 917	109 328	125 913	142 281	148 164	151 239	188 257	215 120	227 320
Swaziland		143	3 059	1 955				1 098	1 352	1 394	1 324	1 531	1 223	1 458	1 137	2 050	2 364	3 022	3 653	4 167	5 877	6 118	6 748	7 749
Togo	208	126	204	174	343	745	596	1 184	1 071	940		1 243		1 005		1 520	1 654	1 623	1 250	1 249	1 409		1 645	1 766
Uganda	1 058	1 170	497	2 029			1 392	1 464	3 066	1 045	14 740	19 016	20 662	21 579	26 994	25 316	27 196	28 349	29 228	31 597	30 372	36 829	40 695	41 805
UR Tanzania	11 483	12 122	11 748	11 753	12 092	13 698	15 452	16 920	18 206	19 262	22 249	25 210	28 462	31 460	34 799	39 847	44 416	46 433	51 231	52 437	54 442	61 603	60 306	61 579
Zambia	5 321	6 162	6 525	6 860	7 272	8 246	8 716	10 025	12 876	14 266	16 863	23 373	25 448	30 496	35 222	35 958	40 417			45 240	49 806	46 259	54 220	53 932
Zimbabwe	4 057	4 051	4 577	3 881	5 694	4 759	5 233	5 848	6 002	6 822	9 132	11 710	16 237	20 125	23 959	30 831	35 735	43 762	47 077	50 138	50 855	56 222	59 170	53 183
Region	219 802	224 102	240 263	258 842	264 928	296 627	301 683	333 842	373 550	365 432	418 530	412 414	432 997	418 995	550 183	504 309	585 773	598 024	687 391	750 780	782 291	851 920	995 791	1 072 671
number reporting	40	41	39	41	37	41	41	43	44	41	43	40	37	41	38	45	44	42	45	41	37	34	41	42
percent reporting	87	89	85	89	80	89	89	93	96	89	93	87	80	89	83	98	96	91	98	89	80	74	89	91

Country data for Africa: case notification rates (per 100 000 population), 1980–2003

	1980	1981	1982	1983	1984	1985	1986	1987	1988	1990	1991	1992	1993	1994	1995	1996	1997	1998	1999	2000	2001	2002	2003
Algeria	14		70	66	62	63	57	48	48	46	44	44	50	49	48	54	57	52	56	61	59	61	62
Angola	144	103	105	85	126	104	110	98	92	110	116	114	81	68	47	138	132	122	118	130	170	228	265
Benin	53	52	49	48	49	51	52	45	46	45	45	49	46	40	43	41	39	39	42	43		43	44
Botswana	270	255	256	264	275	232	218	256	214	217	235	292	316	315	365	418	448	479	510	539	550	577	552
Burkina Faso	38	34	32	42	12	59	13	17	11	17	16		15	9	25	17	15	18	20	19	20	19	20
Burundi	19	15	22	23	40	43	51	53	70	82	85	77	79	64	55	63	88	107	103		101	97	100
Cameroon	28	25	41	36	34	34	21	36	45	51	57	55	56	56	25	22	28	35	52	35	73	70	100
Cape Verde	178	117	132	76	92	82		87	82	63					77	45	48	49			65	43	68
Central African Republic	28	32	61	67	18	20	29	18	29	72	68		2		100	105	127	136	137		68	127	102
Chad	5	6	3	41	29	30	25	20	54	45	49	44	45	51	47	28	30	38	62			61	54
Comoros									43	27	22	19	22	19	20	22	21	20	22	17	19		12
Congo	41	65	193	209	136	125	143	154	166	24	24	44	72	105	123	147	109	119	150	268	275	272	209
Côte d'Ivoire	50	50	54	62	60	55	56	57	56	63	62	68	70	100	83	89	92	97	97	82	103	98	107
DR Congo	18	11	34	43	65	81	84	80	86	57	87	94	88	89	96	101	97	126	125	125	134	138	160
Equatorial Guinea					61	5	0	3	6	74	92	71	81	91	76	78	87	96					
Eritrea										119	119	139	370	489	669	160	248	225	168	179	71	70	114
Ethiopia	112	116	139	146	162	173	189	194	209	181	119	115		178	45	71	97	112	113	139	141	160	166
Gabon	124	111	103	99	83	105	92	100	81	96	92	91	93	96	101	83	122	115	130			156	164
Gambia	37														92	108	114	126	119			134	136
Ghana	47	39	37	22	15	24	29	42	37	42	45	44	52	100	49	58	59	61	54	56	60	57	57
Guinea		39	30	16	23	25	21	22	30	32	36	45	46	46	48	58	58	61	65	67	71	74	77
Guinea-Bissau	81	57	25	44	42	59	144	80	81	114	119	98	139	143	136	137	115	65	88	93		108	110
Kenya	68	59		65		53	49	49	50	50	51	58	79	86	103	125	138	166	191	210	235	254	286
Lesotho	320	293	367	250	207	203	1	15	154	161	188	206	207	261	308	328	373	446	483	546		562	666
Liberia	41	52	42	43		20	11	18	41			94	86	85	65	38		68					
Madagascar	100	80	37	36	86	31	35	36	39	52	49	64	76	80	157	90		97	113		100	99	111
Malawi	77	79	68	70	63	74	82	93	97	131	152	145	174	197	191	201	197	210	220	208	224	207	213
Mali	12	13	3	7	24	20	23	30	30	32	28	33	33	31	30	34	46	37	39	35	39	35	35
Mauritania	471	572	138	135	225	243	122	196	203	260	147	203	183		167	162	156	145	142	116			
Mauritius	14	16	12	15	12	11	12	11	11	11	13	12	15	13	12	10	10	11	13	13	10	11	11
Mozambique	62	56	46	46	40	43	62	83	105	118	120	106	112	111	112	112	112	115	122	118	121	138	152
Namibia						424	373	294	217	190	171	117	354		94	567	569	618	542	563	670	677	593
Niger	13	50	13	11	11	11	8	8	9	68			7	43	22		34	34	39	40			59
Nigeria	15	16	16	15	16	20	18	25	32	23	22	16	12	9	13	15	16	19	22	23	39	32	36
Rwanda	29	26	41	24	25	22	40	51	62	94	49		69		59	66	80	93	90	79	68	73	70
Sao Tome & Principe	139	38		59	48	39	8	51	12	15	101		78	32				75	66	65	63	60	
Senegal	36	45	28	40		17	14	91	81	68	90	96	86	85	91	100	94	92	79	95	89	85	93
Seychelles	25	0	26	24	15	15	35	20	14	58			7		11	20	24	14	27	25	24	36	12
Sierra Leone	23	26	26	9	23	24	10	3	3	16	36	41	66	63	48	79	76	78		85	102	101	106
South Africa	190	201	209	199	195	180	163	166	174	218	206	214	228	225	181	262	297	331	341	344	334	481	505
Swaziland		23	483	299				144	171		176		170		218	246	308	363	406	563	578	631	719
Togo	8	5	8	6	12	25	19	37	33	38	35	34	27	30	39	41	39	29	28	31		34	36
Uganda	8	9	4	15	16	20	9	9	19	85	106	112	113	137	125	130	132	132	139	129	152	163	162
UR Tanzania	61	62	58	57	56	62	68	72	75	85	93	102	109	116	129	140	143	154	154	156	173	166	167
Zambia	89	100	102	104	107	117	120	134	167	206	277	293	342	385	384	421			442	478	438	507	499
Zimbabwe	56	54	59	48	67	54	57	62	61	87	109	147	179	208	263	299	360	381	401	402	441	461	413
Region	**59**	**59**	**61**	**64**	**64**	**69**	**68**	**73**	**80**	**84**	**81**	**83**	**78**	**99**	**89**	**100**	**100**	**112**	**120**	**122**	**130**	**148**	**156**

Country data for Africa: new smear-positive cases, 1993–2003

Number of cases

	1993	1994	1995	1996	1997	1998	1999	2000	2001	2002	2003
Algeria	4 874	6 793	5 735	6 556	7 740	7 462	7 845	8 328	7 953	8 246	8 549
Angola		4 337	3 804	8 016	8 246	7 333	7 379	9 053	11 923	18 087	18 971
Benin	1 653	1 618	1 839	1 868	1 939	1 988	2 192	2 286	2 286	2 415	2 438
Botswana	1 508	1 668	1 903	2 530	2 824	3 112	2 746	3 091	3 057	3 334	3 050
Burkina Faso		561	1 028	1 381	1 126	1 331	1 411	1 560	1 522	1 544	1 703
Burundi	1 861	1 527	1 121	1 533	2 022	2 782	2 924		3 040	2 791	3 017
Cameroon	2 316	1 883	2 896	2 312	3 548	4 374	5 832	3 960	4 695	7 921	10 692
Cape Verde			111	117	103	104			140	111	165
Central African Republic			1 794	1 992	2 267	2 637	2 725		1 382	2 758	2 818
Chad			2 002	870			2 920			3 519	3 599
Comoros			103	107	100	99	112	87			63
Congo		1 691	2 013	2 505	1 984	2 044	2 222	4 218	4 319	4 207	3 477
Côte d'Ivoire	7 012		8 254	8 927	9 093	9 850	10 047	8 497	10 920	9 667	11 411
DR Congo	14 924		20 914	24 125	24 609	33 442	34 923	36 123	42 054	44 518	53 578
Equatorial Guinea			219	209	226	284					
Eritrea					120	135	527	590	702	646	887
Ethiopia		5 752	9 040	13 160	15 957	18 864	21 597	30 510	33 028	36 541	39 698
Gabon		395	486	263	577	889	916			1 033	1 233
Gambia			778	743	820	900	861			1 035	1 040
Ghana		5 778	2 638	6 474	7 254	7 757	6 877	7 316	7 712	7 732	7 714
Guinea	2 082	2 158	2 263	2 844	2 981	3 362	3 563	3 920	4 092	4 300	4 495
Guinea-Bissau			956	922	855	541	704	526		899	963
Kenya	10 149	11 324	13 934	16 978	19 040	24 029	27 197	28 773	31 307	34 337	38 158
Lesotho	1 405	1 330	1 361	1 788	2 398	2 476	2 729	3 041		3 167	3 652
Liberia	1 547		1 154	668		1 190					
Madagascar	6 881	7 366	8 026	8 456		9 639	8 132	8 260	11 092	11 387	12 881
Malawi	5 692	5 988	6 285	6 703	7 587	8 765		8 309		7 686	7 716
Mali		1 740	1 866	2 173	3 178	2 558	2 690	2 527		2 757	3 015
Mauritania			2 074	2 226	2 519		2 051	1 583			
Mauritius			113	99	112	109	122	115	85	86	99
Mozambique	9 526	9 677	10 566	10 478	11 116	12 116	12 825	13 257	13 964	15 236	16 138
Namibia			697	2 849	3 223	3 593	3 751	3 911	4 378	4 535	5 004
Niger	463	1 865	1 492		1 970	2 189	2 631	2 693			4 505
Nigeria			9 476	10 662	11 235	13 161	15 903	17 423	23 410	21 936	28 173
Rwanda	1 723		1 840	2 034	2 820	4 417	4 298	3 681	3 252	3 956	3 710
Sao Tome & Principe	2						30	30	41	42	
Senegal		4 599	5 421	5 940	5 340	5 454	5 011	5 823	6 094	5 796	6 587
Seychelles	2	6	6	11	13	9	10	11	12	9	5
Sierra Leone		1 408	1 454	2 234	2 296	2 262		2 472	2 692	2 938	3 113
South Africa			23 112	42 163	54 073	66 047	72 098	75 967	83 808	98 799	116 364
Swaziland			660	2 226			1 781	1 823	1 279	1 410	1 585
Togo	545		887	913	935	904	904	984		1 203	1 257
Uganda	11 949	14 763	13 631	15 312	17 254	18 222	18 463	17 246	17 291	19 088	20 320
UR Tanzania	15 569	17 164	19 955	21 472	22 010	23 726	24 125	24 049	24 685	24 136	24 899
Zambia		9 620	10 038	12 072	12 072	11 645	11 645	12 927	13 024	16 351	18 934
Zimbabwe	5 331	8 965	11 965	12 072	14 512	14 492	14 414	14 392	15 370	15 941	14 488
Region	**107 012**	**121 005**	**212 910**	**264 650**	**276 022**	**324 648**	**349 133**	**361 053**	**396 632**	**452 100**	**510 164**

Rate (per 100 000 population)

	1993	1994	1995	1996	1997	1998	1999	2000	2001	2002	2003
Algeria	48	25	21	23	27	25	26	28	26	26	27
Angola		41	35	72	72	62	61	73	93	137	139
Benin	32	30	34	33	34	34	36	37	37	37	36
Botswana	102	110	123	159	174	187	162	179	175	188	171
Burkina Faso		6	10	13	10	12	12	13	12	12	13
Burundi	32	26	19	25	33	46	47		47	42	44
Cameroon	18	14	22	17	25	30	39	26	30	50	67
Cape Verde			28	29	25	25			31	24	36
Central African Republic			53	58	65	74	75		37	72	73
Chad			30	13			38			42	42
Comoros			17	17	15	15	16	12			8
Congo		60	69	83	63	63	66	122	122	116	93
Côte d'Ivoire	51		57	61	61	64	65	54	68	59	69
DR Congo	36		47	53	54	71	73	74	84	87	102
Equatorial Guinea			55	51	54	66					
Eritrea					4	4	15	16	18	16	21
Ethiopia		10	16	22	26	30	34	47	49	53	56
Gabon					49	74	74			79	93
Gambia		37	70	64	69	73	68		39	75	73
Ghana			15	36	40	41	36	37		38	37
Guinea		34	31	38	39	43	45	48	50	51	53
Guinea-Bissau	30	30			68	42	53	38		62	65
Kenya	39	42	51	60	66	82	91	94	101	109	119
Lesotho	86	80	81	105	139	141	154	170		176	203
Liberia	75		54	30		46					
Madagascar	53	55	54	60		64		73	67	67	74
Malawi	58	60	58	60	64	64		71	71	65	64
Mali		17		65	72	81	23	21		22	23
Mauritania			18	20	29	23		60			
Mauritius			90		104		80	10	9	7	8
Mozambique	64	63	66	64	66	71	73	74	77	82	86
Namibia			42	168	184	199	203	207	227	231	252
Niger	5	21	17	10	20	22	25	25	20	18	38
Nigeria			10	10	11	12	14	15	20	18	23
Rwanda			36	38	48	60	60	48	40	48	44
Sao Tome & Principe	2						25	20	27	27	
Senegal	3	57	65	70	61	61	55	62	63	59	65
Seychelles			8	15	13	12	13	14	15	11	6
Sierra Leone		35	36	54	55	54		56	59	62	63
South Africa			56	101	128	154	166	173	189	221	258
Swaziland			70	232			173	175	121	132	147
Togo	15		23	23	23	21	20	22	21	25	26
Uganda	63	75	67	73	80	82	81	73	71	76	79
UR Tanzania	54	57	65	68	68	71	71	69	69	67	67
Zambia		105	107	126	114		115	124	123	153	175
Zimbabwe	47	76	100	100	119	115	114	117	120	124	112
Region	**20**	**22**	**37**	**45**	**46**	**53**	**56**	**56**	**60**	**67**	**74**

Notes

Cape Verde
The NTP notes that age and sex data are incomplete.

Ethiopia
The NTP notes that treatment outcome data are provisional.

Gabon
Selected data received in non-standard format. DOTS coverage was assumed to be same as in the previous report.

Kenya
The treatment outcome cohort excludes nomadic patients (roughly 10% of patients registered) who are not evaluated at the end of their treatment regimen.

Madagascar
Data are considered preliminary (83% of expected quarterly reports received). Treatment success for a subset of 11 214 patients on short-course chemotherapy was 74% (with 15% defaulting). Treatment success for a subset of 69 patients on long-course chemotherapy was 67% (with 23% defaulting).

Mali
Some 100 patients classified and registered as new smear-positive were excluded from the cohort analysis of treatment outcomes after a chart audit revealed that the initial smear result for these patients could not be identified.

Mozambique
Age and sex data are not available according to the categories requested. Among smear-positive cases in 2003, 1.9% were in children. Aside from DOTS coverage, an estimate of "access" to TB services is reportedly 57%.

Seychelles
DOTS coverage was not reported, but assumed to be same as in the previous report.

South Africa
Data on age and sex of new smear-positive cases are available as follows:

Age (years)	Male	Female
0–14	38	36
15–19	115	132
20–39	1 143	837
40–59	549	359
60+	81	49

Swaziland
The NTP notes that age and sex data are incomplete.

Uganda
The NTP notes that age and sex data are incomplete.

United Republic of Tanzania
Aside from DOTS coverage, an estimate of "access" is reported in terms of distance from health facility: 70% of the population lives with 5 km from a health unit, and 90% lives within 10 km from a health unit.

THE AMERICAS: SUMMARY OF TB CONTROL POLICIES

	STATUS[a]	MANUAL[b]	MICROSCOPY[c]	SCC[d]	DOT[e]	MONITORING OUTCOME[f]
ANGUILLA	NON-DOTS	YES				
ANTIGUA AND BARBUDA	DOTS	NO				
ARGENTINA	DOTS	YES				
BAHAMAS	DOTS	YES				
BARBADOS						
BELIZE	DOTS	YES				
BERMUDA						
BOLIVIA	DOTS	YES				
BRAZIL	DOTS	YES				
BRITISH VIRGIN ISLANDS	NON-DOTS	NO				
CANADA	DOTS	YES				
CAYMAN ISLANDS	DOTS	YES				
CHILE	DOTS	YES				
COLOMBIA	DOTS	YES				
COSTA RICA	DOTS	YES				
CUBA	DOTS					
DOMINICA						
DOMINICAN REPUBLIC	DOTS	YES				
ECUADOR	DOTS	YES				
EL SALVADOR	DOTS	YES				
GRENADA	NON-DOTS	YES				
GUATEMALA	DOTS	YES				
GUYANA	DOTS	YES				
HAITI	DOTS	YES				
HONDURAS	DOTS	YES				
JAMAICA	DOTS	NO				
MEXICO	DOTS	YES				
MONTSERRAT	DOTS	YES				
NETHERLANDS ANTILLES						
NICARAGUA	DOTS	YES				
PANAMA	DOTS	YES				
PARAGUAY	DOTS	YES				
PERU	DOTS	YES				
PUERTO RICO	DOTS	YES				
SAINT KITTS AND NEVIS	DOTS	YES				
SAINT LUCIA	DOTS	YES				
ST VINCENT & GRENADINES	DOTS	YES				
SURINAME	NON-DOTS	NO				
TURKS & CAICOS ISLANDS	NON-DOTS	NO				
TRINIDAD AND TOBAGO	NON-DOTS	YES				
URUGUAY	DOTS	YES				
US VIRGIN ISLANDS						
USA	DOTS	YES				
VENEZUELA	DOTS	YES				

AMR

- Implemented in all units/areas
- Implemented in some units/areas
- Not implemented
- Unknown

a Status: DOTS status (bold indicates DOTS introduced in 2003. Blank indicates no report received)
b Manual: national TB control manual (recommended)
c Microscopy: use of smear microscopy for diagnosis (core component of DOTS)
d SCC: short course chemotherapy (core component of DOTS)
e DOT: directly observed treatment (core component of DOTS)
f Outcome monitoring: monitoring of treatment outcomes by cohort analysis (core component of DOTS)

Country data for Americas: estimated burden of TB

	Incidence, 1990				Prevalence, 1990				Death, 1990				Incidence, 2003				Prevalence, 2003				Death, 2003			
	All cases incl. HIV+		New ss+ incl. HIV+		All cases incl. HIV+		All cases excl. HIV+		All cases incl. HIV+		All cases excl. HIV+		All cases incl. HIV+		New ss+ incl. HIV+		All cases incl. HIV+		All cases excl. HIV+		All cases incl. HIV+		All cases excl. HIV+	
	number	rate	number	rate	number	rate	number	rate	number	rate	number	rate	number	rate	number	rate	number	rate	number	rate	number	rate	number	rate
Anguilla	3	31	1	14	4	49	4	49	0.4	5	0.4	5	3	25	1	11	5	40	5	40	0.5	5	0.5	5
Antigua & Barbuda	5	8	2	4	8	13	8	13	0.8	1	0.8	1	5	7	2	3	7	10	7	10	0.8	1	0.8	1
Argentina	23 579	72	10 504	32	36 733	113	36 631	113	3 482	11	3 406	10	17 024	44	7 584	20	21 377	56	21 180	55	2 245	6	2 154	6
Bahamas	151	59	67	26	221	87	214	84	25	10	20	8	127	40	56	18	170	54	164	52	21	7	17	6
Barbados	45	18	20	8	70	27	70	27	7	3	6	3	33	12	15	5	38	14	37	14	6	2	5	2
Belize	77	41	34	18	119	64	118	64	12	6	11	6	143	56	63	25	149	58	143	56	14	5	11	4
Bermuda	4	6	2	2	6	9	6	9	0.6	0.8	0.6	1	4	4	2	2	6	7	6	7	0.7	1	0.7	1
Bolivia	19 334	290	8 692	130	30 266	454	30 251	454	2 824	42	2 812	42	19 849	225	8 924	101	26 548	301	26 508	301	2 969	34	2 945	33
Brazil	139 850	94	62 608	42	217 589	146	216 854	146	20 716	14	20 161	14	110 319	62	49 387	28	164 385	92	163 105	91	14 613	8	13 955	8
British Virgin Islands	3	19	1	8	5	29	5	29	0.5	3	0.5	3	3	15	1	7	5	24	5	24	0.6	3	0.6	3
Canada	2 440	9	1 088	4	2 731	10	2 731	10	392	1	392	1	1 745	6	778	2	1 446	5	1 410	4	182	1	174	1
Cayman Islands	1	6	0.6	2	2	9	2	9	0.2	1	0.2	1	2	4	1	2	3	7	3	7	0.3	1	0.3	1
Chile	7 719	59	3 465	26	11 904	91	11 813	90	1 166	9	1 098	8	2 492	16	1 119	7	2 727	17	2 662	17	219	1	200	1
Colombia	20 109	58	8 994	26	31 416	90	31 370	90	2 951	8	2 916	8	23 126	52	10 343	23	35 507	80	35 190	80	3 748	8	3 545	8
Costa Rica	683	22	306	10	1 062	35	1 058	34	101	3	98	3	633	15	284	7	760	18	754	18	63	2	60	1
Cuba	3 332	31	1 499	14	5 220	49	5 218	49	486	5	485	5	1 216	11	547	5	1 452	13	1 451	13	120	1	120	1
Dominica	14	19	6	9	22	30	22	30	2	3	2	3	12	16	6	7	18	23	18	23	2	3	2	3
Dominican Republic	9 873	140	4 382	62	15 205	215	15 079	214	1 496	21	1 402	20	8 363	96	3 712	42	11 035	126	10 779	123	1 462	17	1 296	15
Ecuador	20 776	202	9 327	91	32 421	316	32 357	315	3 057	30	3 008	29	17 995	138	8 078	62	27 295	210	27 198	209	3 608	28	3 531	27
El Salvador	5 136	101	2 296	45	7 958	156	7 916	155	768	15	736	14	3 683	57	1 646	25	5 150	79	5 095	78	606	9	572	9
Grenada	5	6	2	3	8	10	8	10	0.8	0.9	0.8	1	4	5	2	2	6	8	6	8	0.7	1	0.7	1
Guatemala	8 734	100	3 892	44	13 528	155	13 454	154	1 307	15	1 251	14	9 180	74	4 091	33	13 097	106	12 895	104	1 564	13	1 433	12
Guyana	321	44	142	19	463	63	444	61	55	8	41	6	992	130	438	57	1 405	184	1 365	178	187	24	158	21
Haiti	32 632	472	14 113	204	44 747	647	41 753	604	6 146	89	3 882	56	26 867	323	11 619	140	34 529	415	32 174	386	5 898	71	4 182	50
Honduras	5 694	117	2 529	52	8 862	182	8 833	181	843	17	821	17	5 643	81	2 506	36	7 272	105	7 107	102	909	13	812	12
Jamaica	194	8	86	4	304	13	304	13	28	1	28	1	250	8	90	3	250	9	244	9	27	1	24	1
Mexico	40 747	49	18 294	22	63 703	77	63 632	76	5 969	7	5 916	7	34 631	33	15 548	15	46 624	45	46 445	45	4 860	5	4 759	5
Montserrat	1	11	0.5	5	2	18	2	18	0.2	2	0.2	2	0.3	9	0.1	4	0.4	12	0.4	12	0.0	1	0.0	1
Netherlands Antilles	21	11	10	5	33	18	33	18	3	2	3	2	20	9	9	4	41	18	41	18	4	2	4	2
Nicaragua	5 904	154	2 652	69	9 237	242	9 230	241	863	23	858	22	3 426	63	1 539	28	4 279	78	4 264	78	417	8	410	8
Panama	1 691	70	755	31	2 646	110	2 645	110	247	10	246	10	1 496	48	668	21	1 635	52	1 610	52	124	4	117	4
Paraguay	3 188	76	1 429	34	4 994	118	4 993	118	465	11	464	11	4 115	70	1 844	31	6 236	106	6 199	105	755	13	728	12
Peru	86 299	397	38 662	178	134 489	619	134 488	618	12 684	58	12 503	57	50 957	188	22 829	84	63 257	233	62 746	231	6 193	23	5 959	22
Puerto Rico	676	19	303	9	1 059	30	1 059	30	98	3	98	3	235	6	106	3	307	8	306	8	33	1	32	1
Saint Kitts & Nevis	6	14	2	6	9	21	9	21	0.8	2	0.8	2	5	11	2	5	7	16	7	16	0.8	2	0.8	2
Saint Lucia	27	21	12	9	43	32	43	32	4	3	4	3	25	17	11	8	33	22	33	22	3	2	3	2
St Vincent & Grenadines	40	36	18	16	62	56	62	56	6	5	6	5	35	29	16	13	48	40	48	40	5	4	5	4
Suriname	403	100	179	44	618	154	612	152	62	15	57	14	299	69	132	30	452	104	442	102	61	14	53	12
Trinidad & Tobago	168	14	74	6	258	21	256	21	25	2	24	2	123	9	54	4	170	13	163	13	20	2	16	1
Turks & Caicos Islands	3	25	1	11	5	39	5	39	0.4	4	0.4	4	4	20	2	9	6	31	6	31	0.6	3	0.6	3
Uruguay	1 087	35	488	16	1 694	55	1 690	54	161	5	157	5	940	28	422	12	1 127	33	1 121	33	102	3	100	3
US Virgin Islands	17	17	8	8	27	26	27	26	2	2	2	2	13	11	6	5	20	18	20	18	2	2	2	2
USA	28 068	11	12 420	5	31 417	12	31 417	12	4 507	2	4 507	2	13 409	5	5 933	2	10 233	3	9 730	3	1 338	0.0	1 241	0.0
Venezuela	8 417	43	3 767	19	13 171	68	13 171	68	1 229	6	1 225	6	10 711	42	4 793	19	13 489	52	13 355	52	1 416	6	1 352	5
Region	**477 480**	**66**	**213 134**	**29**	**724 584**	**100**	**719 898**	**99**	**72 195**	**10**	**68 652**	**9**	**370 107**	**43**	**165 210**	**19**	**502 605**	**58**	**496 048**	**57**	**53 803**	**6**	**49 983**	**6**

See Explanatory notes, page 151.

Country data for the Americas: notification, detection and DOTS coverage, 2003

Country	Pop (thousands)	All cases Country number	All cases WHO number	All cases WHO rate	New Smear-positive number	New Smear-positive rate	New Pulm confirmed number	New Smear-negative or unknown number	New Extra-pulmonary number	Re-treat Relapse number	Re-treat After failure number	Re-treat After default number	Re-treat Other number	Other number	Detection rate All cases %	Detection rate New ss+ %	DOTS % of pop	DOTS Notif All cases number	DOTS Notif All cases rate	DOTS Notif New ss+ number	DOTS Notif New ss+ rate	DOTS DDR %	DOTS % of pulm cases ss+	non-DOTS All cases number	non-DOTS New ss+ number	non-DOTS % of pulm cases ss+
Anguilla	12	1	1	0									1		0		0									
Antigua & Barbuda	73	1	1	1	1	1									20	45	100	1	1	1	1	45	100			
Argentina	38 428	12 278	10 728	28	4 961	13	5 583	3 653	1 812	102	404		0	1 146	63	65	100	10 728	28	4 961	13	65	56			
Bahamas	314	38	38	12	29	9	32	3	6						30	52	100	38	12	29	9	52	91			
Barbados	270																									
Belize	256	87	99	39	62	24	62	23	2	6		6			69	98	100	99	39	62	24	98	73			
Bermuda	82																									
Bolivia	8 808	10 093	9 836	112	6 344	72	6 344	1 374	1 589	529	44	213		3 946	50	71	100	9 836	112	6 344	72	71	82	63 554	30 877	62
Brazil	178 470	88 522	80 114	45	39 938	22	40 163	23 522	10 584	6 070		4 462			73	81	34	16 560	9	9 061	5	18	65			
British Virgin Islands	21	0	0	0	0	0	0	0	0				0		0	0	0	0						0	0	
Canada	31 510	1 611	1 451	5	592	2	731	185	507	67			0	160	83	76	100	1 451	5	592	2	76	76			
Cayman Islands	40	0	0	0	0	0	0	0	0						0	0	100	0	0	0	0					
Chile	15 805	2 896	2 226	14	1 276	8	484	37	712	201	18	64		13	89	115	100	2 226	14	1 276	8	115	97	10 521	7 217	84
Colombia	44 222	11 640	11 640	26	7 972	18	8 665	1 565	1 666	437					50	77	19	1 119	3	755	2	7	84			
Costa Rica	4 173	604	527	13	346	8	474	61	94	26	5	52		20	83	122	91	498	12	332	8	117	87	29	14	56
Cuba	11 300	807	844	7	511	5	593	179	101	53		4			69	93	100	844	7	511	5	93	74			
Dominica	79																							683	393	68
Dominican Republic	8 745	4 963	4 696	54	2 806	32	2 894	919	551	420	31	236		94	56	76	71	4 013	46	2 413	28	65	77	2 457	1 507	75
Ecuador	13 003	7 568	6 442	50	4 488	35		829	160	653	153	492		369	36	56	50	3 985	31	2 981	23	37	90			
El Salvador	6 515	1 383	1 383	21	870	13	870	269	160	84	8	14			38	53	100	1 383	21	870	13	53	76			
Grenada	80	2	2	2	2	2		0	0						50	112	0							2	2	100
Guatemala	12 347	2 499	2 642	21	1 795	15	2 499	479	225	143	57	17			29	44	100	2 642	21	1 795	15	44	79			
Guyana	765	661	631	82	244	32		328	23	36	6	24			64	56	38	178	23	136	18	31	85	453	108	26
Haiti	8 326	14 070	14 004	168	7 015	84	7 015	5 305	1 383	301		66			52	60	55	9 958	120	5 345	64	46	62	4 046	1 670	45
Honduras	6 941	3 297	3 102	45	1 956	28	1 956	749	105	292	0	2		193	55	78	75	3 102	45	1 956	28	78	72			
Jamaica	2 651	120	120	5	81	3		31	7	1	4	6			60	90	100	120	5	81	3	90	72			
Mexico	103 457	17 366	17 078	29	12 933	13	12 586	929	2 513	703	104	530		2 153	49	83	90	16 157	16	12 577	12	81	94	921	356	84
Montserrat	4	1	1	29	1	29	1	0	0			0			311	690	100		29	1	29	690	100			
Netherlands Antilles	221																									
Nicaragua	5 466	2 283	2 283	42	1 404	26	1 404	480	262	137	17	47		35	67	91	100	2 283	42	1 404	26	91	75	396	175	49
Panama	3 120	1 585	1 585	51	788	25	799	560	181	56	15	162		119	106	118	73	1 189	38	613	20	92	62	1 725	829	56
Paraguay	5 878	2 116	2 175	37	1 166	20	1 179	712	225	72	5				53	63	22	450	8	337	6	18	84			
Peru	27 167	33 238	31 273	115	18 504	68	19 475	5 090	4 361	3 316	476	518		791	61	81	100	31 273	115	18 504	68	81	78			
Puerto Rico	3 879	115	115	3	62	2	102	43	10						49	59	100	115	3	62	2	59	59			
Saint Kitts & Nevis	42	15	14	9			0	1		5		0			22		100	14	9							
Saint Lucia	149	14	14	9	8	5		1		3		0		1	56	71	100	14	9	8	5	71	89			
St Vincent & Grenadines	120	14	14	12	6	5	6	8		4	0	0		10	40	38	100	14	12	6	5	38	43	95	35	43
Suriname	436	111	95	22	35	8	35	46	11	5	1	5			32	26	0							147	77	56
Trinidad & Tobago	1 303	129	147	11	77	6	129	60	6	0	2	25			120	143	0									
Turks & Caicos Islands	21	7	6	29	6	29	6	0	0	0		1					0							6	6	100
Uruguay	3 415	646	643	19	339	10	503	185	71	46	3	0			68	80	100	643	19	339	10	80	65			
US Virgin Islands	111																									
USA	294 043	14 874	14 861	5	5 303	2	11 332	6 529	3 029					13	111	89	100	14 861	5	5 303	2	89	45	107	58	59
Venezuela	25 699	6 501	6 734	26	3 882	15	3 969	1 616	1 003	235	13	154			63	81	99	6 627	26	3 824	15	80	71			
Region	**867 768**	**242 143**	**227 551**	**26**	**125 803**	**14**	**130 377**	**55 971**	**31 771**	**14 000**	**1 366**	**7 101**		**9 063**	**61**	**76**	**78**	**142 409**	**16**	**82 479**	**10**	**50**	**72**	**85 142**	**43 324**	**64**

See Explanatory notes, page 151.

Country data for the Americas: treatment outcomes for cases registered in 2002

	New smear-positive cases – DOTS											New smear-positive cases – non-DOTS											Smear-positive re-treatment cases – DOTS								
	Number of cases notified	regist'd	% of notif regist'd	% cured	% compl-eted	% died	% failed	% default	% trans-ferred	% not eval	% success	Number of cases notified	regist'd	% of notif regist'd	% cured	% compl-eted	% died	% failed	% default	% trans-ferred	% not eval	% success	Number regist'd	% cured	% compl-eted	% died	% failed	% default	% trans-ferred	% not eval	% success
Anguilla	2	4	200	100							100																				
Antigua & Barbuda																														
Argentina	5 498	4 791	87	29	29	6	0	8	4	22	58																				
Bahamas	32	44	138	41	18	25		7	9		59																				
Barbados	5																														
Belize	71	74	104	85		9		5			85																				
Bermuda																														
Bolivia	6 829	6 828	100	81	3	3	1	5	5	2	84	36 536	24 246	66	24	57	6	0	12	1		81	816	62	7	5	3	8	5	9	69
Brazil	4 835	4 606	95	46	29	6	0	8	11		75												640	36	24	7	1	18	13		60
British Virgin Islands																														
Canada	445	787	177	19	62	10		2	2	5	81																				
Cayman Islands																														
Chile	1 412	1 263	89	86		8	0	4	2		86	6 979	2 755	39	52	17	6	2	10	13	0	69									
Colombia	808	961	119	73	11	4	2	7	3		84	111	133	120	42	27	5	1	23	2		69									
Costa Rica	217	215	99	80	5	10	1	5			85																				
Cuba	538	540	100	91	1	6	1	2			92												100	55	8	16	3	10	8		63
Dominica	2																						69	64	16	7	4	3		6	80
Dominican Republic	1 532	2 074	135	63	15	5	1	12	4		78	647	400	62	44	30	4	1	17	5		74	405	46	8	11	6	24	4		55
Ecuador	2 477	1 200	48	70	14	2	3	9	2		84	1 746	1			100						100									
El Salvador	980	978	100	85	3	5	1	6			88												108	69	3	6	2	19	2		71
Grenada																														
Guatemala	1 865	1 843	99	78	5	6	1	7	1	0	84	97	95	98	34	13	12	4	34	4		46	249	60	11	8	4	15	2		71
Guyana	41	98	239	83	2	7	1	6	1		85												47	68	6	19	3	2			74
Haiti	4 681	4 681	100	69	8	5	1	6	6	4	78	1 507	1 507	100	52	13	6	2	18	4	6	65	283	63	5	5	3	11	8	5	69
Honduras	2 956	2 938	99	76	11	6		4	2		87												142	80	10	2		2	6		90
Jamaica	60	63	105	5	44	25		19		6	49												7	43	29	14		14			71
Mexico	11 066	12 850	116	72	12	4	1	7	4		84	489	427	87	58	11	4	2	13	3	10	68	1 516	49	9	7	6	17	7	5	58
Montserrat	1											7																			
Netherlands Antilles						100			100																					
Nicaragua	1 320	1 420	108	73	9	5	1	10	2	2	82												243	70	7	6	2	13	2		77
Panama	568	622	110	53	19	8	1	12	6	6	73	141	151	107	13	53	5		28		2	66	155	32	19	12	9	32	4		51
Paraguay	145	145	100	59	33	4		3	1		92	859	859	100	12	61	5		18	2	2	72	32	56	25	3	5	6	1		81
Peru	20 533	16 142	79	92		2	2	3	1		92												2 560	83		3	5	7			83
Puerto Rico	76	73	96		62	22		11	1	4	62																				
Saint Kitts & Nevis	1	1	100																												
Saint Lucia	8	8	100	13	13	100				75	25												9	33	11	50		50		56	44
St Vincent & Grenadines												41	40	98	60	10	8	3	18	3		70	2								
Suriname												60																			
Trinidad & Tobago												2	3						33	67										
Turks & Caicos Islands																														
Uruguay	308	372	121	82		16	1	1			82												30	83		17					83
US Virgin Islands																						83									
USA	9 938	9 543	96		70	8	0	0	3	19	70	381	368	97	29	49	6	1	16	2		79									
Venezuela	3 063	3 015	98	82		5	0	10	4		82												222	78		6	1	13	2		78
Region	82 312	78 180	95	64	17	5	1	5	3	4	81	49 603	30 985	62	29	49	6	1	13	2	0	78	7 635	64	7	6	4	12	4	2	71

See Explanatory notes, page 151.

Country data for the Americas: re-treatment outcomes for cases registered in 2002

	Relapse – DOTS									After failure – DOTS									After default – DOTS								
	number regist'd	% cured	% compl-eted	% died	% failed	% default	% trans-ferred	% not eval	% success	number regist'd	% cured	% compl-eted	% died	% failed	% default	% trans-ferred	% not eval	% success	number regist'd	% cured	% compl-eted	% died	% failed	% default	% trans-ferred	% not eval	% success
Anguilla																											
Antigua & Barbuda																											
Argentina																											
Bahamas																											
Barbados																											
Belize																											
Bermuda																											
Bolivia	350	40	28	8	1	11	11		69	24	21	21	13	4	17	25		42	266	32	19	6	1	28	15		51
Brazil																											
British Virgin Islands																											
Canada																											
Cayman Islands																											
Chile																											
Colombia	30	60	10	27	3				70	4	75			25				75	66	52	8	12	2	15	12		59
Costa Rica	58	69	19	5	2	3		2	88	4	50		25	25				50	7	29		14	14	14		43	29
Cuba																											
Dominica																											
Dominican Republic	234	55	7	9	4	21	4		62	44	27	14	23	20	16			41	127	36	9	10	6	34	4		46
Ecuador	63	83	3	5		8	2		86	14	57			14	29			57	31	45	3	13		35	3		48
El Salvador																											
Grenada																											
Guatemala	7	57		29	14				57	2	50		50					50	38	71	8	16	3	3	3		79
Guyana	215	65	5	5	2	10	7	6	69										68	59	7		6	13	10	4	66
Haiti																											
Honduras	142	80	10	2		2	6		90	1		100						100	1		100						100
Jamaica	5	60		20		20			60																		
Mexico	794	57	10	6	5	11	3	7	67	176	28	4	4	13	17	34		32	546	44	9	8	5	26	3	5	53
Montserrat																											
Netherlands Antilles	146	74	8	6		8	4		82	23	74	4		17	4			78	74	61	5	8	2	26	4		66
Nicaragua	46	50	24	7		15	4		74	12	58		33	8				58	97	20	20	11		43	4		39
Panama																											
Paraguay																											
Peru	2 263	85		3	5	5	1		85										297	69		3	4	22	2		69
Puerto Rico																											
Saint Kitts & Nevis																			2			50		50	50		
Saint Lucia	9	33	11					56	44																		
St Vincent & Grenadines																											
Suriname																											
Trinidad & Tobago																											
Turks & Caicos Islands																											
Uruguay	27	81		19					81	3	100							100									
US Virgin Islands																											
USA																											
Venezuela	222	78		6	1	13	2		78																		
Region	**4 611**	**73**	**6**	**5**	**4**	**8**	**3**	**2**	**78**	**307**	**35**	**7**	**8**	**13**	**15**	**21**		**42**	**1 620**	**47**	**9**	**7**	**4**	**26**	**5**	**2**	**56**

See Explanatory notes for previous table, page 151.

AMR

Country data for the Americas: trends in DOTS treatment success and detection rates, 1994–2003

DOTS new smear-positive treatment success (%)

Country	1994	1995	1996	1997	1998	1999	2000	2001	2002
Anguilla									
Antigua & Barbuda					50	50	100	100	100
Argentina		59			55	59	54	64	58
Bahamas					72	66		64	59
Barbados									
Belize						88	78	66	85
Bermuda									
Bolivia	66	62	71	77	62	74	79	82	84
Brazil					91	89	73	67	75
British Virgin Islands									
Canada					35	79	80	67	81
Cayman Islands								100	
Chile	83	79	80	77	83	83	82	83	86
Colombia					74	82	80	85	84
Costa Rica						81	76	72	85
Cuba	86	90	92	90	94	91	93	93	92
Dominica			100					100	
Dominican Republic						81	79	85	78
Ecuador									
El Salvador					77	78	79	82	84
Grenada								88	88
Guatemala	62	61	81	73	79	81	86	85	84
Guyana					79	70	91	90	85
Haiti				73			73	75	78
Honduras					93	88	89	86	87
Jamaica		67	72	79	89	74	45	78	49
Mexico			75	65	78	80	76	83	84
Montserrat									
Netherlands Antilles									
Nicaragua	81	80	79	81	82	81	82	83	82
Panama	46	51		51	51	80	67	65	73
Paraguay		83	89	90	92	93	90	86	92
Peru	81	65	68	68	68	77	72	80	62
Puerto Rico					68	77			
Saint Kitts & Nevis					25	50			
Saint Lucia				67	82	89	100	50	25
St Vincent & Grenadines				86		100	100	80	
Suriname									
Trinidad & Tobago									
Turks & Caicos Islands									
Uruguay	83	68	80	77	71	83	85	85	82
US Virgin Islands		50	75		84				
USA		72	71	72	72	76	82	83	70
Venezuela	68	74	80	72	81	82	76	80	82
Region	**77**	**77**	**81**	**81**	**80**	**83**	**81**	**83**	**81**

DOTS new smear-positive case detection rate (%)

Country	1995	1996	1997	1998	1999	2000	2001	2002	2003
Anguilla									
Antigua & Barbuda					44	132	44	89	45
Argentina			4	7	20	30	38	70	65
Bahamas					62	95		56	52
Barbados							39	34	
Belize		100	67			80	92	118	98
Bermuda									
Bolivia	40	78	73	76	75	72	75	76	71
Brazil				4	4	8	8	10	18
British Virgin Islands									
Canada					45	60	61		
Cayman Islands							126	56	76
Chile	70	76	84	91	95	89	102	117	115
Colombia					28	83		8	7
Costa Rica					31	120	87	76	117
Cuba	81	88	87	92	96	98	88	91	93
Dominica			84	51					
Dominican Republic					9	6	9		
Ecuador							5	41	65
El Salvador			45	52	56	56	58	30	37
Grenada							58	58	53
Guatemala	42	56	55	56	56	51	41	46	44
Guyana						10	20	10	31
Haiti			2	12	24	22	30	40	46
Honduras				2	15	62	107	117	78
Jamaica		92	95	91	102	101	84	67	90
Mexico			15	30	39	68	91	70	81
Montserrat									
Netherlands Antilles									690
Nicaragua	72	83	84	86	85	84	90	82	91
Panama	14	55		13	8	43	66	84	92
Paraguay						4	9	8	18
Peru	101	88	94	98	91	87	87	86	81
Puerto Rico		59	73	66	72	61	57	66	59
Saint Kitts & Nevis				174	89				
Saint Lucia			118	85	77	60	52	70	71
St Vincent & Grenadines									
Suriname				18		56	19		38
Trinidad & Tobago									
Turks & Caicos Islands					116				
Uruguay	76	93	94	84	89	80	79	72	80
US Virgin Islands		75							
USA		84	82	84	84	83	84	86	89
Venezuela	73	75	75	78	82	77	67	65	80
Region	**23**	**28**	**30**	**34**	**37**	**44**	**43**	**46**	**50**

Country data for the Americas: age and sex distribution of smear-positive cases in DOTS areas, 2003 (absolute numbers)

	MALE							FEMALE							ALL						
	0-14	15-24	25-34	35-44	45-54	55-64	65+	0-14	15-24	25-34	35-44	45-54	55-64	65+	0-14	15-24	25-34	35-44	45-54	55-64	65+
Anguilla																					
Antigua & Barbuda	0	0	1	0	0	0	0				1				0	0	1	1	0	1	0
Argentina	89	574	565	413	461	366	405	99	516	513	294	241	192	231	188	1 090	1 078	707	702	558	636
Bahamas	0	2	5	6	3	1	3	2	2	2	4	3	2	3	2	4	7	10	6	3	6
Barbados																					
Belize	1	4	8	10	3	2	8	2	6	3	3	2	5	5	3	10	11	13	5	7	13
Bermuda																					
Bolivia	156	1 164	742	501	438	335	442	167	811	549	313	224	196	305	323	1 975	1 291	814	662	532	747
Brazil	118	974	1 218	1 322	1 076	635	587	109	744	797	536	360	272	311	227	1 718	2 015	1 858	1 436	907	898
British Virgin Islands																					
Canada	3	45	58	59	52	39	94	5	37	54	53	23	24	56	8	82	112	112	75	63	150
Cayman Islands																					
Chile	1	77	131	181	183	150	135	8	59	106	81	42	41	80	9	136	237	262	225	191	216
Colombia	13	73	89	61	74	47	78	16	65	67	48	33	35	56	29	138	156	109	107	82	134
Costa Rica	3	31	46	32	37	24	30	4	25	22	21	30	11	16	7	56	68	53	67	35	46
Cuba	2	23	90	91	63	52	79	0	11	14	20	23	13	30	2	34	104	111	86	65	109
Dominica																					
Dominican Republic	49	309	429	290	173	100	96	48	265	250	186	93	68	57	97	574	679	476	266	168	153
Ecuador	18	310	266	194	125	75	96	24	217	140	94	56	44	40	42	527	406	288	181	119	136
El Salvador	7	75	105	103	81	59	89	7	70	71	47	48	44	64	14	145	176	150	129	103	153
Grenada																					
Guatemala	29	175	200	169	156	125	128	24	186	179	157	104	88	75	53	361	379	326	260	213	203
Guyana	0	13	28	36	16	11	6	2	4	13	19	9	6	2	2	17	41	55	25	17	8
Haiti	66	769	774	470	314	162	114	101	859	791	440	289	135	77	167	1 628	1 565	910	603	297	191
Honduras	52	20	344	235	227	161	17	42	15	232	225	236	127	23	94	35	576	460	463	288	40
Jamaica	1	11	9	14	12	4	6	2	7	8	3	3	0	2	3	18	17	16	15	4	8
Mexico	180	1 174	1 429	1 387	1 272	977	1 298	174	830	811	714	798	718	815	354	2 004	2 240	2 101	2 070	1 695	2 113
Montserrat	0	0	1	0	0	0	1								0	0	1	0	0	0	1
Netherlands Antilles																					
Nicaragua	14	179	210	135	103	68	65	42	174	150	91	71	54	48	56	353	360	226	174	122	113
Panama	6	72	93	73	60	54	48	8	49	57	35	28	10	20	14	121	150	108	88	64	68
Paraguay	7	50	31	31	34	21	26	14	30	25	24	16	10	18	21	80	56	55	50	31	44
Peru	101	758	506	355	206	139	165	107	659	380	228	138	106	98	208	1 417	886	583	344	245	263
Puerto Rico	0	3	5	8	10	12	9	0	3	2	3	1	3	3	0	6	7	11	11	15	12
Saint Kitts & Nevis																					
Saint Lucia	0	0	0	1	2	2	2	0	1	1	0	3	2	1	0	1	1	1	5	4	3
St Vincent & Grenadines				2		1					1			1				3		1	1
Suriname																					
Trinidad & Tobago																					
Turks & Caicos Islands																					
Uruguay	3	46	50	35	42	38	26	1	28	24	13	13	6	14	4	74	74	48	55	44	40
US Virgin Islands																					
USA	13	360	518	750	821	480	641	14	268	352	307	264	169	344	27	628	870	1 057	1 085	649	985
Venezuela	37	353	454	446	404	284	314	45	330	347	235	198	139	238	82	683	801	681	602	423	552
Region	969	7 644	8 405	7 410	6 448	4 425	5 009	1 067	6 272	5 960	4 195	3 349	2 520	3 033	2 036	13 916	14 365	11 605	9 797	6 945	8 042

Note: the sum of cases notified by age is less than the number of new smear-positive cases notified for some countries.

AMR

Country data for the Americas: age and sex distribution of smear-positive cases in non-DOTS areas, 2003 (absolute numbers)

	MALE							FEMALE							ALL						
	0-14	15-24	25-34	35-44	45-54	55-64	65+	0-14	15-24	25-34	35-44	45-54	55-64	65+	0-14	15-24	25-34	35-44	45-54	55-64	65+
Anguilla																					
Antigua & Barbuda																					
Argentina																					
Bahamas																					
Barbados																					
Belize																					
Bermuda																					
Bolivia																					
Brazil	264	3 511	4 491	4 712	3 787	1 954	1 470	292	2 838	2 745	2 004	1 316	729	711	556	6 349	7 236	6 716	5 103	2 683	2 181
British Virgin Islands																					
Canada																					
Cayman Islands																					
Chile																					
Colombia	224	611	727	783	779	595	683	158	597	625	464	349	257	365	382	1 208	1 352	1 247	1 128	852	1 048
Costa Rica		2	1		2	4	3			2						2	3		2	4	3
Cuba																					
Dominica																					
Dominican Republic	3	55	89	41	21	16	16	0	36	38	25	23	14	16	3	91	127	66	44	30	32
Ecuador																					
El Salvador																					
Grenada																					
Guatemala																					
Guyana	10	43	83	78	42	16	7	10	31	48	37	18	4	3	20	74	131	115	60	20	10
Haiti	23	233	207	155	92	46	33	21	255	273	166	89	30	31	44	488	480	321	181	76	64
Honduras																					
Jamaica																					
Mexico	7	33	32	30	41	28	54	10	20	15	20	15	25	26	17	53	47	50	56	53	80
Montserrat																					
Netherlands Antilles																					
Nicaragua																					
Panama	4	19	27	20	16	16	15	3	2	18	12	6	12	5	7	21	45	32	22	20	20
Paraguay	4	113	143	78	89	60	65	14	57	46	53	34	30	43	18	170	189	131	123	90	108
Peru																					
Puerto Rico																					
Saint Kitts & Nevis																					
Saint Lucia																					
St Vincent & Grenadines																					
Suriname	0	5	0	10	5	1	5	1	3	2	1	1	0	1	1	8	2	11	6	1	6
Trinidad & Tobago	0	9	13	10	13	10	6	1	2	2	0	8	1	2	1	11	15	10	21	11	8
Turks & Caicos Islands	0	0	2	0	0	0	0	0	0	2	0	2	0	0	0	0	4	0	2	0	0
Uruguay																					
US Virgin Islands																					
USA																					
Venezuela	2	8	5	7	1	0	2	1	10	8	5	6	1	2	3	18	13	12	7	1	4
Region	**541**	**4 642**	**5 820**	**5 924**	**4 888**	**2 746**	**2 359**	**511**	**3 851**	**3 824**	**2 787**	**1 867**	**1 103**	**1 205**	**1 052**	**8 493**	**9 644**	**8 711**	**6 755**	**3 849**	**3 564**

Note: the sum of cases notified by age is less than the number of new smear-positive cases notified for some countries.

Country data for the Americas: smear-positive notification rates (per 100 000 population) by age and sex, 2003

	MALE							FEMALE							ALL						
	0-14	15-24	25-34	35-44	45-54	55-64	65+	0-14	15-24	25-34	35-44	45-54	55-64	65+	0-14	15-24	25-34	35-44	45-54	55-64	65+
Anguilla																					
Antigua & Barbuda																					
Argentina	2	17	19	18	24	25	26	2	6	18	13	12	12	10	2	16	19	15	17	18	17
Bahamas	0	7	19	26	22	11	39	4	7	8	17	19	18	28	2	7	13	22	20	15	33
Barbados																					
Belize	2	15	39	73	34	40	147	4	22	15	22	24	106	92	3	18	27	47	29	72	119
Bermuda																					
Bolivia	9	136	115	111	138	164	252	10	97	84	66	65	86	140	9	116	99	88	100	123	190
Brazil	2	25	39	49	56	51	48	2	21	24	20	18	17	18	2	23	31	34	36	33	31
British Virgin Islands																					
Canada	0	2	3	2	2	2	5	0	2	3	2	1	1	2	0	2	3	2	2	2	4
Cayman Islands																					
Chile	0	6	11	15	21	27	27	0	5	9	7	5	7	11	0	5	10	11	13	16	18
Colombia	3	16	23	29	43	57	79	3	16	19	16	17	23	34	3	16	21	22	29	39	54
Costa Rica	0	8	14	10	19	25	30	1	8	8	7	15	10	13	1	7	11	9	17	17	21
Cuba	0	3	9	9	10	10	14	0	1	1	2	3	2	5	0	2	5	6	7	6	9
Dominica																					
Dominican Republic	4	40	72	57	51	49	57	3	35	43	38	30	34	34	4	38	58	48	40	41	45
Ecuador	1	23	25	24	23	23	31	1	17	13	12	10	13	11	1	20	19	18	16	18	20
El Salvador	1	12	19	33	35	38	59	1	11	13	13	18	25	33	1	11	16	22	26	31	44
Grenada																					
Guatemala	1	13	23	31	43	55	60	1	15	21	28	27	37	32	1	14	22	29	35	46	45
Guyana	9	72	163	241	189	161	79	11	46	86	101	75	48	23	10	59	124	165	127	98	47
Haiti	5	103	168	173	165	123	100	8	115	177	154	128	81	60	7	109	173	163	145	100	78
Honduras	4	3	66	66	103	125	14	3	2	45	64	105	94	17	3	2	56	65	104	109	16
Jamaica	0	4	4	9	11	6	7	1	3	4	1	3	0	2	0	3	4	5	7	3	4
Mexico	1	12	17	24	31	39	57	1	8	9	11	18	26	29	1	10	13	17	24	32	42
Montserrat																					
Netherlands Antilles																					
Nicaragua	1	31	54	53	63	76	84	4	30	37	33	40	55	50	2	30	45	43	51	65	65
Panama	2	32	46	44	53	75	72	2	18	29	23	24	24	27	2	25	37	33	39	49	49
Paraguay	1	27	41	33	51	68	100	3	15	17	23	21	33	50	2	21	29	28	37	50	71
Peru	2	28	23	21	18	19	26	2	25	18	14	12	14	13	2	27	20	18	15	17	19
Puerto Rico	0	1	2	3	5	7	5	0	1	1	1	0	1	1	0	1	1	2	2	4	3
Saint Kitts & Nevis																					
Saint Lucia	0	0	0	11	35	56	59	0	7	8	0	47	51	20	0	3	4	5	41	53	36
St Vincent & Grenadines				25		33					8	13		22				4	19	16	12
Suriname	0	11	0	32	37	11	46	2	7	6	3	6	0	7	1	9	3	18	21	5	24
Trinidad & Tobago	0	7	13	11	18	22	15	1	1	2	0	11	2	4	0	4	7	5	14	12	9
Turks & Caicos Islands																					
Uruguay	1	17	20	17	23	27	15	0	11	10	6	7	4	5	1	14	15	11	15	15	9
US Virgin Islands																					
USA	0	2	3	4	4	4	4	0	1	2	1	1	1	2	0	2	2	2	3	2	3
Venezuela	1	14	23	27	35	41	58	1	14	18	14	17	19	36	1	14	20	21	26	30	46
Region	1	16	22	23	24	24	24	1	14	15	11	11	11	10	1	15	18	17	17	17	16

Note: rates are missing where data for smear-positive cases are missing, or where age- and sex-specific population data are not available.

Country data for the Americas: number of TB cases notified, 1980–2003

	1980	1981	1982	1983	1984	1985	1986	1987	1988	1989	1990	1991	1992	1993	1994	1995	1996	1997	1998	1999	2000	2001	2002	2003
Anguilla	0	0	4	0	0	1	0	0	0	0	0	0	0			2		0	4	3		0	0	0
Antigua & Barbuda	8	3	0	1	3	2	7	0	3	0	1	0	6			0	3	4	4	3		1	4	1
Argentina	16 406	16 693	17 292	17 305	16 359	15 987	14 681	13 368	13 267	12 636	12 309	12 185	12 606	13 887	13 683	13 450	13 397	12 621	12 276	11 871	11 767	11 456	11 548	10 728
Bahamas	70	67	54	58	53	63	52	43	51	52	46	53	63	60	78	57	59	88	75	76	82		44	38
Barbados	64	3	30	17	14	12	7	3	4	3	5	5	6			3	3	5	7	2	3	6	5	
Belize	21	33	44	140	35	25	23	41	28	30	57	89	65	80	59	95	99	107	123	104	106	136	135	99
Bermuda	1	2	5	10	3	3	2	2	1	2	0	3	4			4	0	4	0	0	0	0	0	
Bolivia	4 412	5 072	4 777	5 178	4 131	7 679	6 837	8 960	10 664	12 563	11 166	11 223	9 520	8 614	9 431	14 422	10 194	9 853	10 132	9 863	10 127	10 531	10 201	9 836
Brazil	72 608	86 411	87 822	86 617	88 365	84 310	83 731	81 826	82 395	80 048	74 570	84 990	85 955	75 759	75 759	91 013	87 254	83 309	95 009	78 870	77 899	74 466	81 436	80 114
British Virgin Islands	0	0		1		3			1		0		0	0	0	4	0	3	0	0	0	0	1	0
Canada	2 885	2 554	2 515	2 186	2 345	1 980	2 046	1 972	1 947	2 035	1 997	2 018	2 108	2 012	2 074	1 931	1 868	1 976	1 791	1 806	1 694	1 703	1 556	1 451
Cayman Islands	0	2	0			4	2	0	3	3	3	3		3				0	2	2		0	1	0
Chile	8 523	7 337	6 941	6 989	6 561	6 644	6 854	6 280	6 324	6 728	6 151	5 498	5 304	4 598	4 138	4 150	4 178	3 880	3 652	3 429	3 021	3 006	2 448	2 226
Colombia	11 589	11 483	12 126	13 716	12 792	12 024	11 639	11 437	11 469	11 329	12 447	12 263	11 199	11 043	8 901	9 912	9 702	8 042	9 155	10 999	11 630	11 480	11 376	11 640
Costa Rica	396	521	459	479	393	376	418	434	442	311	230	201	118	313	325	586	636	692	730	851	585	630	543	527
Cuba	1 133	833	815	762	705	680	656	630	628	581	546	514	410	790	1 681	1 553	1 465	1 346	1 234	1 135	1 135	929	896	844
Dominica	20	26	18	16	5	8	35	27	7	13	6	14	13	7	12	8	10	6	5	5		2	2	
Dominican Republic	2 174	1 778	2 457	2 959	3 100	2 335	2 634	2 459	3 081	3 145	2 597	1 837	3 490	4 033	4 337	4 053	6 302	5 381	5 114	5 767	5 291	4 766	4 040	4 696
Ecuador	3 950	3 966	3 880	3 985	4 301	4 798	5 687	5 867	5 497	5 480	8 243	6 879	7 313	7 050	9 685	7 893	8 397	9 435	7 164	5 756	6 908	6 015	5 829	6 442
El Salvador	2 255	2 091	2 171	2 053	1 564	1 461	1 659	1 647	2 378	617	2 367	2 304	2 495	3 347	3 901	2 422	1 686	1 662	1 700	1 623	1 485	1 458	1 550	1 383
Grenada	17	1		6	4	4			4	4	4	1			4	4	2	2	2	5				2
Guatemala	5 624	6 641	7 277	6 013	6 586	6 570	4 806	5 700	5 739	4 900	3 813	2 631	2 517	2 474	2 508	3 119	3 232	2 948	2 755	2 820	2 913	2 419	2 909	2 642
Guyana	124	117	135	149	165	215	190	117	150	120	168	134	182	91	266	296	314	407	318	407	422	422	590	631
Haiti	8 306	6 550	3 337	6 839	5 803	4 959	8 583	8 514	8 054	8 100		10 237				6 212	6 632	10 116	9 770	9 124	10 420	10 224	12 066	14 004
Honduras	1 674	1 696	1 714	1 935	2 120	3 377	4 213	4 227	3 962	4 026	3 647	4 560	4 155	3 745	4 291	4 984	4 176	4 030	4 916	4 568	3 984	4 435	4 579	3 102
Jamaica	176	178	153	157	160	130	88	133	65	86	123	121	111	115	109	109	121	118	121	115	127	121	106	120
Mexico	31 247	32 572	24 853	22 795	14 531	15 017	13 180	14 631	15 371	15 489	14 437	15 216	14 446	15 145	16 353	11 329	20 722	23 575	21 514	19 802	18 434	18 879	17 790	17 078
Montserrat	1	0	0	1		9		13	6	5	1	1	0		0						0			
Netherlands Antilles					7		5															5	7	
Nicaragua	1 300	3 723	3 082	2 773	2 705	2 604	2 617	2 983	2 737	3 106	2 944	2 797	2 885	2 798	2 750	2 842	3 003	2 806	2 604	2 558	2 402	2 447	2 092	2 283
Panama	643	580	580	429	413	614	709	765	770	672	846	863	750	1 146	827	1 300	1 314	1 473	1 422	1 387	1 168	1 711	1 514	1 585
Paraguay	1 354	1 388	1 415	1 800	1 718	1 931	1 628	1 502	1 438	2 270	2 167	2 283	1 927	2 037	1 850	1 745	2 072	1 946	1 831	2 115	1 950	2 073	2 107	2 175
Peru	16 011	21 925	21 579	22 753	22 792	24 438	24 702	30 571	36 908	35 687	37 905	40 580	52 552	51 675	48 601	45 310	41 739	42 062	43 723	40 345	38 661	37 197	36 092	31 273
Puerto Rico	686	521	473	452	418	338	363	303	275	314	159	241		257	274	263	110	257	201	200	174	121	129	115
Saint Kitts & Nevis	7	4	6	3	3	0	0	0	0	0	0	1	4	6	2	5	3	12	5	3	3	2	3	1
Saint Lucia	41	39	37	48	55	21	34	25	32	28	13	25	26		24	11	35	22	20	16	9	15	17	14
St Vincent & Grenadines	78	11	14	4	23	14	9	3	6	3	2	1	4	13	0	13	6	6	8	9	16	10	10	14
Suriname	78	81	56	78	76	50	60	77	77	70	82	47	58	45	53		53	76	85	95	90	80	93	95
Trinidad & Tobago	80	82	62	112	108	112	119	122	108	124	120	141	142	112	129	166	204	260	199	159	198	206	133	147
Turks & Caicos Islands	2	0	2	5	0	4	2	12	2	4	0	0	0	0			8			17		3	3	6
Uruguay	1 874	1 699	1 450	1 359	1 389	1 201	1 082	1 023	951	987	886	759	699	689	666	625	701	708	668	627	645	689	536	643
US Virgin Islands	0	1	1	2	3	1			6	5	4	4			10	4	4							
USA	27 749	27 373	25 520	23 846	22 255	22 201	22 768	22 517	22 436	23 495	25 701	26 283	26 673	25 287	24 361	22 860	21 119	17 314	18 199	17 521	16 362	15 980	15 055	14 861
Venezuela	4 233	4 093	4 159	4 266	4 737	4 822	4 974	4 954	4 557	4 524	5 457	5 216	5 444	5 169	4 877	5 578	5 650	5 984	6 273	6 598	6 466	6 251	6 204	6 734
Region	227 820	248 150	237 316	238 296	226 801	227 022	227 107	233 192	241 834	239 594	231 215	252 221	253 256	166 640	242 018	258 331	256 467	252 536	262 809	240 650	236 183	229 874	233 650	227 551
number reporting	42	42	42	42	42	42	42	42	41	41	41	42	39	33	35	39	39	39	39	39	39	40	43	39
percent reporting	95	95	95	95	95	95	95	95	93	93	93	95	89	75	80	89	89	91	89	89	86	91	98	89

Country data for the Americas: case notification rates (per 100 000 population), 1980–2003

	1980	1981	1982	1983	1984	1985	1986	1987	1988	1989	1990	1991	1992	1993	1994	1995	1996	1997	1998	1999	2000	2001	2002	2003
Anguilla	0	0	57	0	0	14	0	0	0	0	0	0	0			20		0					0	0
Antigua & Barbuda	13	5	0	2	5	3	0	0	5	5	2	0	9			0	4	6	6	4	6	1	6	0
Argentina	58	59	60	59	55	53	48	43	42	39	38	37	38	41	40	39	38	35	34	32	32	31	30	28
Bahamas	33	31	25	26	23	27	22	18	21	21	18	20	24	22	28	20	20	30	25	25	27		14	12
Barbados	26	1	12	7	6	5	3	1	2	2	2	2	2			1	1	2	3	1	1	2	2	
Belize	15	22	29	91	22	15	14	24	16	17	31	47	33	40	28	45	45	48	54	44	44	55	54	39
Bermuda	1	3	7	14	4	4	8	3	1	3	0	4	5			5	0	5	0	0	0	0	0	
Bolivia	82	93	85	91	71	129	112	144	167	193	167	164	136	120	129	193	133	126	127	121	122	124	118	112
Brazil	60	69	67	67	66	62	60	58	57	55	50	56	56		48	57	54	50	57	47	45	43	46	45
British Virgin Islands																		16				0	5	0
Canada	12	10	10	9	9	8	8	7	7	7	7	7	7	7	7	7	6	7	6	6	6	5	5	5
Cayman Islands	0	11	0	5	5	19	5	0	0	8	8	11	4	7		6	0	0	9	6	14	3	0	0
Chile	76	65	60	60	55	55	56	50	50	52	47	41	39	33	30	29	29	27	25	23	20	19	16	14
Colombia	41	39	41	45	41	38	36	35	34	33	36	34	31	30	24	26	25	20	22	27	28	27	26	26
Costa Rica	17	22	18	19	15	14	15	15	15	10	7	6	4	9	10	17	18	19	19	22	15	16	13	13
Cuba	12	9	8	8	7	7	6	6	6	6	5	5	4	7	15	14	13	12	11	10	10	8	8	7
Dominica	27	35	24	22	7	11	48	37	10	18	8	19	18	10	16	11	13	8	7	10	10	8	3	7
Dominican Republic	38	30	41	48	49	36	40	37	45	45	37	26	48	54	57	53	81	68	63	70	63	56	47	54
Ecuador	50	48	46	46	49	53	61	61	56	55	80	66	68	64	87	69	72	80	60	47	56	48	46	50
El Salvador	49	45	46	44	33	31	34	34	48	12	46	44	47	62	70	43	29	28	28	27	24	23	24	21
Grenada	19	1	1	7	5	2	1	2	0	5	0	1	4	0	4	5	0	2	2	6	0	1	1	2
Guatemala	82	95	101	82	87	85	61	70	69	57	44	29	27	26	26	31	32	28	25	25	26	21	24	21
Guyana	16	15	18	20	22	29	25	16	20	16	23	18	25	12	36	40	42	54	42	54	56	55	77	82
Haiti	152	117	58	117	97	81	136	132	122	120		145				83	87	131	125	115	130	126	147	168
Honduras	47	46	45	49	52	81	98	95	86	85	75	91	80	70	78	88	72	68	80	73	62	67	68	45
Jamaica	8	8	7	7	7	6	4	6	3	4	5	5	5	5	4	4	5	5	5	4	5	5	4	5
Mexico	46	47	35	32	20	20	17	19	19	19	17	18	17	17	18	12	22	25	22	20	19	19	17	17
Montserrat	8	0	0	9	61	80	45	118	55	46	9	9	0	0	0									29
Netherlands Antilles																			16	41	0	2	3	
Nicaragua	45	124	99	86	82	77	75	84	75	83	77	71	71	67	64	64	66	60	54	52	47	47	39	42
Panama	33	29	28	21	19	28	32	34	33	28	35	35	30	45	32	49	48	53	50	48	40	57	49	51
Paraguay	43	43	43	53	49	54	44	39	36	55	51	53	43	44	39	36	42	38	35	40	36	37	37	37
Peru	92	123	119	122	120	125	124	150	177	157	174	183	233	225	208	190	172	170	174	158	149	141	135	115
Puerto Rico	21	16	14	14	12	10	11	9	8	9	5	7	10	7	8	7	3	7	5	5	5	3	3	3
Saint Kitts & Nevis	16	9	14	5	7	0	0	0	0	9	0	2	10	14	5	11	7	28	12	7	0	5	7	2
Saint Lucia	36	34	32	41	46	17	28	20	25	22	10	19	19		17	8	25	15	14	11	6	10	11	9
St Vincent & Grenadines	78	11	14	4	22	13	9	3	6	3	2	1	4	12	0	11	5	5	7	8	14	8	8	12
Suriname	22	23	15	21	20	13	15	20	19	18	20	12	14	11	13		13	18	20	23	21	19	22	22
Trinidad & Tobago	7	7	6	10	9	10	10	10	9	10	10	12	12	9	10	13	16	20	16	12	15	16	10	11
Turks & Caicos Islands	27	0	24	58	0	42	20	113	31	34	0	0	22	0		13		22		95		16		29
Uruguay	64	58	49	46	46	40	36	34	31	32	29	24	22	22	21	19	22	22	20	19	19	16	15	19
US Virgin Islands	0	1	1	2	3	1	1	2	0	9	0	4	0	0	10	4	8							
USA	12	12	11	10	9	9	9	9	9	9	10	10	10	10	9	8	8	6	7	6	6	6	5	5
Venezuela	28	26	26	26	28	28	28	27	25	24	28	26	27	25	23	25	25	26	27	28	27	25	25	26
Region	**37**	**40**	**37**	**37**	**34**	**34**	**33**	**34**	**34**	**34**	**32**	**34**	**34**	**22**	**31**	**33**	**32**	**31**	**32**	**29**	**28**	**27**	**27**	**26**

Country data for the Americas: new smear-positive cases, 1993–2003

	Number of cases											Rate (per 100 000 population)										
	1993	1994	1995	1996	1997	1998	1999	2000	2001	2002	2003	1993	1994	1995	1996	1997	1998	1999	2000	2001	2002	2003
Anguilla																						
Antigua & Barbuda			0	2	0		1	3	1	2	1			0	3	0		1	4	1	3	1
Argentina	5 937	5 696	5 698	5 787	5 307	5 186	4 830	4 749	5 595	5 498	4 961	18	17	16	16	15	14	13	13	15	14	13
Bahamas	41	41	38	25	57	30	37	56		32	29	15	15	13	9	20	10	12	18	10	10	9
Barbados					5	4	2	3	6	5						2	2	1	1	2	2	
Belize	50	36	36	46	32	52	48	44	53	71	62	25	17	17	21	14	23	20	18	22	28	24
Bermuda															0	0	0	0	0	0	0	0
Bolivia	6 833	6 905	7 010	6 949	6 458	6 750	6 673	6 458	6 672	6 829	6 344	96	94	94	91	83	85	82	78	79	79	72
Brazil		39 167	45 650	44 503	43 490	43 554	41 619	41 186	38 478	41 371	39 938		25	28	27	26	26	25	24	22	23	22
British Virgin Islands															0	0			0	0	0	0
Canada	542		404	156	487	471	395	506	502	445	592	2		1	1	2	2	1	2	2	1	2
Cayman Islands	2		0	0	0	2	2	5	1	0	0	7		0	0	0	6	6	14	3	0	0
Chile	2 629	1 951	1 561	1 562	1 582	1 576	1 497	1 290	1 355	1 412	1 276	19	14	11	11	11	11	10	8	9	9	8
Colombia	6 987	6 532	7 530	7 572	6 090	6 969	8 329	8 358	8 022	7 787	7 972	19	17	20	19	15	17	20	20	19	18	18
Costa Rica		230	245	302	320	353	458	349	385	328	346		7	7	8	9	9	12	9	10	8	8
Cuba	565	914	834	835	765	746	720	677	562	538	511	5	8	8	8	7	7	6	6	5	5	5
Dominica	6	8	5	7	5	5	5			2		8	11	7	9	7	7	6			3	
Dominican Republic	2 297	3 177	2 787	3 733	3 162	2 669	3 278	2 907	2 622	2 179	2 806	31	42	36	48	40	33	40	35	31	25	32
Ecuador	5 325	6 674	5 890	6 426	7 214	4 900	4 300	5 064	4 439	4 223	4 488	49	60	52	55	61	41	35	41	35	33	35
El Salvador	2 471	2 144		965	882	1 071	1 023	1 008	1 003	980	870	45	39		17	15	18	17	16	16	15	13
Grenada	0	3	2	0	1	2	3	0		0	2	0	4	2	0	1	2	4	0		0	2
Guatemala	2 128	1 994	2 368	2 224	2 218	2 255	2 264	2 052	1 669	1 865	1 795	23	21	24	22	21	21	20	18	14	15	15
Guyana	51	61	85	71	105	85	178	119	174	138	244	7	8	11	10	14	11	24	16	23	18	32
Haiti				3 524	5 497	6 442	6 828	5 887	5 607	6 188	7 015				46	71	83	86	74	69	75	84
Honduras	2 016	2 385	2 306	1 808	1 928	2 311	2 415	2 415	2 839	2 956	1 956	38	44	41	31	32	38	38	37	43	44	28
Jamaica	83	61	93	81	84	90	90	90	75	60	81	3	2	4	3	3	4	4	3	3	2	3
Mexico	8 164	9 726	9 220	8 495	15 440	11 473	11 968	11 676	15 103	11 555	12 933	9	11	10	9	16	12	12	12	15	11	13
Montserrat		0				1	2	0	0	0	1		0				16	41	0	0	0	29
Netherlands Antilles										7											3	
Nicaragua	1 714	1 615	1 568	1 722	1 670	1 648	1 564	1 471	1 510	1 320	1 404	41	38	35	38	36	34	32	29	29	25	26
Panama	1 046	748	1 066	904	592	1 393	432	410	575	709	788	41	29	40	33	21	49	15	14	19	23	25
Paraguay	985	873	748	894	859	850	1 041	900	915	1 004	1 166	21	19	15	18	17	16	20	16	16	17	20
Peru	35 646	33 925	32 096	26 800	27 498	27 707	24 511	22 580	21 685	20 533	18 504	155	145	135	110	111	110	96	87	82	77	68
Puerto Rico	117		128	110	126	106	106	82	71	76	62	3		3	3	3	3	3	2	2	2	2
Saint Kitts & Nevis	2	2	4	2		4	2	0	0	0		5	5	9	5	10	3	5	0	4	2	
Saint Lucia		17	11	22	14	10	9	7	6	1	8		12	8	16		7	6	5	4	5	5
St Vincent & Grenadines	11	0	5	3	2	3	4	9	3	8	6	10	0	5	3	2	3	4	8	3	9	5
Suriname		55	7	39	31	32	36	37	35	41	35		4	1	9	7	8	9	9	8	9	8
Trinidad & Tobago				58	52	82	87	115	152	60	77				5	4	6	7	9	12	5	6
Turks & Caicos Islands							2			2	6							11				6
Uruguay	388	381	349	426	423	374	392	348	340	308	339	12	12	11	13	13	11	12	10	10	10	10
US Virgin Islands			2	5										2	5							
USA	16 046	14 346	8 013	7 401	6 882	6 630	6 252	5 865	5 600	5 380	5 303	6	5	3	3	2	2	2	2	2	2	2
Venezuela	2 849	2 738	3 056	3 195	3 234	3 450	3 670	3 525	3 476	3 444	3 882	14	13	14	14	14	15	15	15	14	14	15
Region	104 931	142 405	138 820	136 657	142 512	139 286	135 068	130 251	129 536	127 357	125 803	14	19	18	17	18	17	16	16	15	15	14

Notes

Brazil

The NTP notes that age and sex data are incomplete and that treatment outcome data are provisional.

Ecuador

Treatment outcomes were available from only 3 provinces.

Guyana

Age and sex data are for all new cases, not just smear-positive.

Peru

Age and sex data are for quarter 3 only.

Uruguay

Treatment outcomes listed under new smear-positive patients are for laboratory-confirmed cases.

USA

The NPT notes that treatment outcome data are provisional. Treatment outcomes listed under new smear-positive cases are for laboratory-confirmed cases.

Africa

The Americas

Eastern Mediterranean

Europe

South-East Asia

Western Pacific

EASTERN MEDITERRANEAN: SUMMARY OF TB CONTROL POLICIES

	STATUS[a]	MANUAL[b]	MICROSCOPY[c]	SCC[d]	DOT[e]	MONITORING OUTCOME[f]
AFGHANISTAN	DOTS	YES				
BAHRAIN	DOTS	YES				
DJIBOUTI	DOTS	YES				
EGYPT	DOTS	YES				
IRAN	DOTS	YES				
IRAQ	DOTS	YES				
JORDAN	DOTS	YES				
KUWAIT	DOTS	YES				
LEBANON	DOTS	YES				
LIBYAN ARAB JAMAHIRIYA	DOTS	YES				
MOROCCO	DOTS	YES				
OMAN	DOTS	YES				
PAKISTAN	DOTS	YES				
QATAR	DOTS	NO				
SAUDI ARABIA	DOTS	YES				
SOMALIA	DOTS	YES				
SUDAN	DOTS	YES				
SYRIAN ARAB REPUBLIC	DOTS	YES				
TUNISIA	DOTS	YES				
UNITED ARAB EMIRATES	DOTS	YES				
YEMEN	DOTS	YES				
WEST BANK AND GAZA STRIP	DOTS					

- Implemented in all units/areas
- Implemented in some units/areas
- Not implemented
- Unknown

a Status: DOTS status (bold indicates DOTS introduced in 2003. Blank indicates no report received)
b Manual: national TB control manual (recommended)
c Microscopy: use of smear microscopy for diagnosis (core component of DOTS)
d SCC: short course chemotherapy (core component of DOTS)
e DOT: directly observed treatment (core component of DOTS)
f Outcome monitoring: monitoring of treatment outcomes by cohort analysis (core component of DOTS)

EMR

Country data for the Eastern Mediterranean: estimated burden of TB

	Incidence, 1990				Prevalence, 1990				Death, 1990				Incidence, 2003				Prevalence, 2003				Death, 2003			
	All cases incl. HIV+		New ss+ incl. HIV+		All cases incl. HIV+		All cases excl. HIV+		All cases incl. HIV+		All cases excl. HIV+		All cases incl. HIV+		New ss+ incl. HIV+		All cases incl. HIV+		All cases excl. HIV+		All cases incl. HIV+		All cases excl. HIV+	
	number	rate	number	rate	number	rate	number	rate	number	rate	number	rate	number	rate	number	rate	number	rate	number	rate	number	rate	number	rate
Afghanistan	45 996	333	20 698	150	95 688	693	95 688	693	10 370	75	10 370	75	79 656	333	35 845	150	160 303	671	160 302	671	22 125	93	22 123	93
Bahrain	332	68	149	30	691	141	691	141	75	15	75	15	330	46	148	20	374	52	373	52	33	5	33	5
Djibouti	3 161	599	1 395	264	7 060	1 338	7 028	1 332	845	160	811	154	5 152	733	2 273	324	7 166	1 020	6 939	988	805	115	690	98
Egypt	23 323	42	10 492	19	48 521	87	48 521	87	5 259	9	5 259	9	20 233	28	9 102	13	26 148	36	26 133	36	2 350	3	2 343	3
Iran	23 179	41	10 424	18	48 221	85	48 221	85	5 226	9	5 226	9	19 423	28	8 735	13	25 165	37	25 137	36	2 259	3	2 246	3
Iraq	15 983	92	7 192	41	33 250	192	33 250	192	3 604	21	3 604	21	39 552	157	17 797	71	59 419	236	59 411	236	8 298	33	8 293	33
Jordan	408	13	184	6	849	26	849	26	92	3	92	3	270	5	121	2	283	5	283	5	27	0.0	27	0.0
Kuwait	848	40	381	18	1 764	82	1 764	82	191	9	191	9	671	27	302	12	774	31	773	31	68	3	67	3
Lebanon	1 158	43	521	19	2 409	89	2 409	89	261	10	261	10	448	12	201	6	492	13	491	13	45	1	45	1
Libyan Arab Jamahiriya	1 333	31	599	14	2 772	64	2 772	64	300	7	300	7	1 156	21	519	9	1 151	21	1 145	21	84	2	83	2
Morocco	32 960	134	14 822	60	68 569	279	68 569	279	7 431	30	7 431	30	34 327	112	15 437	51	32 211	105	32 159	105	3 099	10	3 084	10
Oman	316	17	142	8	657	36	657	36	71	4	71	4	307	11	138	5	350	12	349	12	34	1	34	1
Pakistan	201 031	181	90 388	82	418 218	377	418 218	377	45 325	41	45 325	41	278 392	181	125 172	82	550 948	359	550 424	358	66 503	43	66 037	43
Qatar	248	53	112	24	516	110	516	110	56	12	56	12	372	61	167	27	440	72	439	72	41	7	40	7
Saudi Arabia	9 065	55	4 079	25	18 858	114	18 858	114	2 044	12	2 044	12	9 751	40	4 387	18	13 720	57	13 718	57	1 132	5	1 131	5
Somalia	24 042	336	10 738	150	53 815	751	53 598	748	6 408	89	6 187	86	40 645	411	18 154	184	74 655	755	73 972	748	12 468	126	11 695	118
Sudan	44 706	179	19 756	79	100 764	404	100 558	403	11 818	47	11 607	47	73 802	220	32 614	97	122 277	364	119 285	355	20 960	62	18 067	54
Syrian Arab Republic	8 673	68	3 903	31	18 043	142	18 043	142	1 955	15	1 955	15	7 551	42	3 398	19	9 292	52	9 290	52	814	5	813	5
Tunisia	3 122	38	1 405	17	6 495	79	6 495	79	704	9	704	9	2 170	22	976	10	2 374	24	2 373	24	227	2	227	2
United Arab Emirates	538	26	242	12	1 119	55	1 119	55	121	6	121	6	532	18	239	8	778	26	776	26	62	2	61	2
West Bank and Gaza Strip	771	36	347	16	1 603	74	1 603	74	174	8	174	8	856	24	385	11	1 332	37	1 332	37	150	4	150	4
Yemen	16 431	138	7 386	62	34 182	286	34 182	286	3 705	31	3 705	31	18 514	93	8 323	42	30 299	151	30 257	151	2 353	12	2 332	12
Region	457 623	120	205 352	54	964 066	253	963 610	253	106 036	28	105 570	28	634 112	122	284 434	55	1 119 950	216	1 115 362	215	143 937	28	139 623	27

See Explanatory notes, page 151.

Country data for the Eastern Mediterranean: notification, detection and DOTS coverage, 2003

	Pop thousands	Whole country All cases Country number	WHO number	rate	New cases Smear-positive number	rate	Pulm confirmed number	Smear-negative or unknown number	Extra-pulmonary number	Re-treatment Relapse number	After failure number	After default number	Other number	Other number	Detection rate All cases %	New ss+ %	DOTS % of pop	Notifications All cases number	rate	New ss+ number	rate	DDR %	cases ss+ % of pulm	non-DOTS All cases number	New ss+ number	% of pulm cases ss+
Afghanistan	23 897		13 808	58	6 510	27	6 510	3 440	3 254	604	141				17	18	53	13 808	58	6 510	27	18	65			
Bahrain	724	263	263	36	73	10		66	124		38				80	49	100	263	36	73	10	49	53			
Djibouti	703	3 231	3 231	460	1 202	171		858	987	184		23			63	53	100	3 231	460	1 202	171	53	58			
Egypt	71 931	11 747	11 490	16	5 118	7	5 118	2 764	3 045	563	144				57	56	100	11 490	16	5 118	7	56	65			
Iran	68 920	10 857	10 857	16	5 166	7	5 166	2 366	3 006	319	113	113		113	56	59	100	10 857	16	5 166	7	59	69			
Iraq	25 175	11 656	11 656	46	3 577	14		3 727	3 454	898					29	20	85	11 656	46	3 577	14	20	49			
Jordan	5 473	310	310	6	108	2	119	61	139	2	2	0		10	115	89	100	310	6	108	2	89	64			
Kuwait	2 521	566	566	22	201	8	201	73	288	4		30			84	67	100	566	22	201	8	67	73			
Lebanon	3 653	380	380	10	134	4	156	80	157	9	0	0			85	67	100	360	10	134	4	67	63			
Libyan Arab Jamahiriya	5 551	1 559	1 917	35	764	14		351	795	7	5	131			166	147	100	1 917	35	764	14	147	69			
Morocco	30 566	26 789	26 789	88	12 842	42	13 009	2 271	11 676						78	83	100	26 789	88	12 842	42	83	85			
Oman	2 851	257	257	9	112	4	112	35	103	7	0	0			84	81	100	257	9	112	4	81	76			
Pakistan	153 578	73 130	73 100	48	20 962	14		34 447	12 874	1 633	39	3 145			26	17	63	73 100	48	20 962	14	17	38			
Qatar	610	276	276	45	95	16	276	63	117	1					74	57	100	275	45	95	16	57	60			
Saudi Arabia	24 217	3 317	3 317	14	1 646	7	1 646	546	1 010	115					34	38	100	3 317	14	1 646	7	38	75			
Somalia	9 890	9 278	9 278	94	5 190	52	20 429	2 193	1 388	507		0			23	29	100	9 273	94	5 190	52	29	70			
Sudan	33 610	25 095	25 095	75	10 993	33		7 796	4 666	1 640					34	34	99	25 095	75	10 993	33	34	59			
Syrian Arab Republic	17 800	4 966	4 820	27	1 545	9	1 545	1 026	2 173	76	56	35		55	64	45	100	4 820	27	1 545	9	45	60			
Tunisia	9 832	1 965	1 965	20	890	9		194	840	41					91	91	100	1 965	20	890	9	91	82			
United Arab Emirates	2 995	117	117	4	77	3	77	6	33	1	0	0			22	32	100	117	4	77	3	32	93			
West Bank and Gaza Strip	3 557	37	36	1	15	0		4	17						4	4	100	36	1	15	4	4	79			
Yemen	20 010	10 413	10 413	52	3 793	19		3 435	2 759	426					56	46	98	6 632	33	3 602	18	43	73	3 781	191	8
Region	518 063	192 585	209 941	41	81 013	16	54 364	65 802	52 905	7 037	538	3 477		178	33	28	86	206 160	40	80 822	16	28	56	3 781	191	8

See Explanatory notes, page 151.

EMR

Country data for the Eastern Mediterranean: treatment outcomes for cases registered in 2002

	New smear-positive cases – DOTS											New smear-positive cases – non-DOTS											Smear-positive re-treatment cases – DOTS								
	Number of cases notified	regist'd	% of notif regist'd	% cured	% compl-eted	% died	% failed	% default	% trans-ferred	% not eval	% success	Number of cases notified	regist'd	% of notif regist'd	% cured	% compl-eted	% died	% failed	% default	% trans-ferred	% not eval	% success	Number regist'd	% cured	% compl-eted	% died	% failed	% default	% trans-ferred	% not eval	% success
Afghanistan	6 509	7 780	120	60	27	4	2	5	3		87																					
Bahrain	17	17	100	88		12					88																					
Djibouti	1 253	1 256	100	66	16	1	1	15	1		82												268	43	29	2	3	21	2		73
Egypt	4 889	4 605	94	76	12	2	3	3	3		88																				
Iran	5 335	5 366	101	81	4	6	2	3	3	0	85												599	61	13	8	5	8	5	1	74
Iraq	3 895	3 895	100	86	5	3	2	3	2		91												553	68	7	5	11	8	1		75
Jordan	91	91	100	80	9	5		5			89												12	58	17	17		8			75
Kuwait		206		42	13			25	4	16	55																				
Lebanon	148	147	99	80	11		1	7	1		91												1		100						100
Libyan Arab Jamahiriya	722	716	99	48	13	1	0	17	18	3	61												14							100	
Morocco	12 914	12 830	99	83	6	2	1	8			89												1 727	69	5	5	5	12	5		74
Oman	151	119	79	92		7		1	1		92												1	100							100
Pakistan	15 331	14 314	93	65	13	3	1	14	4	1	77	934											2 871	33	43	4	2	11	5	2	76
Qatar	64	64	100	69	6	6	0	14	19		75																				
Saudi Arabia	1 674	1 365	82	69	7	7		2	2		76												112	51	16	4	2	13	4	11	67
Somalia	4 818	4 818	100	86	3	3	1	3	4		89												411	54	4	5	3	4	30		59
Sudan	10 338	10 993	106	59	19	3	1	7	2	8	78												1 640	51	26	3	0	5	2	12	77
Syrian Arab Republic	1 447	1 447	100	69	18	3	2	7	1		87												167	35	21	7	17	18	7		56
Tunisia	927	913	98	89	3	2	1	2	2		92												53	75		2	9	11	2		75
United Arab Emirates	57	57	100	70	9	4	2	2	2	12	79												3							100	
West Bank and Gaza Strip		10		100							100																				
Yemen	3 870	3 790	98	73	9	4	1	9	4		82	389	334	86	28	49	1	1	15	5		78	393	50	20	5	5	9	5	10	70
Region	**74 450**	**74 799**	**100**	**72**	**12**	**3**	**1**	**8**	**3**	**1**	**84**	**1 323**	**334**	**25**	**28**	**49**	**1**	**1**	**15**	**5**		**78**	**8 825**	**51**	**23**	**4**	**4**	**10**	**5**	**3**	**74**

See Explanatory notes, page 151.

Country data for the Eastern Mediterranean: re-treatment outcomes for cases registered in 2002

	Relapse – DOTS									After failure – DOTS									After default – DOTS								
	number regist'd	% cured	% compl-eted	% died	% failed	% default	% trans-ferred	% not eval	% success	number regist'd	% cured	% compl-eted	% died	% failed	% default	% trans-ferred	% not eval	% success	number regist'd	% cured	% compl-eted	% died	% failed	% default	% trans-ferred	% not eval	% success
Afghanistan																											
Bahrain																											
Djibouti	268	43	29	2	3	21	2		73																		
Egypt																											
Iran	363	71	7	8	4	5	5		79	103	67	3	8	9	8	5	1	70	133	28	38	8	4	15	5	2	66
Iraq	553	68	7	5	11	8	1		75																		
Jordan	9	78	22						100	3			67		33												
Kuwait																											
Lebanon	1		100						100																		
Libyan Arab Jamahiriya	14							100																			
Morocco	1372	71	6	4	4	9	5		78	96	59		10	13	14	4		59	259	56		5	9	24	6		56
Oman	1	100							100																		
Pakistan	2198	28	53	4	1	7	5	1	81										673	48	10	6	3	22	7	4	58
Qatar																											
Saudi Arabia	112	51	16	4	2	13	4	11	67																		
Somalia	411	54	4	5	3	4	30		59																		
Sudan	1640	51	26	3	0	5	2	12	77																		
Syrian Arab Republic	82	41	30	7	7	12	1		72	61	33	11	7	31	16	2		44	24	21	13	4	13	42	8		33
Tunisia	53	75		2	9	11	2		75																		
United Arab Emirates	3							100																			
West Bank and Gaza Strip		68	7	5	5	9	5		76																		
Yemen	393	50	20	5		20		10	70																		
Region	**7 473**	**51**	**26**	**4**	**3**	**8**	**5**	**3**	**77**	**263**	**56**	**4**	**9**	**15**	**12**	**4**	**0**	**59**	**1 089**	**47**	**11**	**6**	**5**	**22**	**7**	**3**	**58**

See Explanatory notes for previous table, page 151.

EMR

Country data for the Eastern Mediterranean: trends in DOTS treatment success and detection rates, 1994–2003

	DOTS new smear-positive treatment success (%)									DOTS new smear-positive case detection rate (%)								
	1994	1995	1996	1997	1998	1999	2000	2001	2002	1995	1996	1997	1998	1999	2000	2001	2002	2003
Afghanistan				45	33	87	86	84	87				6	5	9	14	19	18
Bahrain					13	95	73	87	88			2		14	62	59	11	49
Djibouti		75	77	76	79	72	62	78	82		103	107	90	79	68	61	57	53
Egypt	52		81	82	87	87	87	82	88	43	1	11	17	31	45	49	53	56
Iran			87	84	83	82	85	84	85	47		13	35	53	58	61	60	59
Iraq					83	85	92	89	91				2	6	22	23	23	20
Jordan	90				92	88	90	86	89				73	71	64	71	72	89
Kuwait									55									67
Lebanon	89				73	96	92	91	91	53				90	79	72	68	67
Libyan Arab Jamahiriya					68	67			61					148	113	83	138	147
Morocco	86	90	88	89	88	88	89	87	89	94	94	93	88	88	84	83	84	83
Oman		84	87	91	86	95	93	90	92		114	115	110	85	117	112	109	81
Pakistan	74	70		67	66	70	74	77	77	1	2		4	2	3	5	13	17
Qatar	83	81	72	79	84	74	66	60	75	46	34	28	48	39	34	48	39	57
Saudi Arabia					57	66	73	77	76					22	37	39	38	38
Somalia		86	84	90	88	88	83	86	89		19	24	23	24	25	29	28	29
Sudan				70	65	81	79	80	78		2	1	29	29	34	31	33	34
Syrian Arab Republic			92	88	88	84	79	81	87			8	21	29	42	43	42	45
Tunisia					91	91	91	90	92					96	103	104	92	91
United Arab Emirates							74	62	79						29	28	24	32
West Bank and Gaza Strip									100						10	13		4
Yemen			76	81		83	75	80	82		8	30	37		54	51	47	43
Region	**82**	**87**	**86**	**79**	**76**	**83**	**83**	**83**	**84**	**11**	**9**	**10**	**17**	**17**	**22**	**23**	**27**	**28**

Country data for the Eastern Mediterranean: age and sex distribution of smear-positive cases in DOTS areas, 2003 (absolute numbers)

	MALE							FEMALE							ALL						
	0-14	15-24	25-34	35-44	45-54	55-64	65+	0-14	15-24	25-34	35-44	45-54	55-64	65+	0-14	15-24	25-34	35-44	45-54	55-64	65+
Afghanistan	127	511	436	284	256	288	203	245	1 152	1 287	814	462	305	158	372	1663	1723	1098	718	593	361
Bahrain	0	2	2	1	1	3	4	0	1	0	0	1	1	0	0	3	2	1	2	4	4
Djibouti	10	222	288	132	76	42	24	19	127	123	55	38	28	8	29	349	411	187	114	70	32
Egypt	42	586	814	675	631	404	195	57	463	338	268	282	175	71	99	1049	1152	943	913	579	266
Iran	29	404	524	393	281	292	673	78	445	278	254	304	438	773	107	849	802	647	585	730	1446
Iraq	30	659	876	355	293	168	143	43	258	241	154	160	143	34	73	917	1117	509	453	311	177
Jordan	0	19	20	17	8	13	0	1	6	7	2	3	12	0	1	25	27	19	11	25	0
Kuwait	1	14	39	33	26	11	5	1	16	31	18	2	3	1	2	30	70	51	28	14	6
Lebanon	0	19	26	22	6	5	7	3	14	12	9	5	2	4	3	33	38	31	11	7	11
Libyan Arab Jamahiriya	0	108	266	142	32	25	19	4	43	28	30	25	21	21	4	151	294	172	57	46	40
Morocco	91	2 225	2 347	1 667	1 004	525	550	168	1 455	1 029	633	431	366	351	259	3680	3376	2300	1435	891	901
Oman	0	12	10	20	19	5	11	2	11	6	6	6	6	4	2	23	16	20	25	11	15
Pakistan	278	2 582	2 219	1 763	1 623	1 238	844	613	3 032	2 371	1 595	823	478	478	891	5614	4590	3358	2446	1746	1322
Qatar	1	10	27	17	16	5	5	0	4	6	0	2	0	2	1	14	33	17	18	5	7
Saudi Arabia	5	150	285	200	145	102	107	13	210	181	75	58	51	59	23	360	466	275	203	153	166
Somalia	118	1 054	850	513	319	250	214	106	535	462	333	171	161	104	224	1589	1312	846	490	411	318
Sudan	489	1 195	1 644	1 271	856	645	473	443	881	1 052	879	562	384	219	932	2076	2696	2150	1418	1029	692
Syrian Arab Republic	10	343	279	127	98	75	64	26	242	99	68	48	33	33	36	585	378	195	146	108	97
Tunisia	3	102	166	131	96	67	75	7	58	56	37	35	24	33	10	160	222	168	131	91	108
United Arab Emirates	2	10	8	12	3	2	10	4	9	5	3	3	2	4	6	19	13	15	6	4	14
West Bank and Gaza Strip	0	1	1	1	3	0	2	0	1	0	0	0	0	3	0	2	1	1	6	0	5
Yemen	37	555	551	376	238	148	93	72	451	404	300	196	111	70	109	1006	955	676	434	259	163
Region	1 273	10 783	11 678	8 152	6 030	4 343	3 721	1 910	9 414	8 016	5 527	3 620	2 744	2 430	3 183	20 197	19 694	13 679	9 650	7 087	6 151

Note: the sum of cases notified by age is less than the number of new smear-positive cases notified for some countries.

EMR

Country data for the Eastern Mediterranean: age and sex distribution of smear-positive cases in non-DOTS areas, 2003 (absolute numbers)

	MALE							FEMALE							ALL						
	0-14	15-24	25-34	35-44	45-54	55-64	65+	0-14	15-24	25-34	35-44	45-54	55-64	65+	0-14	15-24	25-34	35-44	45-54	55-64	65+
Afghanistan																					
Bahrain																					
Djibouti																					
Egypt																					
Iran																					
Iraq																					
Jordan																					
Kuwait																					
Lebanon																					
Libyan Arab Jamahiriya																					
Morocco																					
Oman	5	16	22	11	10	8	4	8	15	12	12	7	5	3	13	31	34	23	17	13	7
Pakistan																					
Qatar																					
Saudi Arabia																					
Somalia																					
Sudan																					
Syrian Arab Republic																					
Tunisia																					
United Arab Emirates																					
West Bank and Gaza Strip																					
Yemen	3	26	36	23	12	6	10	2	19	22	17	8	3	4	5	45	58	40	20	9	14
Region	8	42	58	34	22	14	14	10	34	34	29	15	8	7	18	76	92	63	37	22	21

Note: the sum of cases notified by age is less than the number of new smear-positive cases notified for some countries.

Country data for the Eastern Mediterranean: smear-positive notification rates (per 100 000 population) by age and sex, 2003

	MALE							FEMALE							ALL						
	0-14	15-24	25-34	35-44	45-54	55-64	65+	0-14	15-24	25-34	35-44	45-54	55-64	65+	0-14	15-24	25-34	35-44	45-54	55-64	65+
Afghanistan	2	21	26	23	31	56	61	5	52	81	72	60	61	46	4	36	52	47	45	58	54
Bahrain	0	3	2	1	2	20	42	0	2	0	0	4	9	0	0	3	1	1	3	15	21
Djibouti	7	326	592	395	346	280	237	13	87	251	160	162	170	66	10	257	421	275	251	223	144
Egypt	0	8	16	17	20	22	13	0	6	6	7	9	9	4	0	7	11	12	14	15	8
Iran	0	5	10	10	10	21	42	1	5	5	7	11	28	50	0	5	8	8	11	25	46
Iraq	1	25	46	27	34	33	43	1	10	13	12	19	27	9	1	18	30	20	27	30	24
Jordan	0	3	4	5	5	11	0	0	1	2	1	2	11	0	0	2	3	3	4	11	0
Kuwait	0	7	11	9	14	20	23	0	9	15	10	2	9	6	0	8	13	9	11	16	15
Lebanon	0	5	8	9	4	6	7	1	4	4	3	3	2	3	0	5	6	6	4	4	5
Libyan Arab Jamahiriya	0	16	54	46	13	15	17	0	7	6	10	12	16	20	0	11	31	29	13	15	19
Morocco	2	69	88	86	75	80	90	4	46	40	32	32	48	46	3	58	64	59	53	63	66
Oman	1	10	10	12	24	23	47	2	10	10	11	19	28	24	1	10	10	11	22	25	36
Pakistan	1	16	21	23	28	36	30	2	21	24	21	15	14	16	1	18	22	22	22	25	23
Qatar	1	24	40	17	23	24	78	0	10	22	0	8	0	51	1	17	35	12	19	17	68
Saudi Arabia	0	7	12	11	15	23	31	0	10	10	6	9	13	19	0	8	11	9	13	18	25
Somalia	5	110	135	124	118	166	201	4	56	72	78	59	96	82	5	83	103	101	88	129	136
Sudan	7	36	64	73	73	84	85	7	27	42	50	47	47	34	7	32	53	61	60	65	57
Syrian Arab Republic	0	16	20	14	18	25	26	1	12	7	7	8	10	11	1	14	13	11	13	17	18
Tunisia	0	10	19	20	21	27	27	1	6	7	5	8	9	11	0	8	13	13	14	17	18
United Arab Emirates	1	4	2	2	1	2	41	1	4	3	2	3	7	23	0	4	2	2	1	3	34
West Bank and Gaza Strip	0	0	0	1	3	0	4	0	0	0	0	3	0	4	0	0	0	0	3	0	4
Yemen	1	28	48	49	45	51	48	2	24	37	38	36	37	31	1	26	42	43	41	44	39
Region	**1**	**20**	**30**	**28**	**30**	**38**	**40**	**2**	**18**	**22**	**20**	**19**	**24**	**24**	**2**	**19**	**26**	**24**	**25**	**31**	**32**

Note: rates are missing where data for smear-positive cases are missing, or where age- and sex-specific population data are not available.

EMR

Country data for the Eastern Mediterranean: number of TB cases notified, 1980–2003

	1980	1981	1982	1983	1984	1985	1986	1987	1988	1989	1990	1991	1992	1993	1994	1995	1996	1997	1998	1999	2000	2001	2002	2003
Afghanistan	71 685	71 554	41 752	52 502	18 784	10 742	14 351	18 091	16 051	14 386	4 332	23 067	140	114				1 290	3 084	3 314	7 107	10 139	13 794	13 808
Bahrain	219	262	156	232	208	194	142	120	142	122	117	142				43	49	45	83	36	94	120	44	263
Djibouti		2 265	671		1 489	2 262	1 864	1 978	2 030	2 040	2 100	2 900	2 884	3 489	3 311		3 332	3 830	3 785	4 133	3 971	4 198	3 191	3 231
Egypt	1 637	1 306	1 805	1 932	1 572	1 308	1 209	22 063	1 378	1 492	2 142	3 634	8 876	3 426	3 911	11 145	12 338	13 971	12 662	11 763	10 762	10 549	11 177	11 490
Iran	42 717	11 728	9 509	8 589	10 493	8 728	8 032	10 034	9 967	12 005	9 255	14 246	14 121	20 569	13 021	15 936	14 189	12 659	11 794	12 062	11 850	11 780	11 436	10 857
Iraq	11 809	10 614	7 741	6 970	6 807	6 485	6 846	6 517	6 504	8 032	14 684			18 553	19 733	9 697	29 196	26 607	29 410	29 897	9 697	10 478	11 898	11 656
Jordan	298	646	860	856	672	769	592	537	553	484	439	390	504	427	443	498	468	397	380	373	306	342	312	310
Kuwait	847	819	880	855	812	717	611	540	480	468	277	330	282	217	237	336	400	528	564					566
Lebanon		67	75	284	410	1 943	2 257	2 478				884	884		940	983	836	701	640	679	571	516	437	380
Libyan Arab Jamahiriya	718	481	512	610	357	325	276	331	416	265	442	239	1 164			1 440	1 282	1 575	1 575	1 615	1 341	1 824	1 824	1 917
Morocco	24 878	28 637	28 095	26 944	22 279	26 790	27 553	27 159	25 717	26 756	27 658	27 638	25 403	27 626	30 316	29 829	31 771	30 227	29 087	29 854	28 852	28 285	29 804	26 789
Oman	1 872	928	897	802	843	861	1 265	616	477	478	482	442	367	281	304	276	300	298	287	249	321	292	290	257
Pakistan	316 340	324 576	326 492	117 739	91 572	111 419	149 004	179 480	194 323	170 562	156 759	194 323		73 175		13 142	4 307		89 599	20 936	11 050	34 066	52 172	73 100
Qatar	257	213	172	206	203	250	220	248	223	191	184	195		200		304	257	212	253	259	279	284	278	276
Saudi Arabia	10 956	8 263	8 529	7 551	7 163	3 966	3 696	3 029	2 433	2 583	2 415	2 221	2 016	2 386	2 518	2 504	3 920	3 138	3 235	3 507	3 452	3 327	3 374	3 317
Somalia				2 838	2 719	2 722	3 079	7 322	2 728	1 323														9 278
Sudan	32 971	47 431				1 509	2 460	800	693	701	212	16 423	19 503	37 516	23 178	14 320	20 230	20 894	22 318	26 875	24 807	23 997	24 554	25 095
Syrian Arab Republic	1 689	1 908	1 838	1 867	2 111	2 163	3 942	4 290	4 952	5 504	6 018	5 651	5 437		5 127	4 404	5 200	4 972	5 417	5 447	5 090	4 997	4 766	4 820
Tunisia	2 504	2 316	2 554	3 062	2 501	2 510	2 487	2 272	2 309	2 403	2 054	2 064	2 164	2 565	2 376	2 383	2 387	2 211	2 158	2 038	1 945	1 945	1 885	1 965
United Arab Emirates	522	638	597	507	534	568	464	818	339	308	285	234	227		426		507		773	66	115	74	90	117
West Bank and Gaza	191	139	136	136	123	113	63	82	85	145	64	89	97			77	40	18			82			36
Yemen																14 428	14 364	12 007	12 383	13 027	13 651	13 029	11 677	10 413
Region	522 110	514 791	433 271	234 482	171 652	186 344	230 427	288 805	271 800	250 248	229 919	295 112	84 069	190 544	107 864	121 745	145 373	136 226	233 878	171 052	141 122	165 270	190 394	209 941
number reporting	18	20	19	19	20	21	21	21	20	20	19	19	16	14	15	17	19	16	21	19	20	18	19	22
percent reporting	86	95	90	90	95	100	100	100	95	95	90	90	76	67	71	81	90	76	100	90	95	86	90	100

Country data for the Eastern Mediterranean: case notification rates (per 100 000 population), 1980–2003

	1980	1981	1982	1983	1984	1985	1986	1987	1988	1989	1990	1991	1992	1993	1994	1995	1996	1997	1998	1999	2000	2001	2002	2003
Afghanistan	474	480	286	369	136	79	108	138	123	108	31	158	27	21		7		6	15	16	33	46	60	58
Bahrain	63	73	42	60	52	47	36	27	31	26	24	28	27				8	7	13	5	14	17	6	36
Djibouti		667	193		408	593	458	451	429	405	398	535	524	630	593		571	634	604	638	596	617	461	460
Egypt	4	3	4	4	3	3	2	42	3	3	4	6	15	6	6	18	20	22	19	18	16	15	16	16
Iran	109	29	22	19	23	13	16	19	19	22	16	25	24	34	21	26	22	20	18	18	18	18	17	16
Iraq	91	79	56	49	46	43	44	41	40	43	85			98	101	48	140	124	134	132	42	44	49	46
Jordan	13	28	36	34	26	28	21	19	18	16	13	11	14	11	11	12	11	9	8	8	6	7	6	6
Kuwait	62	57	59	55	50	42	33	28	23	22	13	16	14	12	14	20	23	29	29	20	16	15	12	22
Lebanon		3	3	11	15	73	85	93				32	31		31	31	26	21	19	20	16	15		10
Libyan Arab Jamahiriya	24	15	15	17	10	9	7	8	10	6	10	5	26			30	26		31	31	26		34	35
Morocco	128	144	138	129	104	122	122	118	109	111	113	110	100	106	115	111	116	109	103	104	99	96	99	88
Oman	158	74	68	58	58	56	79	37	28	27	26	23	18	14	14	12	13	12	12	10	12	11	10	9
Pakistan	392	389	379	132	99	117	152	177	186	158	141	171		61		11	3		66	15	8	23	35	48
Qatar	112	85	62	68	61	69	57	61	52	42	39	40		40		58	48	39	45	45	48	48	46	45
Saudi Arabia	114	81	79	66	59	31	27	21	16	16	15	13	11	13	14			16	16	16	16	15	14	14
Somalia	170	237		42	41	41	46	107	39	19		64	75	140	28	34	52	57	54	57	65	75	78	94
Sudan	19	21	19	19	20	7	11	3	3	3	1	43	40		85	51	70	71	74	87	79	75	75	75
Syrian Arab Republic							35	37	41	45	47	25	25	30	36	30	35	32	34	34	31	29	27	27
Tunisia	39	35	37	44	35	34	33	29	29	30	25	25		30	27	27	26		24	23	21	20	19	20
United Arab Emirates	51	57	48	38	37	37	28	47	18	16	14	11	10		18		20		29	2	4	3	3	4
West Bank and Gaza Strip	13	9	9	8	7	6	3	4	4	7	3	4	4			3			1					1
Yemen																95	91	74	73	75	76	70	60	52
Region	184	176	143	75	53	56	68	82	75	68	60	76	21	46	26	28	33	30	51	36	29	33	38	41

EMR

Country data for the Eastern Mediterranean: new smear-positive cases, 1993–2003

Number of cases

	1993	1994	1995	1996	1997	1998	1999	2000	2001	2002	2003
Afghanistan					618	1 833	1 669	2 892	4 639	6 509	6 510
Bahrain	82		17	31	22	25	21	94	89	17	73
Djibouti	1 668	1 743		1 744	1 904	1 690	1 564	1 391	1 312	1 253	1 202
Egypt		1 811	4 229	5 084	5 469	4 915	5 094	4 606	4 514	4 889	5 118
Iran		4 615	5 347	5 373	5 253	5 105	5 426	5 866	5 523	5 335	5 166
Iraq	5 240	5 781	3 194	10 320	8 164	8 933	9 908	3 194	3 559	3 895	3 577
Jordan	173	161	187	170	136	110	102	89	94	91	108
Kuwait	148	155	175	153	201	185					201
Lebanon		148	197	198	206	224	249	202	171	148	134
Libyan Arab Jamahiriya				515			803	607			764
Morocco			14 171	14 278	14 134	13 426	13 420	12 872	12 804	12 914	12 842
Oman	123	135	135	164	165	156	120	164	156	151	112
Pakistan	11 020					14 974	6 248	3 285	10 935	16 265	20 962
Qatar			60	46	39	69	58	53	77	64	95
Saudi Arabia	800		2 578	1 849	1 568	1 644	1 680	1 595	1 686	1 674	1 646
Somalia		1 168	1 572	2 894	3 093	3 121	3 461	3 776	4 640	4 729	5 190
Sudan		3 728	8 761	8 978	10 835	10 820	11 047	12 311	11 136	10 338	10 993
Syrian Arab Republic			1 295	1 523	1 423	1 593	1 577	1 584	1 507	1 447	1 545
Tunisia	1 006	983	1 243	1 005		1 196	1 066	1 099	1 077	927	890
United Arab Emirates			9	24		8	31	73	69	57	77
West Bank and Gaza Strip								37	49		15
Yemen			3 681	4 371	4 717	4 896	5 427	5 565	4 968	4 259	3 793
Region	**20 260**	**20 428**	**46 851**	**58 720**	**57 947**	**74 923**	**68 971**	**61 355**	**69 005**	**74 962**	**81 013**

Rate (per 100 000 population)

	1993	1994	1995	1996	1997	1998	1999	2000	2001	2002	2003
Afghanistan					3	9	8	14	21	28	27
Bahrain	15		3	5	4	4	3	14	13	2	10
Djibouti	301	312		299	315	270	241	209	193	181	171
Egypt		3	7	8	9	8	8	7	7	7	7
Iran		8	9	8	8	8	8	9	8	8	7
Iraq	28	29	16	50	38	41	44	14	15	16	14
Jordan	5	4	4	4	3	2	2	2	2	2	2
Kuwait	8	9	10	9	11	9					8
Lebanon		5	6	6	6	7	7	6	5	4	4
Libyan Arab Jamahiriya				11			16	12			14
Morocco			53	52	51	48	47	44	43	43	42
Oman	6	6	6	7	7	6	5	6	6	5	4
Pakistan	9							2	7	11	14
Qatar			11	9	7	11	4	9	13	11	16
Saudi Arabia	4				8	12	10	7	7	7	7
Somalia		16	21	38	40	39	41	43	51	50	52
Sudan		14	31	31	37	36	36	39	35	31	33
Syrian Arab Republic			9	10	9	10	10	10	9	8	9
Tunisia	12	11	14	11		13	11	12	11	10	9
United Arab Emirates			0	1		0	1	3	2	2	3
West Bank and Gaza Strip								1	1		0
Yemen			24	28	29	29	31	31	27	22	19
Region	**5**	**5**	**11**	**13**	**13**	**16**	**15**	**13**	**14**	**15**	**16**

Notes

Bahrain
Of the 263 total TB cases, 73 were in nationals.

Kuwait
Treatment after default cases were included under new smear-positive cases.

Libyan Arab Jamahiriya
"Transfer out" treatment outcomes were all non-nationals who left the country. Among the remaining patients, the success rate was 74%.

Morocco
Among 13 009 new pulmonary laboratory-confirmed cases, 167 cases were smear-negative but culture-positive.

Oman
Treatment outcomes excluded cases in non-nationals who must leave the country after conversion to smear-negative status.

Qatar
From 95 notified cases, 14 were in nationals. Among the cohort of 64 cases evaluated for treatment outcome, 10 were in nationals.

Saudi Arabia
Treatment outcomes excluded 276 cases in non-nationals that left the country, and 33 cases that were not evaluated for other reasons.

Somalia
There is a discrepancy between the population estimate used by the national TB programme (6 992 904) and that used by the UN (9 890 068). Using the country's population estimate, there would be 40 645 estimated TB cases (of which, 18 154 smear-positive cases), and DOTS detection of smear-positive cases would be 40% (instead of 29%).

Sudan
DOTS coverage was not reported, but assumed to be same as in the previous report.

Syrian Arab Republic
Notification data do not include 26 cases diagnosed in prison.

West Bank and Gaza Strip
DOTS coverage was not reported, but assumed to be same as in the previous report.

EMR

Africa

The Americas

Eastern Mediterranean

Europe

South-East Asia

Western Pacific

	STATUS[a]	MANUAL[b]	MICROSCOPY[c]	SCC[d]	DOT[e]	MONITORING OUTCOME[f]
ALBANIA	DOTS	YES				
ANDORRA	DOTS	YES				
ARMENIA	DOTS	YES				
AUSTRIA						
AZERBAIJAN	DOTS	YES				
BELARUS	**DOTS**	YES				
BELGIUM	DOTS	NO				
BOSNIA & HERZEGOVINA	DOTS	YES				
BULGARIA	DOTS	YES				
CROATIA	NON-DOTS					
CYPRUS	DOTS	NO				
CZECH REPUBLIC	DOTS	YES				
DENMARK	**DOTS**	YES				
ESTONIA	DOTS	YES				
FINLAND	NON-DOTS	NO				
FRANCE	NON-DOTS	YES				
GEORGIA	DOTS	YES				
GERMANY	DOTS	YES				
GREECE	NON-DOTS	NO				
HUNGARY	DOTS	YES				
ICELAND	DOTS	NO				
IRELAND	NON-DOTS	YES				
ISRAEL	DOTS	YES				
ITALY	DOTS	YES				
KAZAKHSTAN	DOTS	YES				
KYRGYZSTAN	DOTS	YES				
LATVIA	DOTS	YES				
LITHUANIA	DOTS	YES				
LUXEMBOURG	DOTS	NO				
MALTA	DOTS	YES				
MONACO						
NETHERLANDS	DOTS	YES				
NORWAY	DOTS	YES				
POLAND	DOTS	YES				
PORTUGAL	DOTS	YES				
REPUBLIC OF MOLDOVA	DOTS	YES				
ROMANIA	DOTS	YES				
RUSSIAN FEDERATION	DOTS	YES				
SAN MARINO	DOTS	NO				
SERBIA AND MONTENEGRO	DOTS	YES				
SLOVAKIA	DOTS	YES				
SLOVENIA	DOTS	NO				
SPAIN	NON-DOTS	YES				
SWEDEN	DOTS	YES				
SWITZERLAND	NON-DOTS	YES				
TAJIKISTAN	DOTS	YES				
TFYR MACEDONIA	DOTS	YES				
TURKEY						
TURKMENISTAN	DOTS	YES				
UKRAINE	DOTS	YES				
UNITED KINGDOM	NON-DOTS	YES				
UZBEKISTAN	DOTS	YES				

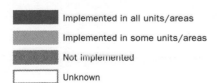

Implemented in all units/areas
Implemented in some units/areas
Not implemented
Unknown

a Status: DOTS status (bold indicates DOTS introduced in 2003. Blank indicates no report received)
b Manual: national TB control manual (recommended)
c Microscopy: use of smear microscopy for diagnosis (core component of DOTS)
d SCC: short course chemotherapy (core component of DOTS)
e DOT: directly observed treatment (core component of DOTS)
f Outcome monitoring: monitoring of treatment outcomes by cohort analysis (core component of DOTS)

Country data for Europe: estimated burden of TB

1990

	Incidence, 1990				Prevalence, 1990				Death, 1990			
	All cases incl. HIV+		New ss+ incl. HIV+		All cases incl. HIV+		All cases excl. HIV+		All cases incl. HIV+		All cases excl. HIV+	
	number	rate	number	rate	number	rate	number	rate	number	rate	number	rate
Albania	879	27	396	12	1 505	46	1 505	46	139	4	139	4
Andorra	19	37	9	16	22	41	22	41	3	6	3	6
Armenia	932	26	419	12	1 569	44	1 569	44	162	5	162	5
Austria	1 535	20	686	9	1 718	22	1 718	22	246	3	246	3
Azerbaijan	2 518	35	1 133	16	4 238	59	4 238	59	437	6	437	6
Belarus	3 894	38	1 745	17	6 533	64	6 525	64	678	7	673	7
Belgium	1 920	19	859	9	2 149	22	2 149	22	308	3	308	3
Bosnia & Herzegovina	4 044	94	1 819	42	6 920	161	6 920	161	638	15	638	15
Bulgaria	2 459	28	1 106	13	4 138	47	4 138	47	427	5	427	5
Croatia	3 578	74	1 610	33	6 123	126	6 123	126	565	12	565	12
Cyprus	34	5	15	2	58	9	58	9	5	0.8	5	0.8
Czech Republic	3 772	37	1 695	16	4 222	41	4 222	41	606	6	606	6
Denmark	802	16	359	7	898	17	898	17	129	3	129	3
Estonia	499	32	222	14	840	53	840	53	87	5	87	5
Finland	882	18	396	8	987	20	987	20	142	3	142	3
France	17 776	31	7 907	14	19 896	35	19 896	35	2 854	5	2 854	5
Georgia	2 087	38	937	17	3 511	64	3 511	64	362	7	362	7
Germany	22 539	28	10 110	13	25 228	32	25 228	32	3 619	5	3 619	5
Greece	3 109	31	1 392	14	3 479	34	3 479	34	499	5	499	5
Hungary	4 181	40	1 881	18	7 154	69	7 154	69	660	6	660	6
Iceland	17	7	8	3	19	8	19	8	7	3	7	3
Ireland	938	27	421	12	1 050	30	1 050	30	151	4	151	4
Israel	833	18	374	8	932	21	932	21	134	3	134	3
Italy	8 092	14	3 593	6	9 057	16	9 057	16	1 299	2	1 299	2
Kazakhstan	9 631	57	4 326	26	16 206	96	16 206	96	1 672	10	1 672	10
Kyrgyzstan	2 290	52	1 030	23	3 854	88	3 854	88	398	9	398	9
Latvia	907	33	406	15	1 525	56	1 525	56	157	6	157	6
Lithuania	1 416	38	637	17	2 382	64	2 382	64	246	7	246	7
Luxembourg	89	24	40	11	100	26	100	26	14	4	14	4
Malta	42	12	19	5	47	13	47	13	7	2	7	2
Monaco	1	5	0.6	2	2	5	2	5	0.2	0.7	0.2	
Netherlands	2 080	14	930	6	2 329	16	2 329	16	334	2	334	2
Norway	456	11	205	5	510	12	510	12	73	2	73	2
Poland	20 251	53	9 106	24	34 655	91	34 655	91	3 195	8	3 195	8
Portugal	7 011	71	3 118	31	7 848	79	7 848	79	1 126	11	1 126	11
Republic of Moldova	2 793	64	1 254	29	4 700	108	4 700	108	485	11	485	11
Romania	17 668	76	7 949	34	29 729	128	29 729	128	3 067	13	3 067	13
Russian Federation	71 540	48	31 875	21	120 377	81	120 377	81	12 417	8	12 417	8
San Marino	3	12	1	5	14		14		0.4		0.4	
Serbia & Montenegro	6 032	59	2 711	27	10 323	102	10 323	102	952	9	952	9
Slovakia	2 187	42	984	19	3 743	71	3 743	71	345	7	345	7
Slovenia	863	45	388	20	1 476	77	1 476	77	136	7	136	7
Spain	24 479	62	10 836	28	27 399	70	27 399	70	3 930	10	3 930	10
Sweden	713	8	320	4	798	9	798	9	115	1	115	1
Switzerland	1 247	18	555	8	1 395	20	1 395	20	200	3	200	3
Tajikistan	5 696	107	2 563	48	9 584	181	9 584	181	989	19	989	19
TFYR Macedonia	1 027	54	462	24	1 757	92	1 757	92	162	8	162	8
Turkey	26 321	46	11 844	21	45 042	78	45 042	78	4 153	7	4 153	7
Turkmenistan	2 163	59	973	27	3 639	99	3 639	99	375	10	375	10
Ukraine	20 214	39	8 983	17	33 892	65	33 841	65	3 525	7	3 491	7
United Kingdom	6 546	12	2 936	5	7 327	13	7 327	13	1 051	2	1 051	2
Uzbekistan	13 924	68	6 260	31	23 429	114	23 429	114	2 417	12	2 417	12
Region	**334 927**	**39**	**149 801**	**18**	**506 317**	**60**	**506 257**	**60**	**55 692**	**7**	**55 653**	**7**

2003

	Incidence, 2003				Prevalence, 2003				Death, 2003			
	All cases incl. HIV+		New ss+ incl. HIV+		All cases incl. HIV+		All cases excl. HIV+		All cases incl. HIV+		All cases excl. HIV+	
	number	rate	number	rate	number	rate	number	rate	number	rate	number	rate
Albania	724	23	326	10	1 060	33	1 060	33	132	4	132	4
Andorra	13	19	6	8	12	17	12	17	1	2	1	2
Armenia	2 146	70	964	32	2 741	90	2 735	89	341	11	338	11
Austria	1 172	14	524	6	970	12	951	12	117	1	114	1
Azerbaijan	6 351	76	2 858	34	9 122	109	9 121	109	914	11	913	11
Belarus	5 206	53	2 333	24	5 919	60	5 868	59	700	7	682	7
Belgium	1 416	14	634	6	1 216	12	1 197	12	148	1	143	1
Bosnia & Herzegovina	2 279	55	1 025	25	2 627	63	2 626	63	333	8	333	8
Bulgaria	3 423	43	1 540	20	3 711	47	3 710	47	466	6	465	6
Croatia	1 909	43	859	19	2 993	68	2 992	68	295	7	295	7
Cyprus	34	4	15	2	35	4	35	4	3	1	3	1
Czech Republic	1 191	12	535	5	1 241	12	1 237	12	135	1	134	1
Denmark	429	8	192	4	343	6	337	6	43	1	42	1
Estonia	658	50	293	22	717	54	702	53	99	7	93	7
Finland	483	9	217	4	504	10	502	10	50	1	50	1
France	7 257	12	3 228	5	7 413	12	7 226	12	759	1	715	1
Georgia	4 244	83	1 906	37	4 869	95	4 849	95	700	14	692	13
Germany	6 749	8	3 027	4	5 521	7	5 472	7	675	1	666	1
Greece	2 148	20	962	9	2 392	22	2 368	22	270	2	262	2
Hungary	2 846	29	1 280	13	3 284	33	3 282	33	380	4	379	4
Iceland	8	3	4	1	8	3	8	3	0.8	1	0.8	
Ireland	459	12	206	5	478	12	474	12	48	1	47	1
Israel	608	9	273	4	498	8	494	8	61	1	60	1
Italy	4 199	7	1 865	3	3 356	6	3 230	6	474	1	447	1
Kazakhstan	22 441	145	10 079	65	23 547	153	23 451	152	3 004	19	2 970	19
Kyrgyzstan	6 391	124	2 874	56	7 210	140	7 200	140	933	18	929	18
Latvia	1 735	75	776	34	1 835	80	1 811	78	255	11	246	11
Lithuania	2 398	70	1 078	31	2 531	73	2 527	73	320	9	319	9
Luxembourg	55	12	25	5	44	10	43	10	5	1	5	1
Malta	23	6	11	3	24	6	24	6	3	1	3	1
Monaco	0.8	2	0.4	1	0.8	2	0.8	2	0.1		0.1	
Netherlands	1 253	8	560	3	1 025	6	1 005	6	125	1	121	1
Norway	250	6	112	2	207	5	205	5	25	1	25	1
Poland	11 878	31	5 342	14	13 302	34	13 283	34	1 587	4	1 581	4
Portugal	4 497	45	2 000	20	3 794	38	3 675	37	492	5	459	5
Republic of Moldova	5 918	139	2 657	62	7 578	178	7 549	177	857	20	843	20
Romania	33 276	149	14 972	67	43 382	194	43 370	194	4 493	20	4 487	20
Russian Federation	160 688	112	71 597	50	229 046	160	225 481	157	29 024	20	26 794	19
San Marino	2	6	0.8	3	2	5	2	5	0.2		0.2	
Serbia & Montenegro	3 648	35	1 639	16	4 647	44	4 636	44	534	5	529	5
Slovakia	1 312	24	591	11	1 569	29	1 569	29	209	4	209	4
Slovenia	366	18	165	8	434	22	434	22	53	3	53	3
Spain	11 237	27	4 974	12	11 345	28	10 932	27	1 178	3	1 082	3
Sweden	393	4	176	2	319	4	316	4	39		39	
Switzerland	529	7	235	3	527	7	515	7	53	1	50	1
Tajikistan	10 508	168	4 729	76	16 671	267	16 670	267	1 983	32	1 983	32
TFYR Macedonia	645	31	290	14	762	37	762	37	114	6	114	6
Turkey	18 555	26	8 349	12	28 872	40	28 870	40	3 166	4	3 165	4
Turkmenistan	3 272	67	1 472	30	4 035	83	4 035	83	477	10	477	10
Ukraine	44 674	92	19 853	41	65 717	135	64 464	133	6 343	13	5 695	12
United Kingdom	7 056	12	3 165	5	7 160	12	7 108	12	706	1	696	1
Uzbekistan	30 001	115	13 487	52	40 754	156	40 688	156	4 093	16	4 063	16
Region	**438 960**	**50**	**196 281**	**22**	**577 371**	**66**	**571 116**	**65**	**67 217**	**8**	**63 941**	**7**

See Explanatory notes, page 151.

Country data for Europe: notification, detection and DOTS coverage, 2003

Country	Pop (thousands)	Notified TB — Country number	WHO number	rate	New — Smear-positive number	rate	Pulm confirmed number	Smear-negative or unknown number	Extra-pulmonary number	Re-treat. Relapse	After failure	After default	Re-treat. Other	Other number	Detection rate All cases %	New ss+ %	DOTS % of pop	DOTS Notif. All cases number	rate	New ss+ number	rate	DDR %	% of pulm cases ss+	non-DOTS All cases number	non-DOTS New ss+ number	% of pulm cases ss+
Albania	3,166	561	543	17	211	7	242	124	192	16		0	6	12	75	65	30	211	6	96	3	29	74	342	115	56
Andorra	71	11	10	14	7	10	7	1	2	0		0	0	1	75	116	100	10	14	7	10	116	88			
Armenia	3,061	1,570	1,538	50	575	19	575	599	263	101		0	32		72	60	100	1,250	41	418	14	43	47	288	157	55
Austria	8,116																									
Azerbaijan	8,370	3,931	3,840	46	1,161	14	1,161	1,871	735	73		0	86	5	60	41	48	1,615	19	808	10	28	57	2,225	353	22
Belarus	9,895	5,963	5,106	52	1,018	10	2,239	3,710	378	0		0	0	857	98	44	70	5,106	52	1,018	10	44	22	0	0	
Belgium	10,318	1,128	1,030	10	362	4	448	406	262			0	64	34	73	57	100	1,030	10	362	4	57	47			
Bosnia & Herzegovina	4,161	1,780	1,740	42	493	12	949	951	205	91		0	0	40	76	48	100	1,740	42	493	12	48	34			
Bulgaria	7,897	3,263	3,069	39	1,254	16	1,260	1,274	424	117		0	194		90	81	100	3,069	39	1,254	16	81	50	1,356	438	37
Croatia	4,428	1,494	1,356	31	438	10	688	756	162	0		0	103	35	71	51	0	0		0						
Cyprus	802	35	35	4	14	2	21	15	6	0		0	0		102	91	100	35	4	14	2	91	48	0	0	
Czech Republic	10,236	1,153	1,101	11	338	3	614	518	245	0		0	25	27	92	63	100	1,101	11	338	3	63	39			
Denmark	5,364	391	378	7	143	3	216	131	93	11		0	40	13	88	75	10	35	1	14	0	75	52			
Estonia	1,323	623	557	42	201	15	339	239	56	61		0	40	26	85	69	100	557	42	201	15	69	46			
Finland	5,207	414	392	8	138	3	230	134	120	0		0	19	3	81	64	0							392	138	51
France	60,144	6,350	5,740	10	2,219	4	2,399	1,919	1,602	0		0	322	288	79	69	0	0		0				5,740	2,219	54
Georgia	5,126	5,993	4,212	82	989	19	989	1,816	1,265	142		0	609	1,172	99	52	96	4,212	82	989	19	52	35			
Germany	82,476	7,184	6,526	8	1,679	2	2,681	3,347	1,313	137		0	159	499	97	55	100	6,526	8	1,679	2	55	33			
Greece	10,976	620	571	5	234	5	340	253	84			0	26	23	27	24	0	0		0				571	234	48
Hungary	9,877	2,745	2,507	25	526	5	874	1,620	176	185		0	25	213	88	41	100	2,507	25	526	5	41	25			
Iceland	290	5	5	2	1	0	2	2	2			0	0		63	28	100	5	2	1	0	28	33			
Ireland	3,956	421	354	9	141	4	146	128	80	5		0	13	54	77	68	100	505	8	150	0	55	38	354	141	52
Israel	6,433	529	505	8	150	2	251	240	107	8			10	14	83	55	100	505	8	150	0	55	38	0	0	
Italy	57,423	4,518	4,234	7	1,481	3	1,865	1,668	1,085	0			153	131	101	79	21	4,234	7	1,481	3	79	47			
Kazakhstan	15,433	32,169	26,936	175	8,665	56	9,331	14,275	978	3,018		0	2,548	2,685	120	86	100	26,936	175	8,665	56	86	38			
Kyrgyzstan	5,138	7,027	6,172	120	1,643	32	967	657	183	205		0	40	7,027	97	57	100	6,172	120	1,643	32	57	100			
Latvia	2,307	1,726	1,686	73	641	28	967	657	183	205		0	40	159	97	83	100	1,686	73	641	28	83	49			
Lithuania	3,444	2,821	2,586	75	912	26	1,171	941	415	318		0	208	27	108	85	98	2,586	75	912	26	85	49			
Luxembourg	453	54	54	12	31	7	50	20	3	3		0	0		98	61	100	54	12	31	7	126	61			
Malta	394	7	6	2	2	1	3	1	3	0		0	0	1	26	28	100	6	2	2	1	19	67			
Monaco	34																									
Netherlands	16,149	1,321	1,282	8	282	2	499	541	441	13		0	12	27	102	50	100	1,282	8	282	2	50	34			
Norway	4,533	339	320	7	52	1	132	149	119	0		0	6	13	128	46	100	320	7	52	1	46	26			
Poland	38,587	10,124	9,677	25	2,983	8	4,774	5,055	441	779		0	12	447	81	56	100	9,677	25	2,983	8	56	37			
Portugal	10,062	4,131	3,861	38	1,742	17	2,196	876	860	183		0	6	135	86	87	100	3,861	38	1,742	17	87	67			
Republic of Moldova	4,267	5,027	3,619	85	1,214	28	2,196	876	1,055	183	221	227	135	4,579	61	46	81	3,261	76	1,029	24	39	100	358	185	100
Romania	22,334	31,623	28,335	127	10,418	47	11,921	10,745	4,008	3,164		0	1,950	1,338	85	70	54	14,909	67	5,757	26	38	52	13,426	4,661	46
Russian Federation	143,246	152,244	124,041	87	28,868	20	29,846	85,332	4,664	5,477		0	22,512	5,691	77	40	25	21,064	15	6,322	4	9	33	102,977	22,546	24
San Marino	28	1	1	4	0	0	0	0	0			0	0		58		100	1	4	0	0					
Serbia & Montenegro	10,527	4,076	3,895	37	611	6	751	823	298	130		1	2	762	107	37	52	1,862	18	611	6	37		2,033		
— Kosovo		1,157	1,127		292												100	1,127		292						
— Serbia & Montenegro		2,919	2,768		319													735		319				2,033		
Slovakia	5,402	983	904	17	200	4	336	458	196	50		0	5	74	69	34	100	904	17	200	4	34	30			
Slovenia	1,984	293	275	14	116	6	205	101	37	21		0	8	10	75	70	100	275	14	116	6	70	53			
Spain	41,060	5,918	5,877	14	2,816	7	2,906	2,731	122	208		0	0	41	52	57								5,877	2,816	51
Sweden	8,876	410	386	4	109	1	211	125	147	5		0	14	10	98	62	100	386	4	109	1	62	47			
Switzerland	7,169	623	554	8	107	1	257	302	145	0		0	42	27	105	45								554	107	26
Tajikistan	6,245	4,883	4,260	68	0	0	0	0	0	0	59	343	0	4,481	41	0	13	882	14					3,378		48
TFYR Macedonia	2,056	697	653	32	200	10	209	250	161	42		0	0	44	101	69	50	483	23	141	7	49	43	170	59	48
Turkey	71,325																									
Turkmenistan	4,867	4,759	3,771	77	1,197	25	1,197	1,569	895	110		0	430	558	115	81	36	1,848	38	715	15	49	53	1,923	482	34
Ukraine	48,523	40,659	37,043	76	12,785	26	1,621	12,858	2,878			0	206	40,659	83	64	15							37,043	12,785	100
United Kingdom	59,251	7,334	6,400	11	1,455	2	1,621	2,067	728			0	0		91	46								6,400	1,455	41
Uzbekistan	26,093	26,172	20,700	79	4,690	18	4,690	12,858	2,167	975		0	1,987	3,485	69	35	52	10,224	39	2,742	11	20	37	10,476	1,948	19
Region	**878,902**	**396,103**	**338,643**	**39**	**95,512**	**11**	**91,809**	**161,308**	**28,632**	**5,706**	**281**	**572**	**31,797**	**76,490**	**77**	**49**	**41**	**142,760**	**16**	**44,673**	**5**	**23**	**41**	**195,883**	**50,839**	**34**

See Explanatory notes, page 151.

EUR

Country data for Europe: treatment outcomes for cases registered in 2002

New smear-positive cases – DOTS

	Number of cases notified	regist'd	% of notif regist'd	% cured	% completed	% died	% failed	% default	% transferred	% not eval	% success
Albania	93	93	100	67	24	1		4		4	90
Andorra	2	3	150	100							100
Armenia	295	295	100	70	9	4	3	2	3	8	79
Austria	220										
Azerbaijan	1 310	748	57	81	3	2	2	9	3		84
Belarus											
Belgium	419	337	80	24	45	9	1	1	1	19	69
Bosnia & Herzegovina	526	526	100	84	11	1	2	1	1		95
Bulgaria	742	742	100	86		3	4	5	2		86
Croatia											
Cyprus	8	8	100	38	38	13			13		75
Czech Republic	329	320	97	59	13	4			2	19	73
Denmark											
Estonia	135	135	100	41	36	10	1	4	4	5	77
Finland	203	203	100	65	2	14	0	9	0	9	67
France	130										
Georgia	987	987	100	35	30	2	3	18	13		65
Germany	1 868	1 329	71	43	26	10	0	2		19	69
Greece	556	549	99	39	16	9	9	5	3	19	55
Hungary	2	2	100	50	50						100
Iceland											
Ireland	271	257	95	72	9	11	0	2	5	1	81
Israel	1 275	185	15	30	49	2	11	4	4	11	79
Italy	9 452	9 185	97	76	1	5	11	5	2		78
Kazakhstan	1 456	1 476	101	78	3	4	7	5	2		82
Kyrgyzstan	636	636	100	74	2	9	1	5	0	8	76
Latvia	634	634	100	72		10	4	9	0	4	72
Lithuania	17		100		60	40					60
Luxembourg	5	5	100								
Malta											
Monaco											
Netherlands	330	296	90	16	51	3		6	1	22	68
Norway	31	35	113	63	17	6		9	6		80
Poland	3 060	2 602	85	75	10	6	1	6	1	1	86
Portugal	1 976	1 902	96	9	73	6	0	5	4	3	82
Republic of Moldova	557	556	100	53	8	8	10	16	4	1	61
Romania	6 086	6 459	106	61	15	5	5	7	1	7	76
Russian Federation	5 179	5 171	100	64	3	13	9	7	4	7	67
San Marino											
Serbia & Montenegro	402	664	165	64	26	3	1	4	1	0	91
Slovakia	202	200	99	35	50	16					85
Slovenia	130	130	100	29	56	8		6			85
Spain											
Sweden	109	108	99		73	6			2	19	73
Switzerland											
Tajikistan	100	107	107	79		5	11	5	1		79
TFYR Macedonia	143	143	100	62	17	1		18		1	79
Turkey	735	735	100	70	7	5	13	4	1		77
Turkmenistan											
Ukraine											
United Kingdom	2 766	2 544	92	66	14	5	8	7			80
Uzbekistan											
Region	**43 112**	**40 307**	**93**	**63**	**13**	**6**	**6**	**6**	**2**	**3**	**76**

New smear-positive cases – non-DOTS

	Number of cases notified	regist'd	% of notif regist'd	% cured	% completed	% died	% failed	% default	% transferred	% not eval	% success
Albania	132	132	100	27	52	2	2	8	1	8	80
Armenia	216										
Azerbaijan	351	401	114	80		3		10	4	4	80
Bulgaria	265	265	100	78		6	1	5	1		78
Croatia	437	204	47	62	8	10	1	9	3	7	70
Denmark	135										
Finland	130										
France	2 276										
Greece	212										
Ireland	100	95	95	5	72	4	2			17	77
Kazakhstan	131										
Lithuania	188	188	100	69		13	6	10		2	69
Republic of Moldova	589	589	100		47					53	47
Romania	4 617	5 141	111	56	15	5	7	8	1	7	70
Russian Federation	22 686										
Spain	3 317										
Switzerland	123										
Tajikistan	587										
TFYR Macedonia	57	57	100	46	39	2	2	5	2	5	84
Turkey	519	519	100	69		6		6	1		69
Ukraine	1 365	1 031	76		62	6	1	6		24	62
Uzbekistan	2 017										
Region	**40 450**	**8 622**	**21**	**47**	**21**	**4**	**4**	**7**	**1**	**15**	**69**

Smear-positive re-treatment cases – DOTS

	Number regist'd	% cured	% completed	% died	% failed	% default	% transferred	% not eval	% success
Albania	10	50	20			20		10	70
Armenia	62	26	5	6	19	3	3	37	31
Azerbaijan	67	57	7	7	13	15			64
Belgium	38	29	47	8				16	76
Bosnia & Herzegovina	58	74	19	2	3	2			93
Bulgaria	293	64	15	4	8	8	1		79
Cyprus	2	100							100
Czech Republic	8	25	25				13	38	50
Denmark	10	20	70	7	4			10	90
Estonia	95	28	5	7	4	21		34	34
Georgia	651	25	11	5	8	20	9	23	36
Germany	164	44	23	11	17	1		21	67
Hungary	110	27	12	15	17	5	2	22	39
Ireland	18	72	11	6			11		83
Israel	22	32	23		14		9	23	55
Italy	3 307	62	2	11	16	6	3		64
Kyrgyzstan	850	26	17	4	7	3	1	42	43
Latvia	192	37	2	16	2	8	1	35	39
Lithuania	295	39		19	9	20		14	39
Netherlands	26	12	27	13		23		38	38
Norway	8	50	25				13		75
Poland	445	64	9	10	2	11	1	3	73
Portugal	247	10	66	8		8	2	6	75
Republic of Moldova	453	30	6	13	20	22	5	3	37
Romania	2 915	31	15	9	11	16	1	18	45
Russian Federation	962	37	9	12	26	9	8		46
Serbia & Montenegro	94	48	32	9	3	9			80
Slovakia	42	48	33	17	2				81
Slovenia	17	24	47	24		6			71
Sweden	13		46		8			46	46
TFYR Macedonia	29	34	34	3	3	21		3	69
Turkey	529	42	21	12	16	8	1		63
Ukraine	519	38	23	10	12	17			61
Region	**12 551**	**42**	**12**	**10**	**12**	**11**	**3**	**10**	**54**

See Explanatory notes, page 151.

Country data for Europe: re-treatment outcomes for cases registered in 2002

	Relapse – DOTS									After failure – DOTS									After default – DOTS								
	number regist'd	% cured	% compl-eted	% died	% failed	% default	% trans-ferred	% not eval	% success	number regist'd	% cured	% compl-eted	% died	% failed	% default	% trans-ferred	% not eval	% success	number regist'd	% cured	% compl-eted	% died	% failed	% default	% trans-ferred	% not eval	% success
Albania	10	50	20		20			10	70																		
Andorra																											
Armenia	40	35	3	10	28	5	3	18	38	22	9	9		5		5	73	18									
Austria																											
Azerbaijan	31	58	10	10	13	10			63	11	36		18	27	18			36	25	64	8	8	8	20			72
Belarus																											
Belgium																											
Bosnia & Herzegovina	58	74	19	2	3	2			93	23	48	33	3	6	10			81	106	78	4	4	9	5			82
Bulgaria	64	70		6	11	8	5		70																		
Croatia																											
Cyprus	1	100							100																		
Czech Republic																											
Denmark	10	20	70	10				10	90																		
Estonia	52	42	10	10	6	13		19	52																		
Finland																											
France	100	43	25	2	8	20	2		68	58	28	9	10	12	24	18		37	164	16	14	6	5	38	21		30
Georgia	84	44	25	13		1		17	69																		
Germany																											
Greece																				10	10	10	30	30	20			20
Hungary	99	29	12	13	16	4	2	23	41																		
Iceland																											
Ireland	18	72	11	6			11		83																		
Israel	19	37	26		16	16	5	16	63	1							100		2						50	50	
Italy																											
Kazakhstan	2 908	63	2	11	15	6	3		65	399	51	3	15	23	6	4		54									
Kyrgyzstan	414	41	4	4	7	3	1	39	46	435	11	29	4	7	3	0	45	40									
Latvia	163	36	1	17	2	5	1	39	37																		
Lithuania	179	46		22	10	13		9	46	37	30		8	5	22		35	30	79	25		16	8	37		14	25
Luxembourg																											
Malta																											
Monaco																											
Netherlands	16	19	31	13		19		31	50																		
Norway	8	50	25				13		75																		
Poland	445	64	9	10	2	11	1	3	73	1		100						100	53	4	55	9		19	4	9	58
Portugal	132	12	67	7		5	2	7	80	87	28	6	22	24	16		3	33	111	15	14	11	17	34	5	3	30
Republic of Moldova	255	38	3	11	20	18	5	3	41										111	19	16	7	6	44	1	6	35
Romania	1 946	37	14	7	10	13	1	18	51	380	23	18	11	14	15	2	18	41									
Russian Federation	962	37	9	12	26	9	8		46																		
San Marino																											
Serbia & Montenegro	94	48	32	9	3	9			80	1			100						2		50			50			50
Slovakia	42	48	33	17	2				81																		
Slovenia	14	29	50	21					79																		
Spain																											
Sweden																											
Switzerland																											
Tajikistan																											
TFYR Macedonia	29	34	34	3	3	21		3	69																		
Turkey																				482	41	23	12	16	7	1		64
Turkmenistan	47	49	2	9	21	19			51																		
Ukraine																											
United Kingdom	519	38	23	10	12	17			61																		
Uzbekistan																											
Region	**8 759**	**48**	**10**	**10**	**13**	**9**	**3**	**8**	**58**	**1 566**	**29**	**17**	**10**	**14**	**9**	**2**	**19**	**46**	**1 145**	**34**	**18**	**10**	**12**	**21**	**4**	**1**	**52**

EUR

See Explanatory notes for previous table, page 151.

Country data for Europe: trends in DOTS treatment success and detection rates, 1994–2003

	DOTS new smear-positive treatment success (%)									DOTS new smear-positive case detection rate (%)								
	1994	1995	1996	1997	1998	1999	2000	2001	2002	1995	1996	1997	1998	1999	2000	2001	2002	2003
Albania					100	67	50	98	90							23	28	29
Andorra					81	88	87	100	100			226	14	59	15	48	33	116
Armenia		83	77	82		77	73	90	79	13	29	50	46	42	51	32	32	43
Austria															58	48	41	28
Azerbaijan			86	87	86	88	91	64	84	5	9	7	7	7	6	0	46	44
Belarus																		
Belgium									69				37	64	68	71	65	57
Bosnia & Herzegovina				93	88	90	94	98	95						23	75	50	48
Bulgaria								87	86							10	47	81
Croatia																		
Cyprus	73	60	66	69	42	78	70	92	75	45		53	94	47	60	61	53	91
Czech Republic					65			73	73		59		65	59			56	63
Denmark																		
Estonia						63	70		77						64	56	61	75
Finland									67									69
France																		
Georgia		58		65	80	61	63	67	65	17	33	63	31	40	31	52	51	52
Germany				54		58	77	67	69				64	66		53	56	55
Greece					80		64		55									
Hungary								46						36	25	37	40	41
Iceland								67	100							74	53	28
Ireland																		
Israel					72	71	78	79	81						6	59	58	55
Italy		80	82	69	79	79	74	40	79		14	9	13	56	32	10	65	79
Kazakhstan						79	79	78	78				4	79	94	93	95	86
Kyrgyzstan			88	76	82	83	82	81	82		3	4	33	61	44		51	57
Latvia		61	64	65	71	74	72	73	76		73	71	74	65	73	76	78	83
Lithuania					79	84	92	75	72					3	2	31	58	85
Luxembourg																41	67	126
Malta		100	100	100	100	75	100	100	60		34	22	45	71	41	26	45	19
Monaco	81																	
Netherlands		72	81	80	65	79	76	87	68	75	48	44	37	47	46	51	57	50
Norway		77	80	44	69	77	70	77	80		66	67	35	16	29	48	26	46
Poland					75	69	72	78	86				2	3	4	3	55	56
Portugal	48	69	74	78	74	85	79	66	82	77	77	67	85	79	84	95	95	87
Republic of Moldova							83	78	61							39	21	39
Romania		65	62	72	85	78	80	67	76			1	84	4	9	10	41	38
Russian Federation				67	68	65	68	67	67				1	2	5	5	7	
San Marino				100								102			115			9
Serbia & Montenegro	96							88	91							26	24	37
Slovakia		64	73	67	85	79	82	87	85	76	81	32	38	34	35	35	33	34
Slovenia		90	87	82	78	88	84	82	85		75	56	62	71	67	70	71	70
Spain							79	62	73							54	59	62
Sweden																		
Switzerland																		
Tajikistan																		
TFYR Macedonia							86	75	79							54	48	49
Turkey								88	79									
Turkmenistan															19	40		49
Ukraine																	2	
United Kingdom																	47	
Uzbekistan													0	2	4	7	22	20
Region	**68**	**69**	**72**	**72**	**76**	**77**	**77**	**75**	**76**	**3**	**3**	**5**	**11**	**11**	**12**	**14**	**22**	**23**

Country data for Europe: age and sex distribution of smear-positive cases in DOTS areas, 2003 (absolute numbers)

Country	MALE							FEMALE							ALL						
	0-14	15-24	25-34	35-44	45-54	55-64	65+	0-14	15-24	25-34	35-44	45-54	55-64	65+	0-14	15-24	25-34	35-44	45-54	55-64	65+
Albania	0	12	8	16	7	12	7	0	7	3	2	6	5	10	0	19	11	18	13	17	17
Andorra	0	0	0	1	2	0	0	0	1	1	1	0	0	0	0	1	1	2	2	0	0
Armenia	2	120	59	64	58	15	18	2	29	31	11	4	2	3	4	149	90	75	62	17	21
Austria	3	147	190	140	77	37	16	1	60	53	41	31	7	5	4	207	243	181	108	44	21
Azerbaijan	0	67	134	243	226	96	60	0	18	39	43	26	21	45	0	85	173	286	252	117	105
Belgium	6	27	33	30	40	17	35	5	20	17	15	11	2	7	11	47	50	45	51	19	42
Bosnia & Herzegovina	4	32	42	49	52	45	50	4	27	37	34	14	30	73	8	59	79	83	66	75	123
Bulgaria	3	99	169	178	200	121	89	7	85	106	63	44	32	58	10	134	275	241	244	153	147
Croatia																					
Cyprus	0	1	4	3	0	0	1	0	0	2	2	1	1	0	0	1	6	5	1	0	1
Czech Republic	0	11	28	42	67	48	50	0	9	15	15	12	7	34	0	20	43	57	79	55	84
Denmark	3	11	20	23	22	12	9	0	6	13	12	6	2	4	3	17	33	35	28	14	13
Estonia	0	7	28	38	35	24	18	0	7	4	11	12	2	15	0	14	32	49	47	26	33
Finland																					
France																					
Georgia	1	112	220	185	111	65	53	1	65	59	56	19	23	17	2	177	279	241	130	88	70
Germany	2	68	107	177	163	103	155	10	61	96	86	43	22	102	12	129	203	263	206	125	257
Greece	0	6	30	89	140	70	38	0	16	26	27	30	11	33	0	22	56	116	170	81	71
Hungary	0	0	0	0	0	0	1								0	0	0	0	0	0	1
Iceland																					
Ireland	2	9	12	22	10	6	25	1	13	13	13	5	1	18	3	22	25	35	15	7	43
Israel	19	79	219	168	80	61	146	6	63	121	77	24	13	91	25	142	340	245	104	74	237
Italy																					
Kazakhstan	0	182	298	238	145	60	70	0	177	227	105	61	29	36	0	359	525	343	206	89	106
Kyrgyzstan	0	36	74	141	106	59	32	0	31	42	42	35	17	26	0	67	116	183	141	76	58
Latvia	1	35	116	175	174	107	60	0	35	49	37	38	20	50	1	70	165	212	212	127	110
Lithuania	0	2	10	7	1	2	2	0	2	1	1	0	0	0	0	4	11	8	1	2	2
Luxembourg	0	0	1	0	1	0	0	0	0	0	0	0	0	0	0	0	1	0	1	0	0
Malta																					
Monaco																					
Netherlands	2	35	50	38	17	15	15	0	16	30	12	10	3	5	2	51	80	50	27	18	20
Norway	0	3	3	4	4	2	2	0	4	9	4	2	0	1	0	7	12	8	6	2	3
Poland	2	93	234	436	653	305	349	3	91	108	152	132	65	358	5	184	342	588	785	370	707
Portugal	11	134	297	333	227	99	148	7	99	163	82	39	27	47	18	233	460	415	266	126	195
Republic of Moldova	11	131	180	202	139	53	25	1	88	58	54	37	9	21	2	219	238	256	206	62	46
Romania	21	435	850	921	1 061	437	346	32	380	437	284	220	100	224	53	815	1 287	1 205	1 281	537	570
Russian Federation	0	487	1 026	1 407	1 228	420	236	0	233	401	339	282	92	163	0	720	1 427	1 746	1 510	512	399
San Marino																					
Serbia & Montenegro	1	51	64	70	113	54	61	1	44	58	38	28	20	54	2	95	122	108	141	74	115
Slovakia	1	6	8	31	36	19	25	1	8	9	10	3	4	38	2	14	17	41	39	23	63
Slovenia	0	3	9	23	22	7	15	0	5	5	4	3	4	16	0	8	14	27	25	11	31
Spain																					
Sweden	0	8	14	12	4	5	20	0	10	18	6	2	0	10	0	18	32	18	6	5	30
Switzerland																					
Tajikistan																					
TFYR Macedonia	1	17	17	26	13	12	8	0	11	14	8	4	1	4	1	28	31	34	22	13	12
Turkey	3	98	146	104	57	24	11	5	71	79	60	21	15	21	8	169	225	164	78	39	32
Turkmenistan																					
Ukraine																					
United Kingdom	9	338	455	297	178	129	131	29	297	323	191	112	118	135	38	635	778	488	290	247	266
Uzbekistan																					
Region	98	2 902	5 155	5 933	5 504	2 541	2 327	116	2 089	2 667	1 938	1 317	704	1 724	214	4 991	7 822	7 871	6 821	3 245	4 051

EUR

Note: the sum of cases notified by age is less than the number of new smear-positive cases notified for some countries.

Country data for Europe: age and sex distribution of smear-positive cases in non-DOTS areas, 2003 (absolute numbers)

	MALE							FEMALE							ALL						
	0-14	15-24	25-34	35-44	45-54	55-64	65+	0-14	15-24	25-34	35-44	45-54	55-64	65+	0-14	15-24	25-34	35-44	45-54	55-64	65+
Albania	0	16	11	16	9	10	12	2	6	5	4	8	7	10	2	22	16	20	17	17	22
Andorra																					
Armenia	10	0	39	11	46	34	0	0	0	0	2	8	7	0	10	0	39	13	54	41	0
Austria																					
Azerbaijan	0	65	68	75	36	29	4	0	12	7	21	17	19	0	0	77	75	96	53	48	4
Belarus																					
Belgium																					
Bosnia & Herzegovina																					
Bulgaria																					
Croatia	0	15	27	68	80	42	60	1	14	19	18	10	15	69	1	29	46	86	90	57	129
Cyprus																					
Czech Republic																					
Denmark																					
Estonia																					
Finland	0	2	3	8	19	17	29	0	2	10	3	6	5	31	0	4	13	11	25	22	60
France	18	129	249	223	190	127	210	16	114	129	79	44	32	159	34	243	378	302	234	159	369
Georgia																					
Germany																					
Greece	2	20	28	25	23	25	36	0	7	9	7	2	5	18	2	27	37	32	25	30	54
Hungary																					
Iceland																					
Ireland	0	10	11	13	14	7	11	0	4	7	6	4	1	10	0	14	18	19	18	8	21
Israel																					
Italy																					
Kazakhstan																					
Kyrgyzstan	0	7	0	3	0	3	0	0	1	0	4	0	0	6	0	8	0	7	0	3	6
Latvia																					
Lithuania																					
Luxembourg																					
Malta																					
Monaco																					
Netherlands																					
Norway																					
Poland																					
Portugal																					
Republic of Moldova	0	21	21	50	37	9	0	0	13	13	10	3	7	1	0	34	34	60	40	16	1
Romania	16	315	715	774	892	399	248	26	287	333	186	192	96	180	42	602	1 048	960	1 084	495	428
Russian Federation	0	1 641	3 786	4 572	4 696	1 594	822	0	923	1 352	1 198	999	370	535	0	2 564	5 138	5 770	5 695	1 964	1 357
San Marino																					
Serbia & Montenegro																					
Slovakia																					
Slovenia																					
Spain	7	153	334	305	219	132	222	6	138	218	113	51	29	87	13	291	552	418	270	161	309
Sweden	0	11	7	19	10	4	11	1	10	10	4	0	3	3	1	21	17	23	10	7	14
Switzerland	0	3	6	9	10	5	9	0	5	2	1	5	0	4	0	8	8	10	15	5	13
Tajikistan																					
TFYR Macedonia																					
Turkey																					
Turkmenistan	0	50	119	108	55	13	3	0	23	60	24	21	6	3	0	73	179	132	76	19	3
Ukraine	10	850	2 033	2 808	2 634	983	617	29	514	745	557	363	221	421	39	1 364	2 778	3 365	2 997	1 204	1 038
United Kingdom	13	101	182	128	81	59	92	14	108	148	88	47	17	55	27	209	330	216	128	76	147
Uzbekistan	0	149	373	298	234	124	89	0	63	265	162	98	54	39	0	212	638	460	332	178	128
Region	76	3 558	8 012	9 513	9 285	3 616	2 475	95	2 244	3 332	2 487	1 878	894	1 628	171	5 802	11 344	12 000	11 163	4 510	4 103

Note: the sum of cases notified by age is less than the number of new smear-positive cases notified for some countries.

Country data for Europe: smear-positive notification rates (per 100 000 population) by age and sex, 2003

	MALE							FEMALE							ALL						
	0-14	15-24	25-34	35-44	45-54	55-64	65+	0-14	15-24	25-34	35-44	45-54	55-64	65+	0-14	15-24	25-34	35-44	45-54	55-64	65+
Albania	0	10	7	13	10	20	21	0	5	3	3	9	11	18	0	7	5	8	9	16	19
Andorra																					
Armenia	4	40	43	31	55	56	15	1	10	14	5	6	8	2	2	25	29	17	29	30	7
Austria																					
Azerbaijan	0	27	45	31	30	39	9	0	9	9	8	12	13	2	0	18	26	19	21	25	5
Belarus	0	8	20	32	33	25	12	0	2	6	5	3	4	5	0	5	13	18	18	13	7
Belgium	1	4	5	4	5	3	5	1	3	3	2	2	0	1	1	4	4	3	3	2	2
Bosnia & Herzegovina	1	10	13	13	17	26	26	1	9	12	9	4	15	27	1	9	13	11	10	20	26
Bulgaria	1	17	28	33	36	28	16	1	16	18	12	7	6	8	1	16	23	22	21	16	11
Croatia	0	5	9	22	24	19	21	0	5	6	6	3	6	15	0	5	8	14	14	12	18
Cyprus	0	2	7	5	0	0	2	0	0	0	4	4	0	0	0	1	6	4	1	0	1
Czech Republic	0	2	3	6	9	8	9	0	1	2	2	2	1	4	0	1	3	4	5	4	6
Denmark	1	4	5	6	6	3	3	0	2	4	3	2	1	1	0	3	4	4	4	2	2
Estonia	0	7	31	44	42	38	25	0	7	4	12	12	2	11	0	7	18	27	26	18	15
Finland	0	1	1	2	5	5	9	0	1	3	1	2	2	6	0	1	2	1	3	3	7
France	0	3	6	5	5	4	5	0	3	3	2	1	1	3	0	3	5	3	3	3	4
Georgia	0	27	59	49	36	32	19	0	16	16	14	5	9	4	0	22	38	31	20	20	10
Germany	0	1	2	2	3	2	3	0	1	2	1	1	0	1	0	1	2	2	2	1	2
Greece	0	3	3	3	3	4	4	0	1	1	1	0	1	2	0	2	2	2	2	2	3
Hungary	0	1	4	14	19	14	7	0	2	3	4	4	2	4	0	2	4	9	11	7	5
Iceland	0	0	0	0	0	0	7	0							0	0	0	0	0	0	3
Ireland	0	3	4	5	6	4	6	0	1	2	2	2	1	4	0	2	3	4	4	2	5
Israel	0	2	2	6	3	3	9	0	3	3	3	1	0	5	0	2	3	5	2	1	7
Italy	0	3	5	4	2	2	3	0	2	3	2	1	0	1	0	2	4	3	1	1	2
Kazakhstan	0	36	76	74	65	61	55	0	35	58	32	25	25	21	0	35	67	53	44	42	34
Kyrgyzstan	0	20	47	87	75	53	27	0	18	27	25	21	11	10	0	19	37	55	46	29	16
Latvia	0	13	50	69	86	71	34	0	14	21	14	16	10	15	0	14	35	40	49	36	22
Lithuania	0	8	29	17	3	9	8	0	8	3	3	0	0	0	0	8	16	10	2	4	3
Luxembourg	0	0	4	0	3	0	0								0	0	2	0	2	0	0
Malta																					
Monaco																					
Netherlands	0	4	4	3	1	2	2	0	2	3	1	1	0	0	0	3	4	2	1	1	1
Norway	0	1	1	1	1	1	1	0	2	3	1	1	0	0	0	2	2	1	1	0	0
Poland	0	3	8	17	22	19	19	0	3	4	5	4	3	12	0	3	6	11	13	10	14
Portugal	1	20	36	47	36	20	23	1	15	20	11	6	5	5	1	18	28	29	20	12	12
Republic of Moldova	0	38	65	86	73	41	16	0	26	23	20	13	8	8	0	32	44	52	41	22	11
Romania	2	42	82	115	129	81	45	3	39	42	32	26	17	22	3	41	62	74	76	47	32
Russian Federation	0	18	47	55	56	36	17	0	10	18	14	11	6	5	0	14	33	34	32	19	9
San Marino																					
Serbia & Montenegro	0	6	8	10	15	11	10	0	6	8	5	4	4	6	0	6	8	8	9	7	8
Slovakia	0	1	2	8	9	8	11	0	2	3	3	1	1	10	0	2	5	5	5	5	10
Slovenia	0	2	6	15	14	7	14	0	4	3	3	4	4	9	0	3	5	9	8	5	11
Spain	0	6	9	9	8	6	8	0	5	6	4	2	1	2	0	6	8	6	5	4	4
Sweden	0	2	2	2	1	1	3	0	2	3	1	0	0	1	0	2	3	1	1	0	2
Switzerland	0	3	2	3	2	1	2	0	3	2	1	0	1	0	0	3	2	2	1	1	1
Tajikistan																					
TFYR Macedonia	0	12	15	24	21	19	18	0	10	10	6	7	1	7	0	11	13	15	14	9	12
Turkey																					
Turkmenistan	0	29	69	68	58	42	15	1	19	37	26	20	21	16	0	24	53	46	38	31	16
Ukraine	0	22	58	81	84	45	25	0	14	22	15	10	7	9	1	18	40	47	44	23	14
United Kingdom	0	3	5	3	2	2	2	0	3	4	2	1	1	1	0	3	4	2	2	1	2
Uzbekistan	0	17	41	36	40	53	41	1	13	29	21	19	33	23	0	15	35	28	29	43	30
Region	0	10	20	24	26	15	10	0	7	9	7	5	4	4	0	8	15	15	15	9	7

Note: rates are missing where data for smear-positive cases are missing, or where age- and sex-specific population data are not available.

Country data for Europe: number of TB cases notified, 1980–2003

	1980	1981	1982	1983	1984	1985	1986	1987	1988	1989	1990	1991	1992	1993	1994	1995	1996	1997	1998	1999	2000	2001	2002	2003
Albania	1 050	954	978	891	975	916	989	915	759	695	653	628			707	641	738	655	694	733	604	555	594	543
Andorra										12	23	24	21	15	24		17	19	8	10	12	10	5	10
Armenia	756	924	759	702	774	768	832	766	651	649	590	741	235	590	753	1 157	928	1 026	1 455	1 488	1 333	1 389	1 433	1 538
Austria	2 191	2 061	1 942	1 825	1 765	1 442	1 377	1 390	1 402	1 334	1 521	1 426	1 354	1 267	1 264	1 399	1 375	1 369	1 307	1 085	1 185	1 013	1 044	
Azerbaijan	3 080	3 180	3 217	3 176	3 506	3 772	3 804	3 677	3 340	2 989	2 620	2 771	2 821	3 036	2 839	1 630	2 480	4 635	4 672	4 654	5 187	4 898	5 142	3 840
Belarus	5 954	6 198	5 468	5 509	5 065	4 873	4 128	3 911	3 769	3 708	3 039	3 745	2 414	4 134	4 348	4 854	5 598	5 985	6 150	7 339	6 799	5 505	5 139	5 106
Belgium	2 687	2 837	2 652	2 190	2 149	1 956	1 893	1 772	1 588	1 648	1 577	1 462	1 335	1 503	1 521	1 380	1 348	1 263	1 203	1 124	1 278	1 321	1 211	1 030
Bosnia & Herzegovina	4 421	4 376	4 678	4 468	4 691	4 666	4 605	4 522	4 093	4 176	4 073	3 546	600	680	1 595	2 132	2 220	2 869	2 711	2 923	2 476	2 469	1 691	1 740
Bulgaria	3 280	3 007	2 999	2 892	2 856	2 555	2 530	2 352	2 387	2 301	2 256	2 606	3 096	3 213	5 296	3 245	3 109	3 437	4 117	3 530	3 349	3 862	3 335	3 069
Croatia	3 999	4 021	3 718	3 632	3 612	3 605	3 355	3 326	2 973	2 861	2 576	2 158	2 189	2 279	2 217	2 114	2 174	2 054	2 118	1 765	1 630	1 376	1 443	1 356
Cyprus	69	69	86	73	39	61	48	35	39	23	29	43	39	37	37	36	24	47	45	39	33	40	20	35
Czech Republic	4 962	4 312	4 146	4 016	3 653	3 117	2 553	2 196	2 047	1 905	1 937	2 079	1 986	1 864	1 960	1 834	1 969	1 834	1 805	1 605	1 414	1 291	1 156	1 101
Denmark	430	394	378	348	302	312	299	322	304	328	350	334	359	411	495	448	484	554	529	587	587	494	403	378
Estonia	614	560	563	587	546	541	522	446	471	422	423	406	403	532	623	624	683	744	820	754	791	708	620	557
Finland	2 247	2 204	2 170	1 882	1 791	1 819	1 546	1 419	1 078	970	772	771	700	542	553	661	645	573	629	565	527	460	449	392
France	17 199	16 459	15 425	13 831	12 302	11 290	10 535	10 241	9 191	9 027	9 030	8 510	8 605	9 551	9 093	8 723	7 656	6 832	5 981	6 052	6 122	5 814	5 709	5 740
Georgia	2 098	2 124	2 168	1 881	1 855	1 822	1 833	1 810	1 598	1 609	1 537		2 130	3 741		1 625	3 522	8 446	6 302	4 793	4 397	4 006	4 490	4 212
Germany	29 991	27 083	25 397	22 977	20 243	20 074	17 906	17 102	16 282	15 385	14 653	13 474	14 113	14 161	12 982	12 198	11 814	11 163	10 440	9 974	9 064	6 959	6 931	6 526
Greece	5 412	7 334	5 193	3 880	1 956	1 556	1 566	1 193	907	1 068	877	762	920			939	945	767	1 152	936	703	503	570	571
Hungary	5 412	5 322	5 181	5 028	4 472	4 852	4 522	4 125	4 016	3 769	3 588	3 658	3 960	4 209	4 163	4 339	4 403	4 240	3 999	3 532	3 073	2 923	2 720	2 507
Iceland	25	23	25	24	26	13	13	12	16	18	18	15	16	12	18	12	11	10	17	10	16	12	8	5
Ireland	1 152	1 018	975	924	837	804	602	581	534	672	624	640	604	598	544	458	434	416	424	455	386	393	375	354
Israel	249	227	232	222	257	368	239	184	226	160	234	505	345	419	395	398	369	422	656	490	557	546	485	505
Italy	3 311	3 182	3 850	4 253	3 472	4 113	4 077	3 278	3 610	3 996	4 246	3 719	4 685	4 734	5 816	5 627	4 155	4 596	5 727	4 429	3 501	4 287	3 925	4 234
Kazakhstan	14 442	13 876	13 808	13 357	12 563	12 423	13 090	13 286	13 501	13 307	10 969	10 821	10 920	10 425	10 519	11 310	13 944	16 109	20 623	24 979	25 843	26 224	27 546	26 936
Kyrgyzstan	1 973	2 085	2 051	1 981	2 022	2 094	2 122	2 088	2 159	2 132	2 306	2 515	2 582	2 427	2 726	3 393	4 093	5 189	5 706	6 376	6 205	6 654	6 613	6 172
Latvia	1 194	1 140	1 077	1 072	1 054	1 223	982	948	938	857	906	943	955	994	1 131	1 541	1 761	2 003	2 182	2 711	1 982	2 000	1 803	1 686
Lithuania	1 636	1 599	1 495	1 477	1 420	1 453	1 412	1 372	1 339	1 381	1 471	1 556	1 598	1 895	2 135	2 362	2 608	2 926	3 016	2 800	2 657	2 598	2 414	2 586
Luxembourg	71	45			46		45	48	16	45	48	48	25	35	33	32	41	38	44	37	44	31	31	54
Malta	24	26	13	24	15	11	14	14	12	16	13	26	30	26	25		28	11	16	22	16	16	24	6
Monaco	1						2	1	1				1	1	1		0	0	0	3	0	0	0	
Netherlands	1 701	1 734	1 514	1 423	1 400	1 362	1 238	1 227	1 341	1 317	1 369	1 345	1 465	1 587	1 811	1 619	1 678	1 486	1 341	1 398	1 244	1 408	1 355	1 282
Norway	499	461	448	396	373	374	343	307	294	255	285	290	288	256	242	236	217	205	244	213	221	276	243	320
Poland	25 807	24 087	23 685	23 411	22 527	21 650	20 603	19 757	18 537	16 185	16 136	16 496	16 551	16 828	16 653	15 958	15 358	13 967	13 302	12 168	10 931	10 153	10 069	9 677
Portugal	6 873	7 249	7 309	7 052	6 908	6 889	6 624	7 099	6 363	6 664	6 214	5 980	5 927	5 447	5 619	5 577	5 248	5 110	5 260	4 599	4 227	4 320	4 381	3 861
Republic of Moldova	2 781	2 852	3 197	2 858	2 554	2 732	3 022	2 810	2 510	2 281	1 728	1 910	1 835		2 626	2 925	2 922	2 908	2 625	2 711	2 935	3 608	3 769	3 619
Romania	13 553	13 602	13 588	13 570	12 952	12 677	12 860	13 361	14 137	14 676	16 256	15 482	18 097	20 349	21 422	23 271	24 189	23 903	25 758	26 107	27 470	28 580	29 752	28 335
Russian Federation	74 270	73 369	72 236	73 280	74 597	64 644	71 764	70 132	67 553	62 987	50 641	50 407	53 148	63 591	70 822	84 980	111 075	119 123	110 935	134 360	140 677	132 477	128 873	124 041
San Marino																								
Serbia & Montenegro	6 232	6 381	6 274	6 443	6 454	6 246	6 126	6 042	5 583	5 045	4 194	4 502	3 771	3 843	3 606	2 798	4 017	4 062	3 028	2 646	2 864	4 556	4 232	3 895
Slovakia	2 465	2 304	2 263	2 252	2 152	1 989	2 022	1 830	1 651	1 501	1 448	1 620	1 733	1 799	1 760	1 540	1 503	1 298	1 282	1 100	1 010	986	975	904
Slovenia	1 085	939	982	925	896	923	816	792	760	768	722	583	640	646	526	525	563	481	449	423	368	359	338	275
Spain	4 853	5 552	7 961	8 987	10 078	10 749	13 755	9 468	8 497	8 058	7 600	9 007	9 703	9 441		8 764	8 331	9 347	8 927	8 393	7 993	6 851	7 283	5 877
Sweden	926	875	784	832	754	702	640	545	536	595	557	521	610	616	537	564	497	456	446	479	417	394	375	386
Switzerland	1 160	1 193	1 167	1 097	946	961	881	1 018	1 201	1 104	1 278	1 134	987	930	924	830	765	747	750	756	544	539	591	554
Tajikistan	2 647	2 631	2 628	2 509	2 427	2 485	2 610	2 727	2 474	2 621	2 460	2 116	1 671	1 712	892	2 029	1 647	2 143	2 448	2 553	2 779	3 508	4 052	4 260
TFYR Macedonia													1 602	652	728	786	724	693	620	557	641	648	686	653
Turkey	36 716	39 992	26 457	28 634	27 589	30 960	31 029	30 531	27 884	26 669	24 468	25 166	25 455			22 981	20 212	25 685	25 501	22 088	18 038	17 263	18 043	
Turkmenistan	1 677	1 625	1 559	1 541	1 604	1 607	1 614	1 956	1 904	2 169	2 325	2 358	2 074	2 751		1 939	2 072	3 438	3 839	4 092	4 038	3 948	3 671	3 771
Ukraine	26 095	25 646	24 710	24 216	24 356	24 058	22 946	22 145	20 744	20 182	16 465	16 713	18 140	19 964	20 622	21 459	23 414	28 344	27 763	32 879	32 945	36 784	40 175	37 043
United Kingdom	10 488	9 290	8 436	7 814	7 026	6 666	6 841	5 732	5 793	5 998	5 908	6 088	6 411	6 481	6 196	6 176	6 238	6 355	6 176	6 183	6 220	6 027	6 889	6 400
Uzbekistan	9 163	9 682	8 697	8 817	8 544	8 717	9 427	9 794	10 134	10 632	9 414		9 370	9 774	14 890	9 866	11 919	13 352	14 558	15 080	15 750	17 391	20 588	20 700
Region	**348 921**	**346 104**	**324 580**	**319 220**	**308 401**	**298 933**	**302 602**	**290 606**	**277 143**	**267 232**	**242 429**	**231 651**	**248 519**	**242 425**	**243 691**	**289 949**	**322 165**	**353 336**	**349 800**	**373 765**	**373 081**	**368 433**	**373 670**	**338 643**
number reporting	48	48	48	48	48	48	48	48	48	49	50	49	49	47	46	50	51	51	51	51	51	51	51	49
percent reporting	94	94	94	94	94	94	94	94	94	96	98	96	96	92	90	98	100	100	100	100	100	100	100	94

Country data for Europe: case notification rates (per 100 000 population), 1980–2003

	1980	1981	1982	1983	1984	1985	1986	1987	1988	1989	1990	1991	1992	1993	1994	1995	1996	1997	1998	1999	2000	2001	2002	2003
Albania	39	35	35	31	34	31	33	29	24	21	20	19	36	25	22	20	23	21	22	24	19	18	19	17
Andorra										24	44	44	36	25	38		26	29	12	15	18	15	7	14
Armenia	24	29	24	22	24	23	25	22	19	18	17	21	17	17	16	35	28	32	46	47	43	45	47	50
Austria	29	27	26	24	23	19	18	18	18	17	20	18	17	16	16	17	17	17	16	13	15	12	13	14
Azerbaijan	50	51	51	49	53	57	56	54	48	42	36	38	38	40	37	21	31	58	58	58	64	60	62	46
Belarus	62	64	56	56	51	49	41	39	37	36	30	36	23	40	42	47	55	59	61	73	68	55	52	52
Belgium	27	29	27	22	22	20	19	18	16	17	16	15	13	15	15	14	13	12	12	11	12	13	12	10
Bosnia & Herzegovina	113	111	117	111	115	113	110	106	94	96	95	85	15	18	45	62	65	81	74	76	62	61	41	42
Bulgaria	37	34	34	32	32	29	28	26	27	26	26	30	36	38	63	39	37	41	50	43	41	48	42	39
Croatia	91	92	85	83	82	81	74	72	63	59	53	45	46	49	49	47	49	47	48	40	37	31	33	31
Cyprus	11	11	14	12	6	9	7	5	6	3	4	3	6	5	5	5	3	6	6	5	4	5	3	4
Czech Republic	48	42	40	39	35	30	25	21	20	18	19	20	19	18	19	18	19	18	18	16	14	13	11	11
Denmark	8	8	7	7	6	6	6	6	6	6	7	6	7	8	10	9	9	11	10	11	11	9	8	7
Estonia	42	38	38	39	36	35	34	29	30	27	27	26	26	35	42	43	48	53	59	55	58	52	46	42
Finland	47	46	45	39	37	37	31	29	22	20	15	15	14	11	11	13	13	11	12	11	10	10	9	8
France	32	30	28	25	22	20	19	18	16	16	16	15	15	17	16	15	13	12	10	10	10	10	10	10
Georgia	41	42	42	36	35	34	34	34	29	30	28		39	69		30	66	159	119	91	84	77	87	82
Germany	38	35	33	30	26	26	23	22	21	19	18	17	18	18	16	15	14	14	13	12	11	8	8	8
Greece	56	75	53	39	20	16	16	12	9	11	9	7	9			9	9	7	11	9	6	5	5	5
Hungary	51	50	48	47	42	46	43	39	38	36	35	35	38	41	41	42	43	42	40	35	31	29	27	25
Iceland	11	10	10	11	11	5	5	5	6	7	7	6	6	4	7	4	4	4	6	4	5	4	3	2
Ireland	34	30	28	26	24	23	17	16	15	19	18	18	17	17	15	13	12	11	11	12	10	10	10	9
Israel	7	6	6	6	6	9	6	4	5	4	5	11	7	8	8	7	7	7	11	8	9	9	10	8
Italy	6	6	7	8	6	7	7	6	6	7	7	7	8	8	10	10	7	8	10	8	6	7	7	7
Kazakhstan	97	92	90	86	80	78	81	81	82	80	65	64	65	62	63	68	85	99	129	158	165	169	178	175
Kyrgyzstan	54	56	54	51	51	52	52	50	51	49	52	57	58	54	60	74	89	111	120	132	126	133	131	120
Latvia	48	45	43	42	41	47	38	36	35	32	33	35	36	38	44	62	72	82	90	79	84	85	77	73
Lithuania	48	47	43	42	40	41	39	38	36	37	39	42	43	52	59	66	74	83	86	80	76	75	70	75
Luxembourg	20	12	11	11	13	11	12	13	4	12	13	13	6	9	8	8	10	9	10	9	10	7	7	12
Malta	7	8	4	7	4	3	4	4	3	4	4	7	8	7	7	3	3	3	4	6	4	0	6	4
Monaco	4	0	0	0	0	4	7	7	3	3	3	0	3		3	3	0	0	0	9	0	0	0	
Netherlands	12	12	11	10	10	9	8	8	9	9	9	9	10	10	12	10	11	10	9	9	8	9	8	8
Norway	12	11	11	10	9	9	8	7	7	6	7	7	6	6	6	5	5	6	6	5	5	6	5	7
Poland	73	67	65	64	61	58	55	52	49	43	42	43	43	44	43	41	40	36	34	31	28	26	26	25
Portugal	70	74	74	71	69	69	66	71	64	67	63	60	60	55	57	56	53	51	53	46	42	43	44	38
Republic of Moldova	69	70	78	69	61	65	71	66	58	52	40	44	42	56	60	67	68	67	61	63	69	84	88	85
Romania	61	61	61	60	57	56	55	58	61	63	70	67	78	89	94	103	107	106	114	116	122	127	133	127
Russian Federation	54	53	51	52	52	45	50	48	46	43	34	34	36	43	48	57	75	81	76	92	97	91	89	87
San Marino											4	4		12	8	8			0	0	4	0	6	4
Serbia & Montenegro	65	66	65	66	66	63	62	61	56	50	41	44	37	37	34	27	38	38	29	25	27	43	40	37
Slovakia	50	46	45	44	42	39	39	35	32	29	28	31	33	34	33	29	28	24	24	20	19	18	18	17
Slovenia	59	51	53	50	48	49	43	42	40	40	38	30	33	33	27	26	28	23	23	21	18	18	17	14
Spain	13	15	21	24	26	28	36	24	22	21	19	23	25	24		22	21	23	22	21	20	17	18	14
Sweden	11	11	9	10	9	8	8	6	6	7	7	6	7	7	6	6	6	5	5	5	5	4	4	4
Switzerland	18	19	18	17	15	15	13	15	18	16	19	16	14	13	13	12	11	10	10	11	8	8	8	8
Tajikistan	67	65	63	58	55	54	55	56	49	51	46	39	30	12	16	35	28	36	41	42	46	57	65	68
TFYR Macedonia													83	88	37	40	37	35	31	28	32	32	34	32
Turkey	80	85	55	58	54	60	59	56	50	47	42	43	43	69		36	32	39	39	33	26	25	26	
Turkmenistan	59	55	52	50	51	50	49	58	55	61	63	63	53	38	40	46	48	78	86	90	87	84	77	77
Ukraine	52	51	49	48	47	45	45	43	40	39	32	32	35	35		42	46	56	55	66	66	75	82	76
United Kingdom	19	17	15	14	13	12	12	10	10	11	10	11	11	11	11	11	11	11	11	11	11	10	12	11
Uzbekistan	57	59	52	51	48	48	51	51	52	53	46		44	45	67	43	51	56	60	62	63	69	80	79
Region	**44**	**43**	**40**	**39**	**38**	**36**	**36**	**35**	**33**	**32**	**28**	**27**	**29**	**28**	**28**	**33**	**37**	**41**	**40**	**43**	**43**	**42**	**43**	**39**

EUR

Country data for Europe: new smear-positive cases, 1993–2002

Number of cases

	1993	1994	1995	1996	1997	1998	1999	2000	2001	2002	2003
Albania	15	250	139	173	241	212	168	171	171	225	211
Andorra		24		8	17		4		3	2	7
Armenia		319	436	327	400	475	576	621	572	511	575
Austria			662	580	370		323	324	262	220	
Azerbaijan	499	513	669	990	981	727	763	890	927	1 661	1 161
Belarus	1 493	1 775	1 845	2 117	2 273	5 047	2 769	2 547	2 341		1 018
Belgium	484	427	400	364	434	418	403	409	472	419	362
Bosnia & Herzegovina			865	927	803	640	786	759	800	526	493
Bulgaria		3 096	1 087	903	1 037	1 325	1 697	2 524	897	1 007	1 254
Croatia			1 204	1 228	1 073	1 129	748	0	421	437	438
Cyprus			6	3	19		9	4		8	14
Czech Republic	548	524	487	586	481	545	449	420	391	329	338
Denmark	243	120	128	97	114	132	172	171	127	135	143
Estonia	303	347	369	240	269	299	274	255	212	203	201
Finland			244	240	186	188	179	205	150	130	138
France	4 455	3 196	3 449	3 002	2 430		2 325	1 815	2 398	2 276	2 219
Georgia			221	482	595	547	746	601	1 014	987	989
Germany	4 730	4 177	3 852	3 689	3 346	3 124	2 918	0	1 935	1 868	1 679
Greece					285	313	143	235	213	212	234
Hungary	1 905	1 357	796	1 066	702	667	660	412	546	556	526
Iceland		6	2	1	4	2	2	1	3	2	1
Ireland				339	123	116	117	138	123	100	141
Israel	150	129		147	207	221	170	17	172	164	150
Italy		1 441	1 413	1 738	1 903	2 361	1 277	687	1 361	1 275	1 481
Kazakhstan			3 022	4 290	4 332	6 180	6 977	8 903	9 079	9 452	8 665
Kyrgyzstan		681	832	991	1 536	830	1 642	1 296		1 587	1 643
Latvia	470		504	575	634	668	588	637	661	636	641
Lithuania	688		979	1 121	1 200	787	787	776	935	822	912
Luxembourg				29	31	24	21	21	11	17	31
Malta	13	6	5	5	3	6	9	5	3	5	2
Monaco				0	0	0	2	0	0	0	
Netherlands	1 063		575	358	312	254	308	289	307	330	282
Norway		86	62	103	100	49	21	37	59	31	52
Poland	7 606	4 000	6 955	6 819	3 497	3 502	3 177	3 180	3 155	3 060	2 983
Portugal	2 072		2 019	1 938	1 628	2 016	1 801	1 863	2 042	1 976	1 742
Republic of Moldova	615	704	665	219	397	477	609	651	1 060	1 146	1 214
Romania	9 339	10 385	10 469	10 359	11 666	10 841	10 317	10 202	11 184	10 703	10 418
Russian Federation		30 389	37 512	42 534	42 094	42 219	21 744	27 467	26 605	27 865	28 868
San Marino				0	1	0	0	1	0	0	0
Serbia & Montenegro	882	409	1 497	1 783	1 702	1 873	2 517	0	461	402	611
Slovakia			788	760	283	303	246	236	226	202	200
Slovenia	361	294	303	221	156	157	165	145	139	130	116
Spain	312		2 605			1 906		3 423	2 456	3 317	2 816
Sweden	528	106	102	90	94	97	117	118	105	109	109
Switzerland		507	185	172	144	165	98	118	116	123	107
Tajikistan			1 042	232	373	435	0	434	719	687	0
TFYR Macedonia			319	209	192	179	122	167	164	200	200
Turkey	472		4 383	2 816	3 439	3 692	4 124	4 315	4 444	0	
Turkmenistan			544	557	764	790	964	1 017	1 243	1 254	1 197
Ukraine	8 314	8 471	8 263	7 827	9 533	10 586	10 412	10 738		0	12 785
United Kingdom	283	270	2 735	4 147	844	1 342	797	1 204	946	1 365	1 455
Uzbekistan		7 487		3 350	3 388	3 504	3 977	3 825	4 608	4 783	4 690
Region	**45 771**	**83 568**	**104 639**	**110 752**	**106 636**	**111 391**	**89 199**	**94 275**	**86 239**	**83 455**	**95 512**

Rate (per 100 000 population)

	1993	1994	1995	1996	1997	1998	1999	2000	2001	2002	2003
Albania		8	4	5	8	7	5	5	5	7	7
Andorra		38	12		26	2	6	2	4	3	
Armenia		9	13	10	12	15	18	20	19	17	19
Austria			8	7	5		4	4	3	3	
Azerbaijan	7	7	9	13	12	9	9	11	11	20	14
Belarus	15	17	18	21	22	50	27	25	23		10
Belgium	5	4	4	4	4	4	4	4	5	4	4
Bosnia & Herzegovina			25	27	23	17	20	19	20	13	12
Bulgaria		37	13	11	13	16	21	31	11	13	16
Croatia			27	28	24	26	17	0	9	10	10
Cyprus			1		2	3	1	1		1	
Czech Republic	5	5	5	6	5	5	4	4	4	3	3
Denmark	5	2	2	2	2	2	3	3	2	3	3
Estonia	20	24	26	17	19	21	20	19	16	15	15
Finland			5	5	4	4	3	4	3	3	3
France	8	6	6	5	4		4	3	4	4	4
Georgia			4	9	11	10	14	11	19	19	19
Germany	6	5	5	5	4	4	4	0	2	2	2
Greece					3	3	1	2	2	2	2
Hungary	19	13	8	10	7	7	7	4	5	6	5
Iceland		2	1	0	1	1	1	0	1	1	0
Ireland				9	3	3	3	4	3	3	4
Israel	3	2		3	4	4	3	0	3	3	2
Italy		3	2	3	3	4	2	1	2	2	3
Kazakhstan			18	26	27	39	44	57	58	61	56
Kyrgyzstan		15	18	21	33	17	34	26	0	31	32
Latvia	18		20	23	26	28	25	27	28	27	28
Lithuania	19		27	32	34	22	22	21	27	24	26
Luxembourg				7	7	6	5	5	2	4	7
Malta	4	2	1	1	1	2	2	1	1	1	1
Monaco				0	0	0	6	0	0	0	
Netherlands	7		4	2	2	2	2	2	2	2	2
Norway		2	1	2	2	1	0	1	1	1	1
Poland	20	10	18	18	9	9	8	8	8	8	8
Portugal		21	20	20	16	20	18	19	20	20	17
Republic of Moldova	14	16	15	5	9	11	14	15	25	27	28
Romania	41	46	46	46	52	48	46	45	50	48	47
Russian Federation		20	25	29	29	29	15	19	18	19	20
San Marino				0	4	0	0	1	0	0	0
Serbia & Montenegro	17	8	14	17	16	18	24	0	4	4	6
Slovakia			15	14	5	6	5	4	4	4	4
Slovenia	18	15	15	11	8	8	8	7	7	7	6
Spain	4	1	7			5		8	6	8	7
Sweden	8	7	1	1	1	1	1	1	1	1	1
Switzerland		7	3	2	2	2	1	2	2	2	1
Tajikistan			18	4	6	7	0	7	12	11	0
TFYR Macedonia			16	11	10	9	6	8	8	10	10
Turkey	12		7	4	5	6	6	6	6	0	
Turkmenistan			13	13	17	18	21	22	26	26	25
Ukraine	16	16	16	15	19	21	21	22	26	0	26
United Kingdom	0	0		7	1	2	1	2	2	2	2
Uzbekistan		34	12	14	15	15	16	15	18	19	18
Region	**5**	**10**	**12**	**13**	**12**	**13**	**10**	**11**	**10**	**10**	**11**

Notes

Belarus

Treatment outcomes for the 2002 cohort of laboratory-confirmed cases were not included in this annex. Among 2145 cases, 1661 patients were cured, 0 completed treatment, 136 died, 194 failed, 44 defaulted, 0 transferred, and 110 were still on treatment.

Belgium

Treatment outcomes listed under smear-positive cases are for all laboratory-confirmed cases.

Cyprus

Data refer only to the Republic of Cyprus, i.e. the northern area is excluded (roughly 40% of the island).

Georgia

Regions Afkhazia and South Osetia are not represented in the data.

Israel

Treatment and re-treatment outcomes listed under smear-positive cases are based on cohorts of culture-positive cases, where cure is based on culture results.

Kazakhstan

Under new smear-positive outcomes, the cohort excluded 185 cases of TB (2% of the cohort) because of resistance to TB drugs, intolerance to TB drugs, deterioration of condition, and loss to follow-up. Under relapse outcomes, 526 cases of TB (18% of cohort) were similarly excluded.

Latvia

Outcomes of "transfer-in" patients are matched against "transfer-out" patients at national level to eliminate unknown outcomes because of transfer. Remaining unknowns are given the outcome "default".

Serbia and Montenegro

Reporting of cases were by site of disease were not available for the entire country. Re-treatment outcomes are from Kosovo only.

Spain

The NTP notes that notification data are provisional. "Pulmonary" refers to respiratory cases, while "extra-pulmonary" include only meningeal cases.

Sweden

DOTS coverage was not reported, but assumed to be same as in the previous report.

Tajikistan

The NTP notes that age and sex data are incomplete.

Turkey

NTP reported to WHO at the time this report was going to press. Data are therefore not shown in the annexes, and not reflected in results. DOTS coverage in 2003 was reported as 2%. The country had 18 590 TB cases in 2003, and 17 923 WHO notifications (among which, 446 cases were reported under DOTS). Among 4245 non-DOTS new smear-positive cases registered in 2002, 79% were successfully treated.

United Kingdom

The NTP notes that notification and treatment outcome data are provisional. WHO notifications were revised from 6400 to 6697 cases at the time this report was going to press. Treatment outcome data do not include Scotland.

EUR

Africa

The Americas

Eastern Mediterranean

Europe

South-East Asia

Western Pacific

SOUTH-EAST ASIA: SUMMARY OF TB CONTROL POLICIES

	STATUS[a]	MANUAL[b]	MICROSCOPY[c]	SCC[d]	DOT[e]	MONITORING OUTCOME[f]
BANGLADESH	DOTS	YES				
BHUTAN	DOTS	YES				
DPR KOREA	DOTS	YES				
INDIA	DOTS	YES				
INDONESIA	DOTS	YES				
MALDIVES	DOTS	YES				
MYANMAR	DOTS	YES				
NEPAL	DOTS	YES				
SRI LANKA	DOTS	YES				
THAILAND	DOTS	YES				
TIMOR-LESTE	DOTS					

SEAR

Implemented in all units/areas

Implemented in some units/areas

Not implemented

Unknown

a Status: DOTS status (bold indicates DOTS introduced in 2003. Blank indicates no report received)
b Manual: national TB control manual (recommended)
c Microscopy: use of smear microscopy for diagnosis (core component of DOTS)
d SCC: short course chemotherapy (core component of DOTS)
e DOT: directly observed treatment (core component of DOTS)
f Outcome monitoring: monitoring of treatment outcomes by cohort analysis (core component of DOTS)

Country data for South-East Asia: estimated burden of TB

1990

	Incidence, 1990				Prevalence, 1990				Death, 1990			
	All cases incl. HIV+		New ss+ incl. HIV+		All cases incl. HIV+		All cases excl. HIV+		All cases incl. HIV+		All cases excl. HIV+	
	number	rate	number	rate	number	rate	number	rate	number	rate	number	rate
Bangladesh	269 193	246	121 126	111	810 699	741	810 699	741	71 342	65	71 342	65
Bhutan	3 526	208	1 586	94	10 618	626	10 618	626	934	55	934	55
DPR Korea	35 493	178	15 972	80	106 891	536	106 891	536	9 406	47	9 406	47
India	1 420 446	168	634 211	75	4 263 735	504	4 260 935	503	377 611	45	374 964	44
Indonesia	519 763	285	233 706	128	1 565 313	860	1 565 313	860	137 748	76	137 748	76
Maldives	388	180	175	81	1 169	542	1 169	542	103	48	103	48
Myanmar	69 260	171	30 847	76	208 022	514	207 910	513	18 402	45	18 296	45
Nepal	39 361	211	17 636	95	118 501	636	118 493	636	10 435	56	10 427	56
Sri Lanka	10 186	61	4 582	27	30 677	182	30 677	182	2 700	16	2 700	16
Thailand	77 404	142	34 377	63	226 398	416	225 061	414	21 069	39	19 805	36
Timor-Leste	4 115	556	1 850	250	12 393	1 674	12 393	1 674	1 091	147	1 091	147
Region	2 449 136	190	1 096 068	85	7 354 416	570	7 350 160	569	650 840	50	646 817	50

2003

	Incidence, 2003				Prevalence, 2003				Death, 2003			
	All cases incl. HIV+		New ss+ incl. HIV+		All cases incl. HIV+		All cases excl. HIV+		All cases incl. HIV+		All cases excl. HIV+	
	number	rate	number	rate	number	rate	number	rate	number	rate	number	rate
Bangladesh	360 767	246	162 331	111	719 411	490	719 339	490	83 533	57	83 467	57
Bhutan	2 492	110	1 121	50	4 378	194	4 377	194	467	21	466	21
DPR Korea	40 277	178	18 124	80	42 429	187	42 428	187	3 549	16	3 549	16
India	1 788 043	168	798 338	75	3 085 876	290	3 054 470	287	352 085	33	329 915	31
Indonesia	627 047	285	281 946	128	1 483 735	675	1 482 607	674	143 178	65	142 168	65
Maldives	142	45	64	20	125	39	125	39	7	2	7	2
Myanmar	84 546	171	37 655	76	92 429	187	90 475	183	12 410	25	11 748	24
Nepal	53 139	211	23 809	95	80 074	318	79 556	316	7 399	29	7 138	28
Sri Lanka	11 530	60	5 187	27	16 956	89	16 948	89	1 685	9	1 680	9
Thailand	89 351	142	39 683	63	130 418	208	127 792	203	12 152	19	10 853	17
Timor-Leste	4 323	556	1 944	250	5 872	754	5 863	753	747	96	742	95
Region	3 061 657	190	1 370 201	85	5 661 702	351	5 623 979	348	617 211	38	591 734	37

See Explanatory notes, page 151.

Country data for South-East Asia: notification, detection and DOTS coverage, 2003

	Pop	| New cases — All cases (Country no.)	All cases WHO no.	rate	Smear-positive number	rate	New cases Pulm confirmed number	Smear-negative or unknown number	Extra-pulmonary number	Re-treatment Relapse number	After failure number	After default number	Other number	Other number	Detection rate All cases %	New ss+ %	DOTS % of pop	DOTS Notif. All cases number	rate	New ss+ number	rate	DDR %	% of pulm cases ss+	non-DOTS Notif. All cases number	New ss+ number	% of pulm cases ss+
	thousands	number	number	rate	number	rate	number	number	number	number	number	number	number	number	%	%	pop	number	rate	number	rate	%	cases ss+	number	number	cases ss+
Bangladesh	146 736	88 156	88 156	60	53 618	37	56 123	24 913	7 120	2 505					24	33	99	88 156	60	53 618	37	33	68			
Bhutan	2 257	1 026	1 026	45	360	16	443	284	344	38	19	11			41	32	100	1 026	45	360	16	32	56			
DPR Korea	22 664	51 280	41 810	184	17 392	77		18 112	4 606	1 700	1 105	833		7 532	104	96	80	39 396	174	16 445	73	91	49	2 414	947	46
India	1 065 462	1 188 754	1 073 065	101	433 271	41	419 668	459 424	132 253	48 117	12 206	61 295	42 288		60	54	67	836 768	79	372 088	35	47	55	236 297	61 183	28
Indonesia	219 883	178 260	178 260	81	92 566	42		77 561	4 047	4 086	0	0			28	33	98	178 260	81	92 566	42	33	54			
Maldives	318	137	137	43	68	21	0	26	40	3					96	106	100	137	43	68	21	106	72			
Myanmar	49 485	78 195	75 744	153	27 448	55		26 006	17 793	4 494	964	1 487		2 194	90	73	95	75 744	153	27 448	55	73	51			
Nepal	25 164	33 831	30 925	123	14 348	57		8 894	5 619	2 064	300	412			58	60	94	30 925	123	14 348	57	60	62			
Sri Lanka	19 065	9 477	8 998	47	4 321	23	4 764	2 650	1 811	216	47	161		271	78	83	74	7 307	38	3 652	19	70	64	1 691	669	53
Thailand	62 833	54 504	54 504	87	28 459	45		17 596	6 756	1 693					61	72	100	54 504	87	28 459	45	72	62			
Timor-Leste	778	3 217	2 760	355	1 027	132		1 240	473	20	8	18		431	64	53	78	2 760	355	1 027	132	53	45			
Region	**1 614 648**	**1 686 837**	**1 555 385**	**96**	**672 878**	**42**	**480 998**	**636 706**	**180 865**	**64 936**	**14 649**	**64 217**	**42 288**	**10 428**	**51**	**49**	**77**	**1 314 983**	**81**	**610 079**	**38**	**45**	**56**	**240 402**	**62 799**	**29**

See Explanatory notes, page 151.

Country data for South-East Asia: treatment outcomes for cases registered in 2002

	New smear-positive cases – DOTS											New smear-positive cases – non-DOTS											Smear-positive re-treatment cases – DOTS								
	Number of cases		% of notif regist'd	% cured	% compl-eted	% died	% failed	% default	% trans-ferred	% not eval	% success	Number of cases		% of notif regist'd	% cured	% compl-eted	% died	% failed	% default	% trans-ferred	% not eval	% success	Number regist'd	% cured	% compl-eted	% died	% failed	% default	% trans-ferred	% not eval	% success
	notified	regist'd										notified	regist'd																			
Bangladesh	45 741	46 811	102	81	3	5	1	7	3	0	84	1 070											4 360	66	3	4	2	10	3	12	69
Bhutan	364	390	107	76	10	3	3	2	5	1	86												85	40	15	2	7	2	2	31	55
DPR Korea	14 290	14 290	100	85	3	2	5	3	2		88	4 286	1 355	32	70	9	4	5	5	7		79	1 097	75	6	6	6	4	3		81
India	245 135	244 859	100	86	1	4	3	6	0		87	150 698	41 368	27	41	17	2	1	30	9		58	84 078	68	3	7	6	14	1	0	72
Indonesia	76 230	76 230	100	72	15	2	1	5	3	3	86												3 731	60	17	2	3	5	3	8	78
Maldives	60	60	100	95		3	2				95												4	75			25				75
Myanmar	24 162	23 922	99	71	10	5	2	9	2	0	81												8 036	65	10	8	4	10	4	0	75
Nepal	13 307	13 307	100	84	2	5	2	5	2	0	86	407	407	100	68	10	4	1	9	1	8	78	2 663	80	2	7	4	4	3	0	82
Sri Lanka	3 643	3 643	100	79	2	4	1	12	2	0	81	654	654	100	68	12	4		12	2	2	80	379	54	6	9	2	26	2	1	60
Thailand	25 593	26 559	104	69	5	11	2	10	4		74												1 990	55	6	17	7	9	6		62
Timor-Leste	1 090	1 091	100	71	10	6	1	10	2		81																				
Region	449 615	451 162	100	81	4	4	2	6	1	1	85	157 115	43 784	28	42	17	2	2	28	9	0	59	106 423	68	4	7	6	13	1	1	72

See Explanatory notes, page 151.

Country data for South-East Asia: re-treatment outcomes for cases registered in 2002

	Relapse – DOTS									After failure – DOTS									After default – DOTS								
	number regist'd	% cured	% compl-eted	% died	% failed	% default	% trans-ferred	% not eval	% success	number regist'd	% cured	% compl-eted	% died	% failed	% default	% trans-ferred	% not eval	% success	number regist'd	% cured	% compl-eted	% died	% failed	% default	% trans-ferred	% not eval	% success
Bangladesh	2485	66	3	4	1	7	2	16	69	365	69	2	4	3	14	4	4	72	1510	67	2	4	3	15	3	6	69
Bhutan	37	65	14	5	11		5		78	19	26	21	8	5	5		42	47	29	17	14		3	3	3	62	31
DPR Korea	638	78	5	5	6	4	3		83	268	69	6	8	8	4	4		76	191	76	7	6	3	4	3		83
India	34 317	73	3	7	6	12	1		75	8 727	57	3	8	15	16	1		60	41 034	67	4	7	5	16	1	0	71
Indonesia										1				100													
Maldives	3	100							100																		
Myanmar	3 762	67	9	8	3	9	3		76	300	71	1	7	14	5	2	0	71	465	75	3	8	2	8	3		79
Nepal	1 898	83	2	7	3	3	3	0	84	30	43	10	13	13	17		3	53									
Sri Lanka	208	62	5	9	2	20	2		67										141	45	6	9	1	38	1	1	50
Thailand	1 416	58	7	17	6	8	5		64	574	49	6	17	9	12	7		55									
Timor-Leste																											
Region	**44 764**	**72**	**3**	**7**	**5**	**11**	**1**	**1**	**75**	**10 284**	**58**	**3**	**9**	**14**	**15**	**1**	**0**	**61**	**43 370**	**67**	**4**	**7**	**5**	**16**	**1**	**0**	**71**

See Explanatory notes for previous table, page 151.

SEAR

Country data for South-East Asia: trends in DOTS treatment success and detection rates, 1994–2003

	DOTS new smear-positive treatment success (%)									DOTS new smear-positive case detection rate (%)								
	1994	1995	1996	1997	1998	1999	2000	2001	2002	1995	1996	1997	1998	1999	2000	2001	2002	2003
Bangladesh	73	71	72	78	80	81	83	84	84	7	14	18	23	23	23	25	29	33
Bhutan	71	97	96	85	90	85	90	93	86	28	24	23	22	26	29	31	32	32
DPR Korea					91	94	91	91	88					2	26	53	79	91
India	83	79	79	82	84	82	84	85	87	0	1	1	2	7	12	24	31	47
Indonesia	94	91	81	54	58	50	87	86	86	1	5	7	12	18	19	20	27	33
Maldives	95	97	93	94	94	94	97	97	95	96	97	94	94	101	81	79	87	106
Myanmar		66	79	82	82	81	82	81	81		26	26	29	32	48	56	65	73
Nepal			85	87	89	87	86	88	86		6	11	16	44	56	56	57	60
Sri Lanka	77	79	80	76	76	84	77	80	81	63	61	71	75	75	68	73	71	70
Thailand			78	62	68	77	69	75	74		0	5	21	39	46	73	65	72
Timor-Leste								73	81								59	53
Region	80	74	77	72	72	73	83	84	85	2	4	6	8	14	18	27	33	45

Country data for South-East Asia: age and sex distribution of smear-positive cases in DOTS areas, 2003 (absolute numbers)

	MALE							FEMALE							ALL						
	0-14	15-24	25-34	35-44	45-54	55-64	65+	0-14	15-24	25-34	35-44	45-54	55-64	65+	0-14	15-24	25-34	35-44	45-54	55-64	65+
Bangladesh	320	5 166	7 275	8 058	6 947	5 501	4 142	544	4 298	4 282	3 258	2 086	1 150	591	864	9 464	11 557	11 316	9 033	6 651	4 733
Bhutan	9	62	50	20	25	20	13	14	57	39	17	13	15	6	23	119	89	37	38	35	19
DPR Korea	81	1 101	2 173	2 541	2 340	1 327	562	90	792	1 542	1 531	1 316	723	326	171	1 893	3 715	4 072	3 656	2 050	888
India	1 890	42 830	54 948	56 283	47 204	30 256	16 242	4 120	31 332	31 895	19 662	11 520	6 903	3 379	6 010	74 162	86 843	75 945	58 724	37 159	19 621
Indonesia	532	9 570	12 647	10 925	9 558	6 720	3 615	608	8 734	10 127	7 889	6 085	3 907	1 649	1 140	18 304	22 774	18 814	15 643	10 627	5 264
Maldives	1	14	7	4	9	9	4	0	8	5	1	5	1	0	1	22	12	5	14	10	4
Myanmar	107	2 536	4 408	4 427	3 269	1 974	1 296	154	1 781	2 442	2 003	1 491	943	617	261	4 317	6 850	6 430	4 760	2 917	1 913
Nepal	122	2 039	1 658	1 619	1 769	1 639	735	189	1 283	1 107	873	609	486	220	311	3 322	2 765	2 492	2 378	2 125	955
Sri Lanka	11	286	399	609	665	421	315	2	250	181	148	149	103	103	23	536	580	757	814	524	418
Thailand	41	1 636	4 615	4 259	3 497	2 740	3 241	49	944	1 678	1 350	1 279	1 264	1 866	90	2 580	6 293	5 609	4 776	4 004	5 107
Timor-Leste	5	130	135	107	98	66	41	13	98	116	76	76	43	17	18	228	251	183	174	109	58
Region	3 119	65 370	88 315	88 852	75 381	50 673	30 206	5 783	49 577	53 414	36 808	24 629	15 538	8 774	8 912	114 947	141 729	125 660	100 010	66 211	38 980

Note: the sum of cases notified by age is less than the number of new smear-positive cases notified for some countries.

Country data for South-East Asia: age and sex distribution of smear-positive cases in non-DOTS areas, 2003 (absolute numbers)

	MALE							FEMALE							ALL						
	0-14	15-24	25-34	35-44	45-54	55-64	65+	0-14	15-24	25-34	35-44	45-54	55-64	65+	0-14	15-24	25-34	35-44	45-54	55-64	65+
Bangladesh																					
Bhutan																					
DPR Korea	5	53	106	137	129	85	72	3	31	81	76	79	46	44	8	84	187	213	208	131	116
India	521	4 421	6 810	7 304	5 661	3 483	1 776	625	3 179	4 422	3 658	2 535	1 419	606	1 146	7 600	11 232	10 962	8 196	4 902	2 382
Indonesia																					
Maldives																					
Myanmar																					
Nepal																					
Sri Lanka	1	25	68	85	126	74	74	2	55	37	38	38	29	17	3	80	105	123	164	103	91
Thailand																					
Timor-Leste																					
Region	527	4 499	6 984	7 526	5 916	3 642	1 922	630	3 265	4 540	3 772	2 652	1 494	667	1 157	7 764	11 524	11 298	8 568	5 136	2 589

Note: the sum of cases notified by age is less than the number of new smear-positive cases notified for some countries.

Country data for South-East Asia: smear-positive notification rates (per 100 000 population) by age and sex, 2003

	MALE							FEMALE							ALL						
	0-14	15-24	25-34	35-44	45-54	55-64	65+	0-14	15-24	25-34	35-44	45-54	55-64	65+	0-14	15-24	25-34	35-44	45-54	55-64	65+
Bangladesh	1	34	62	93	123	183	178	2	30	39	40	39	37	24	2	32	51	68	82	109	100
Bhutan	2	27	33	19	33	38	29	3	25	26	17	17	27	12	2	26	30	18	25	32	19
DPR Korea	3	64	115	148	227	135	100	3	48	85	92	129	68	43	3	56	100	120	178	100	67
India	1	45	71	91	106	108	70	3	36	46	36	30	26	14	2	41	59	65	69	67	40
Indonesia	2	44	67	74	94	108	71	2	41	54	54	60	56	26	2	43	60	64	77	80	46
Maldives	1	41	32	25	90	152	69	0	24	24	7	49	19	0	1	33	28	17	69	89	36
Myanmar	1	52	106	147	151	149	123	2	37	58	64	65	66	49	2	45	82	105	107	106	83
Nepal	2	80	90	122	198	276	169	4	54	63	67	68	78	44	3	67	77	95	133	174	102
Sri Lanka	1	17	30	47	68	63	58	1	18	15	14	19	21	18	1	17	22	31	46	44	38
Thailand	1	29	83	93	107	137	194	1	17	29	27	36	59	89	1	23	56	59	70	96	135
Timor-Leste	3	131	265	224	300	331	363	9	111	319	168	248	211	142	6	121	287	197	275	270	250
Region	1	44	72	91	109	117	85	3	35	47	41	38	35	22	2	40	60	67	75	76	51

Note: rates are missing where data for smear-positive cases are missing, or where age- and sex-specific population data are not available.

SEAR

Country data for South-East Asia: number of TB cases notified, 1980–2003

	1980	1981	1982	1983	1984	1985	1986	1987	1988	1989	1990	1991	1992	1993	1994	1995	1996	1997	1998	1999	2000	2001	2002	2003
Bangladesh	39 774	42 644	49 870	52 961	45 679	41 802	45 599	45 355	44 280	45 191	48 673	56 052	31 400	54 001	48 276	56 437	63 471	63 420	72 256	79 339	75 557	76 302	81 963	88 156
Bhutan	1 539	2 657	720	1 017	904	1 073	1 582	608	1 126	1 525	1 154	996	140	108	1 159	1 299	1 271	1 211	1 292	1 174	1 140	1 037	1 089	1 026
DPR Korea	0								0									11 050	1 152	12 287	34 131	29 284	40 159	41 810
India	705 600	769 540	923 095	1 075 098	1 109 310	1 168 804	1 279 536	1 403 122	1 457 288	1 510 500	1 519 182	1 555 353	1 121 120	1 081 279	1 114 374	1 218 183	1 290 343	1 132 859	1 102 002	1 218 743	1 115 718	1 085 075	1 060 951	1 073 065
Indonesia	25 235	32 461	33 000	31 809	32 432	17 681	16 750		97 505	105 516	74 470	60 808	98 458	62 966	49 647	35 529	24 647	22 184	40 497	69 064	84 591	92 792	155 188	178 260
Maldives	73	112	111	143	123	91	111	115	85	203	152	123	92	175	249	231	212	173	176	153	132	139	125	137
Myanmar	12 744	12 461	12 069	11 012	11 045	10 506	10 840	11 986	9 348	10 940	12 416	14 905	17 000	19 009	15 583	18 229	22 201	17 122	14 756	19 626	30 840	42 838	57 012	75 744
Nepal	1 020	337	1 459	700	190	52	252	1 012	1 603	11 003	10 142	8 983		13 161	15 572	19 804	22 970	24 158	24 135	27 356	29 519	29 519	30 359	30 925
Sri Lanka	6 212	6 288	7 334	6 666	6 376	5 889	6 596	6 411	6 092	6 429	6 666	6 174	6 802	6 809	6 132	5 710	5 366	6 542	6 925	7 157	8 413	7 499	8 939	8 998
Thailand	45 704	49 452	48 553	65 413	69 240	77 611	52 152	51 835	50 021	44 553	46 510	43 858	47 697	49 668	47 767	45 428	39 871	30 262	15 850	29 413	34 187	49 656	49 581	54 504
Timor-Leste																							2 760	2 760
Region	837 901	915 952	1 076 211	1 244 819	1 275 299	1 323 509	1 413 418	1 520 444	1 667 348	1 735 860	1 719 365	1 747 252	1 322 709	1 287 176	1 298 759	1 400 850	1 470 352	1 308 981	1 279 041	1 464 312	1 414 228	1 414 141	1 485 366	1 552 625
number reporting	9	8	8	8	8	8	8	7	9	8	8	8	7	8	8	8	8	9	9	9	9	9	10	11
percent reporting	100	89	89	89	89	89	89	78	100	89	89	89	78	89	89	89	89	100	100	100	100	100	100	100

Country data for South-East Asia: case notification rates (per 100 000 population), 1980–2003

	1980	1981	1982	1983	1984	1985	1986	1987	1988	1989	1990	1991	1992	1993	1994	1995	1996	1997	1998	1999	2000	2001	2002	2003
Bangladesh	47	49	56	58	48	43	46	45	43	42	44	50	27	46	40	46	50	49	55	59	55	54	57	60
Bhutan	117	197	52	72	62	72	104	39	70	92	68	58	8	6	65	72	69	64	66	59	55	49	50	45
DPR Korea									0									51	5	56	153	131	178	184
India	102	109	129	147	148	153	164	176	179	182	179	180	127	121	122	131	136	117	112	122	110	105	101	101
Indonesia	17	21	21	20	20	11	10		55	59	41	33	52	33	26	18	12	11	20	33	40	43	71	81
Maldives	46	69	66	83	69	50	59	59	42	97	70	55	40	74	102	92	82	65	64	54	45	46	40	43
Myanmar	38	36	34	31	30	28	29	31	24	27	31	36	41	45	36	41	50	38	32	42	65	89	117	153
Nepal	7	2	9	4	1	0	1	6	9	63	54	47		66	76	95	107	110	107	119	126	123	123	123
Sri Lanka	43	43	49	44	41	38	42	40	37	33	40	36	39	39	35	32	30	36	38	39	45	40	47	47
Thailand	99	105	101	134	139	153	101	99	95	83	86	80	85	88	84	79	68	51	27	49	56	81	80	87
Timor-Leste																							374	355
Region	**80**	**85**	**98**	**111**	**111**	**113**	**119**	**125**	**134**	**137**	**133**	**133**	**99**	**94**	**93**	**99**	**102**	**89**	**86**	**96**	**92**	**90**	**94**	**96**

Country data for South-East Asia: new smear-positive cases, 1993–2003

	Number of cases											Rate (per 100 000 population)										
	1993	1994	1995	1996	1997	1998	1999	2000	2001	2002	2003	1993	1994	1995	1996	1997	1998	1999	2000	2001	2002	2003
Bangladesh	18 993	1 710	20 524	29 674	33 117	37 737	37 821	38 484	40 777	46 811	53 618	16	1	17	23	26	29	28	28	29	33	37
Bhutan		352	367	308	284	270	315	347	359	364	360		20	20	17	15	14	16	17	17	17	16
DPR Korea					3 980	403	5 073	16 440	14 429	18 576	17 392					18	2	23	74	64	82	77
India	225 256	226 543	264 515	290 953	274 877	278 275	345 150	349 374	384 827	395 833	433 271	25	25	28	31	28	28	35	34	37	38	41
Indonesia	62 966	49 647	31 768	11 790	19 492	32 280	49 172	52 338	53 965	76 230	92 566	33	26	16	6	10	16	24	25	25	35	42
Maldives	126	125	114	106	95	88	88	65	59	60	68	53	51	46	41	36	32	31	22	20	19	21
Myanmar			8 681	9 716	9 695	10 089	11 458	17 254	21 161	24 162	27 448			20	22	21	22	24	36	44	49	55
Nepal	6 679	10 442	8 591	10 365	11 323	11 306	13 410	13 683	13 683	13 714	14 348	33	51	41	48	52	50	58	58	57	56	57
Sri Lanka	3 335	3 405	3 049	2 958	3 506	3 761	3 911	4 314	4 316	4 297	4 321	19	19	17	16	19	21	21	23	23	23	23
Thailand		20 260	20 273	16 997	13 214	7 962	14 934	17 754	28 363	25 593	28 459		35	35	29	22	13	25	29	46	41	45
Timor-Leste										1 090	1 027										148	132
Region	317 355	312 484	357 882	372 867	369 583	382 171	481 332	510 053	561 939	606 730	672 878	23	22	25	26	25	26	32	33	36	38	42

Notes

Bangladesh
There is a discrepancy between the population estimate used by the national TB programme (137 059 519) and that used by the UN (146 736 131). Using the country's population estimate, there would be 336 976 estimated TB cases (of which, 162 331 smear-positive cases), and DOTS detection of smear-positive cases would be 35% (instead of 33%).

Bhutan
Estimates of the population vary widely, from 800 000 to over 2 million. The UN population estimate is 2.2 million.

India
DOTS coverage reached 73% by the end of 2003, but it was 67% calculated on a quarter-by-quarter basis (starting from 60% in the first quarter). Cases notified under DOTS included 31 341 cases (of which 13 603 were new smear-positive) in patients receiving non-rifampicin regimens.

Myanmar
DOTS coverage was 95% in 2003, but reached 100% by end of the year.

Nepal
Data refer to a mid-July to mid-July calendar.

Thailand
Data refer to an October–September calendar.

Timor-Leste
DOTS coverage was not reported, but assumed to be same as in the previous report.

Africa

The Americas

Eastern Mediterranean

Europe

South-East Asia

Western Pacific

WESTERN PACIFIC: SUMMARY OF TB CONTROL POLICIES

	STATUS[a]	MANUAL[b]	MICROSCOPY[c]	SCC[d]	DOT[e]	MONITORING OUTCOME[f]
AMERICAN SAMOA	DOTS	YES				
AUSTRALIA	DOTS	YES				
BRUNEI DARUSSALAM	DOTS	YES				
CAMBODIA	DOTS	YES				
CHINA	DOTS	YES				
CHINA, HONG KONG SAR	DOTS	YES				
CHINA, MACAO SAR	DOTS	NO				
COOK ISLANDS	DOTS	YES				
FIJI	DOTS	YES				
FRENCH POLYNESIA	DOTS	YES				
GUAM	DOTS	YES				
JAPAN	DOTS	YES				
KIRIBATI	DOTS	YES				
LAO PDR	DOTS	YES				
MALAYSIA	DOTS	YES				
MARSHALL ISLANDS	DOTS	YES				
MICRONESIA	DOTS	YES				
MONGOLIA	DOTS	YES				
NAURU	DOTS	NO				
NEW CALEDONIA	DOTS	YES				
NEW ZEALAND	DOTS	YES				
NIUE	DOTS	YES				
NORTHERN MARIANA IS	DOTS	YES				
PALAU	DOTS	YES				
PAPUA NEW GUINEA	DOTS	YES				
PHILIPPINES	DOTS	YES				
REP. KOREA	**DOTS**	**YES**				
SAMOA	DOTS	YES				
SINGAPORE	DOTS	YES				
SOLOMON ISLANDS	DOTS	YES				
TOKELAU	NON-DOTS	NO				
TONGA	DOTS	YES				
TUVALU	NON-DOTS	NO				
VANUATU	DOTS	YES				
VIET NAM	DOTS	NO				
WALLIS & FUTUNA IS	DOTS	YES				

WPR

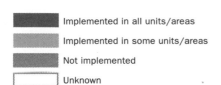

Implemented in all units/areas

Implemented in some units/areas

Not implemented

Unknown

a Status: DOTS status (bold indicates DOTS introduced in 2003. Blank indicates no report received)
b Manual: national TB control manual (recommended)
c Microscopy: use of smear microscopy for diagnosis (core component of DOTS)
d SCC: short course chemotherapy (core component of DOTS)
e DOT: directly observed treatment (core component of DOTS)
f Outcome monitoring: monitoring of treatment outcomes by cohort analysis (core component of DOTS)

Country data for the Western Pacific: estimated burden of TB

	Incidence, 1990				Prevalence, 1990				Death, 1990				Incidence, 2003				Prevalence, 2003				Death, 2003			
	All cases incl. HIV+		New ss+ incl. HIV+		All cases incl. HIV+		All cases excl. HIV+		All cases incl. HIV+		All cases excl. HIV+		All cases incl. HIV+		New ss+ incl. HIV+		All cases incl. HIV+		All cases excl. HIV+		All cases incl. HIV+		All cases excl. HIV+	
	number	rate	number	rate	number	rate	number	rate	number	rate	number	rate	number	rate	number	rate	number	rate	number	rate	number	rate	number	rate
American Samoa	24	52	11	23	68	145	68	145	5	11	5	11	18	30	8	13	34	54	34	54	4	6	4	6
Australia	1 067	6	478	3	1 195	7	1 195	7	171	1	171	1	1 128	6	505	3	1 142	6	1 132	6	113	1	111	1
Brunei Darussalam	159	62	72	28	443	172	443	172	33	13	33	13	195	54	88	25	217	61	217	61	17	5	17	5
Cambodia	56 202	577	24 848	255	154 356	1 584	153 874	1 579	12 009	123	11 593	119	71 830	508	31 758	225	107 836	762	105 008	742	13 493	95	11 469	81
China	1 345 828	116	605 046	52	3 748 967	325	3 748 967	325	282 443	24	282 443	24	1 334 066	102	599 758	46	3 203 059	246	3 200 204	245	235 864	18	233 918	18
China, Hong Kong SAR	6 326	111	2 845	50	17 611	309	17 608	309	1 329	23	1 327	23	5 439	77	2 446	35	5 554	79	5 548	79	468	7	467	7
China, Macao SAR	348	93	156	42	969	260	969	260	73	20	73	20	382	82	172	37	414	89	413	89	45	10	44	10
Cook Islands	10	52	4	23	27	145	27	145	2	11	2	11	5	30	2	13	11	59	11	59	1	6	1	6
Fiji	376	52	169	23	1 047	145	1 047	145	79	11	79	11	249	30	112	13	318	38	317	38	38	4	37	4
French Polynesia	102	52	46	23	283	145	283	145	21	11	21	11	73	30	33	13	94	39	94	38	11	5	11	5
Guam	189	141	85	63	525	392	525	392	40	30	40	30	98	60	44	27	171	105	170	105	19	12	19	12
Japan	64 322	52	28 927	23	71 939	58	71 895	58	10 323	8	10 313	8	39 927	31	17 956	14	53 210	42	53 154	42	4 973	4	4 960	4
Kiribati	101	141	45	63	282	392	282	392	21	30	21	30	53	60	24	27	53	60	53	60	4	4	4	4
Lao PDR	7 376	178	3 318	80	20 547	497	20 547	497	1 548	37	1 548	37	8 891	157	3 999	71	18 504	327	18 494	327	1 482	26	1 475	26
Malaysia	21 380	120	9 591	54	59 540	334	59 536	334	4 488	25	4 485	25	25 785	106	11 567	47	33 128	136	32 945	135	4 044	17	3 942	16
Marshall Islands	63	141	28	63	174	392	174	392	13	30	13	30	32	60	14	27	32	60	32	60	2	4	2	4
Micronesia	136	141	61	63	378	392	378	392	28	30	28	30	66	60	29	27	68	62	68	62	6	6	6	6
Mongolia	4 875	220	2 194	99	13 581	613	13 581	613	1 023	46	1 023	46	5 025	194	2 261	87	6 149	237	6 147	237	834	32	833	32
Nauru	5	52	2	23	14	145	14	145	1	11	1	11	4	30	2	13	5	36	5	36	0.5	4	0.5	4
New Caledonia	241	141	108	63	671	392	671	392	51	30	51	30	137	60	61	27	236	103	235	103	26	11	26	11
New Zealand	356	11	160	5	398	12	398	12	57	2	57	2	413	11	185	5	420	11	418	11	41	1	41	1
Niue	1	52	0.5	23	1	145	1	145	0.3	11	0.3	11	0.6	30	0.3	13	1	59	1	59	0.1	6	0.1	6
Northern Mariana Is	62	141	28	63	172	392	172	392	13	30	13	30	48	60	21	27	53	67	53	67	6	8	6	8
Palau	21	141	10	63	60	392	60	392	4	30	4	30	12	60	6	27	16	76	16	76	2	8	2	8
Papua New Guinea	10 992	267	4 925	120	30 621	744	30 621	744	2 307	56	2 307	56	13 437	235	6 020	105	30 240	529	30 108	527	2 782	49	2 700	47
Philippines	205 495	336	92 457	151	572 431	937	572 431	937	43 126	71	43 126	71	236 885	296	106 580	133	366 171	458	366 079	458	38 872	49	38 811	49
Rep. Korea	36 762	86	16 539	39	102 406	239	102 406	239	7 715	18	7 715	18	41 664	87	18 744	39	56 522	118	56 409	118	4 715	10	4 690	10
Samoa	83	52	37	23	232	145	232	145	17	11	17	11	53	30	24	13	79	44	78	44	9	5	9	5
Singapore	1 763	58	789	26	1 967	65	1 963	65	283	9	282	9	1 749	41	783	18	1 806	42	1 786	42	198	5	193	5
Solomon Islands	449	141	202	63	1 250	392	1 250	392	94	30	94	30	286	60	129	27	288	60	288	60	21	4	21	4
Tokelau	0.8	52	0.4	23	2	145	2	145	0.2	11	0.2	11	0.5	30	0.2	13	0.9	59	0.9	59	0.1	6	0.1	6
Tonga	52	52	23	23	144	145	144	145	11	11	11	11	31	30	14	13	45	44	45	44	5	6	5	6
Tuvalu	5	52	2	23	13	145	13	145	1.0	11	1.0	11	3	30	1	13	6	59	6	59	0.6	6	0.6	6
Vanuatu	210	141	95	63	586	392	586	392	44	30	44	30	127	60	57	27	150	71	150	71	18	8	18	8
Viet Nam	133 660	202	59 924	91	372 326	563	372 326	563	28 051	42	28 051	42	144 942	178	64 982	80	194 970	240	193 762	238	18 750	23	18 116	22
Wallis & Futuna Is	7	52	3	23	20	145	20	145	1	11	1	11	4	30	2	13	4	30	4	30	0.3	2	0.3	2
Region	**1 899 047**	**125**	**853 229**	**56**	**5 175 246**	**341**	**5 174 709**	**341**	**395 426**	**26**	**394 995**	**26**	**1 933 054**	**112**	**868 388**	**50**	**4 081 006**	**236**	**4 073 485**	**235**	**326 862**	**19**	**321 957**	**19**

See Explanatory notes, page 151.

Country data for the Western Pacific: notification, detection and DOTS coverage, 2003

	Pop	All cases (Country no.)	All cases (WHO no.)	All cases rate	New Smear-pos no.	New Smear-pos rate	New Pulm confirmed no.	New Smear-neg/unknown no.	New Extra-pulmonary no.	Relapse no.	Re-treat After failure no.	Re-treat After default no.	Re-treat Other no.	Other no.	Detection All cases %	Detection New ss+ %	DOTS % of pop	DOTS Notif All cases no.	DOTS Notif All cases rate	DOTS Notif New ss+ no.	DOTS Notif New ss+ rate	DOTS DDR %	DOTS % pulm ss+	non-DOTS All cases no.	non-DOTS New ss+ no.	non-DOTS % pulm ss+
	thousands	number	number	rate	number	rate	number	number	number	number	number	number	number	number	%	%	pop	number	rate	number	rate	%	cases ss+	number	number	cases ss+
American Samoa	62	3	3	5	2	3	0	0	0	1		5			16	24	100	3	5	2	3	24	100			59
Australia	19 731	982	949	5	113	5	38	316	457	23					84	22	63	590	3	48	0	0	15	359	65	
Brunei Darussalam	358	211	206	58	121	34	136	41	40	4	0	1	1	3	106	138	100	206	58	121	34	138	75			
Cambodia	14 144	28 386	28 216	199	18 923	134	18 923	4 307	4 252	754	51	28		91	39	60	100	28 216	199	18 923	134	60	81			
China	1 304 196	683 577	615 868	47	267 414	21	267 414	248 805	30 768	38 881			67 709		46	45	91	553 677	42	257 287	20	43	55	62 191	10 127	19
China, Hong Kong SAR	7 049	6 035	5 624	80	1 779	25	3 399	2 932	594	319	0	6		549	103	73	100	4 461	63	1 426	20	58	38	1 163	353	36
China, Macao SAR	464	382	371	80	138	30	224	154	47	32	0	0		5	97	80	100	350	75	130	28	76	47	21	8	50
Cook Islands	18	0	0	0	0	0	0	0	0	0					0	0	100	0	0	0	0					
Fiji	839	179	179	21	70	8	36	49	55	5					72	63	100	179	21	70	8	63	59			
French Polynesia	244	51	50	20	21	9	39	19	7	5	0	0		1	69	65	100	50	20	21	9	65	53			
Guam	163	61	22	14	0	0		15		0					23	0	100	22	14	0	6	40				
Japan	127 654	31 638	31 638	25	10 843	8	17 316	13 621	6 160	1 014					79	60	64	21 350	17	7 212	6	40	44	10 288	3 631	46
Kiribati	88	278	284	324	99	113		71	110	4					540	419	100	284	324	99	113	419	58			
Lao PDR	5 657	2 824	2 780	49	1 882	33	2 277	495	317	86	5	39			31	47	85	2 780	49	1 882	33	47	79			
Malaysia	24 425	15 912	15 671	64	7 989	33		5 811	1 465	406	20	175		46	61	69	100	15 671	64	7 989	33	69	58			
Marshall Islands	53	60	60	113	20	38	20	22	18	0	0	0			189	140	100	50	113	20	38	140	48			
Micronesia	109	109	99	91	27	25	41	51	21	0	0	3		7	151	92	90	39	91	27	25	92	35			
Mongolia	2 594	4 007	3 918	151	1 541	59	1 541	812	1 419	146	58	31			78	68	100	3 918	151	1 541	59	68	65			
Nauru	13	3	3	23	1	8	1	1	1	0	0	0			77	57	100	3	23	1	8	57	50			
New Caledonia	228	36	36	16	14	6	19	9	12	1					26	23	100	36	16	14	6	23	61			
New Zealand	3 875	424	386	10	106	3	181	125	136	19				38	94	57	100	386	10	106	3	57	46			
Niue	2	0	0	0	0	0	0	0	0	0	0	0			0	0	90	0	0	0	0					
Northern Mariana Is	79	45	45	57	16	20	30	19	10	0	0	0			95	75	100	45	57	16	20	75	46			
Palau	20	9	9	44	5	24		2	2	0	0	0			73	90	100	9	44	5	24	90	71			
Papua New Guinea	5 711	18 405	18 405	322	3 231	57	3 231	7 038	6 769	1 367	359	713		724	137	54	46	5 607	98	921	16	15	30	12 798	2 310	32
Philippines	79 999	134 375	134 375	168	72 670	91	72 670	55 942	1 693	4 070					57	68	100	134 375	168	72 670	91	68	57			
Rep. Korea	47 700	40 500	33 888	71	10 976	23	13 062	18 399	1 312	3 201				5 540	81	59	100	13 463	28	4 379	9	23	37	20 425	6 597	37
Samoa	178	27	27	15	12	7	20	8	173	0	0	0			51	51	100	27	15	12	7	51	60			
Singapore	4 253	1 588	1 616	38	586	14	947	645	173	184	12	16			92	75	100	791	15	341	8	44	54	825	245	41
Solomon Islands	477	293	293	61	138	29	138	107	43	5	0	0			103	107	100	293	61	138	29	107	56			
Tokelau	2	0	0	0	0	0	0	0	0	0	0	0			0	0	0	0	0	0	0					
Tonga	104	16	16	15	11	11	11	3	2	0	0	0			52	80	100	16	15	11	11	80	79	30	0	0
Tuvalu	11	30	30	283	11	0	11	0	8	5	1	0		1	954	0	100	16		11	0					
Vanuatu	212	104	104	49	40	19	40	45	18	0	1	0		1	82	70	100	104	49	40	19	70	47			
Viet Nam	81 377	93 421	92 741	114	55 937	69	0	16 791	14 564	5 449	491	189		1	64	86	100	92 741	114	55 937	69	86	77			
Wallis & Futuna Is	15	18	15	102	7	48	11	7	0	1	0	1		2	343	356	90	15	102	7	48	356	50			
Region	1 732 104	1 045 572	987 927	57	454 732	26	401 765	376 679	70 506	85 982	998	1 208	67 709	7 008	51	52	90	879 827	51	431 396	25	50	58	108 100	23 336	27

See Explanatory notes, page 151.

WPR

Country data for the Western Pacific: treatment outcomes for cases registered in 2002

	New smear-positive cases – DOTS											New smear-positive cases – non-DOTS											Smear-positive re-treatment cases – DOTS								
	Number of cases notified	regist'd	% of notif regist'd	% cured	% compl-eted	% died	% failed	% default	% trans-ferred	% not eval	% success	Number of cases notified	regist'd	% of notif regist'd	% cured	% compl-eted	% died	% failed	% default	% trans-ferred	% not eval	% success	Number regist'd	% cured	% compl-eted	% died	% failed	% default	% trans-ferred	% not eval	% success
American Samoa	1	1	100		100						100																					
Australia	127	180	142	21	57	10		1	6	4	78	83	139	167	9	68	11			12		77	17	24	47	18			12		71
Brunei Darussalam	112	77	69	60	25	13		3			84												10	50	20	20		10			70
Cambodia	17 258	17 396	101	89	3	4	0	2	1		92	14 733	13 681	93	85	7	1	1	2	1	2	92	875	86	3	6	1	3	1		89
China	180 239	180 239	100	90	3	4	1	1	2	3	93	389	363	93	0	1	1	0	0	98		1	46 932	83	5	3	4	2	1		88
China, Hong Kong SAR	1 501	1 529	102	71	8	5	8	3	5		79												246	59	9	7	12	9	4	2	68
China, Macao SAR	135	138	102	87	2	5		1	2	2	89	12	12	100			75		25				47	62	26	4		4	4		87
Cook Islands	1	1	100	100							100																					
Fiji	75	73	97	85		5		8	1		85												2	100								100
French Polynesia	28	28	100		82	7		11			82																					
Guam	31	28	90	68		25			7		68												3	100								100
Japan	6 172	6 602	107	52	24	12	4	2	6		76	4 635	2 985	64	17	16	2	4	0	60		34	743	47	24	11	7	3	8		71
Kiribati	82	82	100	87	7	4	2		4		94												3	33	67				3		100
Lao PDR	1 829	1 738	95	67	11	7	0	11	5		78												117	54	12	9	7	9	3	6	66
Malaysia	7 958	7 424	93	76		8		11	5		76																					
Marshall Islands	18	20	111	90	10						100																					
Micronesia	22	22	100	91					9		91												3	55	15	33		33		33	69
Mongolia	1 670	1 671	100	83	4		5	3	3	0	87												226	55	15	8	11	7	5	5	0
Nauru	2	2	100	50		50					50																					
New Caledonia	21	20	95	45	40	5		10			85												1	100								100
New Zealand	88	93	106	60	60	5			3	31	60												3		67					33	67
Niue	1	2	200	50	50						100																					
Northern Mariana Is	21	21	100	71		5			24		71																					
Palau	9	8	89	38	38	25				38	38																					
Papua New Guinea	926	930	100	39	14	3	1	16	5	22	53												82	26	26	12	9	16	12		51
Philippines	65 148	59 453	91	77	11	3	1	5	3	0	88	11 345	1 345								100		1 576	66	2	2	2	5	20	2	68
Rep. Korea	4 743	4 743		81	2	1	2	3	10	1	83																					
Samoa	19	19	100	84		11		6	5		87																					
Singapore	311	449	144		87	7		6			87	238	449	189	65	65	29		6	0		65	87		70	11	1	17			70
Solomon Islands	108	108	100	71	19	4		5	2		90												2	100								100
Tokelau																																
Tonga	23	24	104	75	8	17					83	7	8			25	25		25		25	25	1	100								100
Tuvalu																																
Vanuatu	31	38	123	63	16	11	5	3	3		79												2	100						2		100
Viet Nam	56 698	56 590	100	90	2	3	1	1	2		92												6 079	79	6	5	5	2	2		85
Wallis & Futuna Is	1	5	500	100							100												6	83		3	4			17	83
Region	340 666	339 754	100	84	6	2	1	2	2	2	91	31 442	18 982	60	64	10	2	1	2	12	9	74	57 071	81	6	3	4	2	2	2	87

See Explanatory notes, page 151.

Country data for the Western Pacific: re-treatment outcomes for cases registered in 2002

	Relapse – DOTS									After failure – DOTS									After default – DOTS								
	number regist'd	% cured	% completed	% died	% failed	% default	% transferred	% not eval	% success	number regist'd	% cured	% completed	% died	% failed	% default	% transferred	% not eval	% success	number regist'd	% cured	% completed	% died	% failed	% default	% transferred	% not eval	% success
American Samoa																											
Australia	17	24	47	18			12		71																		
Brunei Darussalam	10	50	20	20		10			70																		
Cambodia	807	88	3	5	1	2	1		91																		
China																											
China, Hong Kong SAR	239	61	8	7	12	9	3		69										7		43		14	14	29		43
China, Macao SAR	45	64	27	2		2	4		91										2			50		50			
Cook Islands	2	100							100																		
Fiji																											
French Polynesia	8		75	25					75																		
Guam	3	100							100																		
Japan	743	47	24	11	7	3	8		71																		
Kiribati	3	33	67						100																		
Lao PDR	117	54	12	9	7	9	3	6	66																		
Malaysia																											
Marshall Islands																											
Micronesia																			3			33	33			33	
Mongolia	134	61	12	8	6	7	5	1	73	66	50	15	5	23	6	2		65	26	35	27	12	4	12	12		62
Nauru																											
New Caledonia	1	100							100																		
New Zealand	3		67					33	67																		
Niue																											
Northern Mariana Is																											
Palau																											
Papua New Guinea	82	26	26	12	9	16	12		51																		
Philippines	1 415	67	2	2	2	4	20	2	69										161	58	4	6	2	14	21	1	62
Rep. Korea																											
Samoa																											
Singapore	65		78	12	2	8			78										22		45	9		45			45
Solomon Islands	2	100							100																		
Tokelau																											
Tonga	1	100							100																		
Tuvalu																											
Vanuatu	1	100							100										1	100							100
Viet Nam	5 446	81	6	5	4	2	2		87	472	57	1	6	18	4	4		68	161	71	7	6	6	8	2		78
Wallis & Futuna Is	5	80						20	80										1	100							100
Region	**9 149**	**74**	**8**	**5**	**4**	**3**	**6**	**0**	**82**	**538**	**65**	**3**	**6**	**18**	**4**	**4**		**67**	**384**	**57**	**10**	**4**	**4**	**13**	**11**	**1**	**67**

See Explanatory notes for previous table, page 151.

WPR

Country data for the Western Pacific: trends in DOTS treatment success and detection rates, 1994–2003

	DOTS new smear-positive treatment success (%)									DOTS new smear-positive case detection rate (%)								
	1994	1995	1996	1997	1998	1999	2000	2001	2002	1995	1996	1997	1998	1999	2000	2001	2002	2003
American Samoa		100			50	100	100	100	100			64		34	23	23	12	24
Australia			66	66	75	84	74	66	78				23	30	24	20	25	9
Brunei Darussalam					85	76	63	56	84					123	100	111	129	138
Cambodia	84	91	94	91	95	93	91	92	92	40	34	44	47	53	49	47	55	60
China	94	96	96	96	97	96	95	96	93	15	28	32	32	29	31	31	30	43
China, Hong Kong SAR					85	78	76	78	79					60	59	57	60	58
China, Macao SAR	75			81		78	89	86	89	86	155	194	163		93	91	79	76
Cook Islands				50		80		100	100				32			75	39	
Fiji	90	86		87	90	92	85	85	85	47	49	49	56	51	50	61	65	63
French Polynesia		67	95	100	74	85	97	80	82		94	107	91	91	82		84	65
Guam						94	93	71	68						85		67	
Japan						76	70	75	76						22	29	33	40
Kiribati					83	88	91	86	94			34	170	203	196	244	329	419
Lao PDR		70	55	62	75	84	82	77	78		24	33	40	45	40	40	46	47
Malaysia		69				90	78	79	76	64	69				73	73	69	69
Marshall Islands					83	82	91	86	100				59	96	66	94	119	140
Micronesia		80	78			95	93	100	91	18	30				43	24	71	92
Mongolia		78	78	86	84	86	87	87	87	7	31	31	54	67	62	73	74	68
Nauru						50	25	100	50						216	110	112	57
New Caledonia	62	75			70	77	89	84	85	24	31			30	28	28	33	23
New Zealand							30	9	60						41	37	48	57
Niue									100								364	
Northern Mariana Is						80	81	74	71						117	85	96	75
Palau	64	67	75					100	38	115	53	97					156	90
Papua New Guinea		60	82	93	72	66	63	67	53		4	1	7	4	7	8	16	15
Philippines	80		71	83	84	87	88	88	88	0	0	3	10	20	48	57	62	68
Rep. Korea	71	76		82					83	34	65	56	58					23
Samoa	50	80	100		86	94	92	77	84	48	30	48		63	49	43	77	51
Singapore	88	86	73	92	92	95	85	88	87	57	26				13	22	39	44
Solomon Islands		65						89	90		55	71	91	63	76	85	81	107
Tokelau																		
Tonga	89	75	82	75	94	80	93	92	83	48	78	64	97	63	98	54	161	80
Tuvalu																		
Vanuatu						88	88	88	79					36	40	77	52	70
Viet Nam	91	91	90	85	93	92	92	93	92		60	79	83	84	83	84	88	86
Wallis & Futuna Is								100	100							100		356
Region	**90**	**91**	**93**	**93**	**95**	**94**	**92**	**93**	**91**	**16**	**28**	**32**	**33**	**31**	**37**	**38**	**39**	**50**

Country data for the Western Pacific: age and sex distribution of smear-positive cases in DOTS areas, 2003 (absolute numbers)

	MALE 0-14	15-24	25-34	35-44	45-54	55-64	65+	FEMALE 0-14	15-24	25-34	35-44	45-54	55-64	65+	ALL 0-14	15-24	25-34	35-44	45-54	55-64	65+
American Samoa	0	4	3	1	6	1	12	0	6	7	2	2	2	2	0	10	10	3	8	3	14
Australia	0	5	25	17	8	8	9	0	9	14	11	4	5	6	0	14	39	28	12	13	15
Brunei Darussalam																					
Cambodia	37	805	1 514	2 183	1 848	1 729	1 487	46	691	1 287	1 975	2 208	1 857	1 256	83	1 496	2 801	4 158	4 056	3 586	2 743
China	1 059	24 199	31 471	30 210	31 370	26 330	31 210	1 350	18 143	18 414	14 147	11 578	8 661	9 145	2 409	42 342	49 885	44 357	42 948	34 991	40 355
China, Hong Kong SAR	3	94	78	119	167	150	337	8	75	113	86	55	37	104	11	169	191	205	222	187	441
China, Macao SAR	0	8	8	16	25	9	23	0	7	7	10	7	4	5	0	15	15	26	33	13	28
Cook Islands																					
Fiji	2	9	7	6	9	5	6	0	5	6	4	4	7	0	2	14	13	10	13	12	6
French Polynesia	0	2	2	1	2	4	3	1	3	1	1	1	0	1	1	5	3	2	3	4	4
Guam	0	2	1	3	4	7	5	1	3	1	4	2	1	5	1	5	2	7	6	8	10
Japan	1	130	335	368	713	956	2 502	2	133	272	153	177	199	1 271	3	263	607	521	890	1 155	3 773
Kiribati	5	13	5	9	6	6	4	5	20	4	12	7	3	4	10	33	9	21	13	9	4
Lao PDR	6	94	186	240	233	202	200	7	78	105	160	161	115	95	13	172	291	400	394	317	295
Malaysia	216	1 211	2 010	2 073	1 798	1 438	1 661	136	969	1 044	857	669	584	626	412	2 180	3 054	2 930	2 467	2 022	2 227
Marshall Islands	6	4	4	7	7	2	4	4	9	7	4	6	1	2	10	13	11	11	13	3	6
Micronesia	0	3	2	2	0	2	1	4	4	4	1	1	2	1	4	7	6	3	1	4	2
Mongolia	10	206	217	171	93	55	39	19	254	233	148	45	32	19	29	460	450	319	138	87	58
Nauru	0	0	0	0	0	0	0	0	0	0	0	0	0	0	0	0	0	0	0	0	0
New Caledonia	0	1	1	1	1	0	3	0	0	2	2	0	1	3	0	1	3	3	1	1	6
New Zealand	5	9	10	6	6	8	9	7	18	8	1	10	4	5	12	27	18	7	16	12	14
Niue	0	0	0	0	1	0	0	1	3	0	2	1	0	2	1	3	0	2	2	0	2
Northern Mariana Is	0	2	2	2	1	0	2	1	0	0	2	1	0	0	1	2	2	4	2	0	2
Palau	0	0	1	1	1	1	2	0	0	0	1	0	0	0	0	0	1	2	1	1	2
Papua New Guinea	15	164	132	83	56	28	6	24	167	148	51	25	17	5	39	331	280	134	81	45	11
Philippines	356	6 360	9 302	11 458	10 713	6 445	3 648	300	3 218	4 551	4 761	4 000	2 858	2 018	656	9 578	13 853	16 219	14 713	9 303	5 666
Rep. Korea	10	401	564	557	493	377	481	13	285	291	174	133	150	450	23	686	855	731	626	527	931
Samoa	0	2				1		0		2	2	2	2	1	0	2	2	2	2	3	1
Singapore	0	10	15	44	70	56	65	0	4	13	13	13	8	30	0	14	28	57	83	64	95
Solomon Islands	4	14	9	12	14	8	0	9	14	14	16	13	10	1	13	28	23	28	27	18	1
Tokelau	0														0						
Tonga		1	1	1	1	0	2		1	0	1	1	2	0		2	1	2	2	2	2
Tuvalu																					
Vanuatu	1	2	4	7	5	2	3	0	4	4	3	2	1	2	1	6	8	10	7	3	5
Viet Nam	49	3 475	7 036	8 486	7 965	5 066	7 793	66	1 659	2 262	2 327	2 574	2 283	4 896	115	5 134	9 298	10 813	10 539	7 349	12 689
Wallis & Futuna Is	0	0	2	2	2	0	0	0	1	1	0	0	0	0	0	3	3	2	2	0	0
Region	1 785	37 230	52 945	56 086	55 619	42 897	49 449	2 063	25 784	28 810	24 929	21 699	16 846	19 957	3 848	63 014	81 755	81 015	77 318	59 743	69 406

Note: the sum of cases notified by age is less than the number of new smear-positive cases notified for some countries.

WPR

Country data for the Western Pacific: age and sex distribution of smear-positive cases in non-DOTS areas, 2003 (absolute numbers)

	MALE							FEMALE							ALL						
	0-14	15-24	25-34	35-44	45-54	55-64	65+	0-14	15-24	25-34	35-44	45-54	55-64	65+	0-14	15-24	25-34	35-44	45-54	55-64	65+
American Samoa																					
Australia	0	10	7	1	5	4	18	0	3	6	1	3	2	5	0	13	13	2	8	6	23
Brunei Darussalam																					
Cambodia																					
China	74	926	1 289	1 394	1 215	913	817	57	668	834	636	523	327	320	131	1 594	2 123	2 030	1 738	1 240	1 137
China, Hong Kong SAR	5	10	12	21	28	27	136	2	9	20	15	8	4	56	7	19	32	36	36	31	192
China, Macao SAR	0	1	1	0	1	0	4	0	0	0	1	0	0	0	0	1	1	1	1	0	4
Cook Islands																					
Fiji																					
French Polynesia																					
Guam																					
Japan	0	80	186	182	350	432	1 229	0	70	123	93	77	114	695	0	150	309	275	427	546	1 924
Kiribati																					
Lao PDR																					
Malaysia																					
Marshall Islands																					
Micronesia																					
Mongolia																					
Nauru																					
New Caledonia																					
New Zealand																					
Niue																					
Northern Mariana Is																					
Palau																					
Papua New Guinea																					
Philippines																					
Rep. Korea	12	331	644	708	714	615	991	19	396	502	327	232	231	875	31	727	1 146	1 035	946	846	1 866
Samoa	1	7	13	24	27	24	69	0	2	13	17	7	13	28	1	9	26	41	34	37	97
Singapore																					
Solomon Islands																					
Tokelau																					
Tonga																					
Tuvalu	4	2	0	1	6	0	0	0	3	0	0	0	0	0	4	5	0	2	6	0	0
Vanuatu																					
Viet Nam																					
Wallis & Futuna Is																					
Region	96	1 367	2 152	2 331	2 346	2 015	3 264	78	1 151	1 498	1 091	850	691	1 979	174	2 518	3 650	3 422	3 196	2 706	5 243

Note: the sum of cases notified by age is less than the number of new smear-positive cases notified for some countries.

Country data for the Western Pacific: smear-positive notification rates (per 100 000 population) by age and sex, 2003

	MALE							FEMALE							ALL						
	0-14	15-24	25-34	35-44	45-54	55-64	65+	0-14	15-24	25-34	35-44	45-54	55-64	65+	0-14	15-24	25-34	35-44	45-54	55-64	65+
American Samoa	0	1	1	0	1	0	3	0	1	1	0	0	0	1	0	1	1	1	1	0	1
Australia	0	15	72	64	39	96	165	0	28	38	43	27	98	108	0	21	55	54	34	96	136
Brunei Darussalam	1	50	185	321	425	706	1077	2	44	154	253	405	523	466	1	47	170	285	414	598	673
Cambodia	1	23	28	29	39	56	73	1	19	17	14	16	19	18	1	21	22	22	28	38	44
China																					
China, Hong Kong SAR																					
China, Macao SAR																					
Cook Islands	1	11	11	11	22	21	42														
Fiji									6	10	7	10	28	17	1	8	10	9	16	25	19
French Polynesia		8	10	5	15	50	54	4	13	5	6	8	0	17		11	8	6	12	26	35
Guam	0	15	8	22	39	120	103	0	24	9	36	22	20	101	2	20	9	28	31	73	102
Japan	0	3	5	7	12	16	37	0	3	4	3	3	3	14	0	3	5	5	7	10	24
Kiribati	1	16	47	87	128	190	212	1	14	26	55	84	93	87	1	15	36	71	105	138	145
Lao PDR	5	53	105	126	147	209	323	5	44	56	53	56	87	109	5	49	81	90	102	149	208
Malaysia																					
Marshall Islands	0	25	28	35	0	102	57	20	34	53	17	23	96	46	9	29	41	26	11	99	51
Micronesia	2	72	96	99	102	106	92	5	90	104	84	48	59	35	3	81	100	91	75	82	59
Mongolia																					
Nauru	0	5	5	6	8	12	49	0	0	11	12	0	0	44	0	3	8	9	4	6	46
New Caledonia	1	3	4	2	2	4	4	2	7	3	0	4	2	2	1	5	4	1	3	3	3
New Zealand																					
Niue																					
Northern Mariana Is																					
Palau																					
Papua New Guinea	1	28	30	25	27	25	8	2	32	33	16	13	17	8	2	30	32	21	21	21	8
Philippines	2	77	147	250	339	344	276	2	40	74	104	124	147	121	2	59	111	177	230	243	190
Rep. Korea	0	19	28	30	39	50	94	1	19	19	12	12	18	57	1	19	24	21	26	34	72
Samoa	0	10	9	17	28	29	88	0	11	17	30			22	0	11	13	24			41
Singapore	0	6	9	17	28	43	88	0	2	9	7	6	11	32	0	4	9	12	17	27	57
Solomon Islands	4	28	24	55	97	84	0	9	30	40	71	91	112	16	6	29	32	63	94	98	8
Tokelau																					
Tonga	0	9	13	19	29	0	72	0	10	0	19	25	69	0	0	9	7	19	27	37	34
Tuvalu																					
Vanuatu	2	9	28	63	65	44	86	0	19	27	26	28	24	60	1	14	27	44	47	34	73
Viet Nam	0	41	103	158	236	297	385	1	20	33	42	74	125	207	0	31	68	99	153	208	289
Wallis & Futuna Is																					
Region	**1**	**27**	**36**	**43**	**55**	**68**	**86**	**1**	**20**	**21**	**20**	**22**	**27**	**29**	**1**	**23**	**29**	**31**	**39**	**48**	**55**

Note: rates are missing where data for smear-positive cases are missing, or where age- and sex-specific population data are not available.

WPR

Country data for the Western Pacific: number of TB cases notified, 1980–2003

	1980	1981	1982	1983	1984	1985	1986	1987	1988	1989	1990	1991	1992	1993	1994	1995	1996	1997	1998	1999	2000	2001	2002	2003
American Samoa	2	6	6	8	12	5	8	9	13	5	9	3	1	4	4		0	6	3	4	3	3	2	3
Australia	1 457	1 386	1 270	1 219	1 299	1 088	906	907	954	952	1 016	950	1 011	991	1 057	1 073	0	1 145	899	1 073	1 043	980	1 013	949
Brunei Darussalam	196	285	245	276	256	238	212	189	126	128	143	180		160				160		272	307	216	230	206
Cambodia	2 576	1 980	8 158	7 572	10 241	10 145	10 325	9 106	10 691	7 906	6 501	10 903	16 148	13 270	15 172	14 603	14 857	15 629	16 946	19 266	18 891	19 170	24 610	28 216
China	0	98 654		117 557	151 564	226 899	265 095	251 600	304 639	310 607	375 481	345 000	320 426	344 218	363 804	515 764	504 758	466 394	445 704	449 518	454 372	470 221	462 609	615 868
China, Hong Kong SAR	8 065	7 729	7 527	7 301	7 843	7 545	7 432	7 269	7 021	6 704	6 510	6 283	6 545	6 537	6 319	0	6 501	7 072	7 673	7 512	7 578	7 262	6 244	5 624
China, Macao SAR	1 101	585	233	455	671	571	420	389	320	274	343	329	294	285		402	570	575	465		449	465	388	371
Cook Islands	37	10	19	29	20	36	17	16	20	1		8	12	6	4		0	0	1	3	2	2	1	0
Fiji	210	180	163	185	165	230	199	173	162	218	226	247	240	183	280	203	200	171	166	192	144	183	150	179
French Polynesia	76	66	65	78	80	78	85	80	63	73	59	49	83	78	89		86	91	105	93	62	62	64	50
Guam	55	41	49	48	54	37	49	34	41	75			60	70	94						54	63	51	22
Japan	70 916	65 867	63 940	62 021	61 521	58 567	56 690	56 496	54 357	53 112	51 821	50 612	48 956	48 461	44 425	43 078	42 122	42 190	44 016	40 800	39 384	35 489	32 828	31 638
Kiribati	146	187	193	127	111	103	129	110	208	121	68	91	100	99	253		327	464	276	255	252	189	196	284
Lao PDR	7 630		4 706	4 700	6 528	4 258	1 514	3 468	7 279	2 952	1 826	1 951	994	2 093	1 135	830	1 440	1 923	2 153	2 434	2 234	2 418	2 621	2 780
Malaysia	11 218	10 970	11 944	11 634	10 577	10 569	10 735	11 068	10 944	10 686	11 702	11 059	11 420	12 285	11 708	11 778	12 691	13 539	14 115	14 908	15 057	14 830	14 389	15 671
Marshall Islands	6	7	12	15	12	15	37	32	11	7	68	26	52	61	173	172	59	107	49	41	34	56	51	60
Micronesia	0		67	73	75	66	60	98	77	68	367	350	111	151			126	107	123		91	104	127	99
Mongolia	1 161	1 094	1 340	1 512	1 651	2 992	2 818	2 432	2 541	2 237	1 577	1 611	1 502	1 433	1 730	2 780	3 457	2 987	2 915	3 348	3 109	3 526	3 829	3 918
Nauru	0	2	8	0	0	0	8	6	8	0	7	1			4			0		2	4	3	5	3
New Caledonia	108	128	120	171	144	104	98	74	111	128	143	140	140	104	97	87	104	88	90	78	94	61	65	36
New Zealand	474	448	437	415	404	359	320	296	295	303	348	335	317	274	352	391	352	321	365	447	344	377	329	386
Niue	1	0	2	3	1	0	5		3	0	0		2	1	2	0	2	0		1	0	0	4	0
Northern Mariana Is	17	26	75	74	58	64	16	56	27	28	28		67		46	48	51	93	97	66	75	58	53	45
Palau	17	10	17	14	20	26	13	38	17	3		6	4	25	41	19	5	15		32			11	9
Papua New Guinea	2 525	2 508	2 742	2 955	3 505	3 453	2 877	2 251	4 261	3 396	2 497	3 401	2 540	7 451	5 335	8 041	5 097	7 977	11 291	13 067	12 121	15 897	5 324	18 405
Philippines	112 307	116 821	104 715	106 300	151 863	151 028	153 129	163 740	183 113	217 272	317 008	207 371	236 172	178 134	180 044	119 186	165 453	195 767	162 360	145 807	119 914	107 133	118 408	134 375
Rep. Korea	89 803	98 532	100 878	91 572	85 669	87 169	88 789	87 419	74 460	70 012	63 904	57 864	48 070	46 999	38 155	42 117	39 315	33 215	34 661	32 075	21 782	37 268	34 967	33 888
Samoa	59	49	43	41	37	43	65	29	29	37	44	44	26	49	45	45	31	32	22	31	43	22	31	27
Singapore	2 710	2 425	2 179	2 065	2 143	1 952	1 760	1 616	1 666	1 617	1 591	1 841	1 778	1 830	1 677	1 889	1 951	1 977	2 120	1 805	1 728	1 536	1 516	1 616
Solomon Islands	266	313	324	302	337	377	292	334	372	488	382	309	364	367	332	352	299	318	295	289	302	292	256	293
Tokelau	0	1	0	0	0	2	0	9		0	1	1	1		0	2				0		0		0
Tonga	64	49	45	50	54	49	35	24	14	36	23	20	29	33	23	20	22	21	30	22	24	12	29	16
Tuvalu	33	18	12	23	9	32	27	22	24	26	23	30	30	28	19	36			18	14	16	16	13	30
Vanuatu	178	92	173	196	188	124	131	90	118	144	140	230	193	114	152	79	126	184	178	120	152	175	101	104
Viet Nam	43 062	43 506	51 206	43 185	43 875	46 941	47 557	55 505	52 463	52 270	50 203	59 784	56 594	52 994	51 763	55 739	74 711	77 838	87 468	88 879	89 792	90 728	95 044	92 741
Wallis & Futuna Is	23	24	5	17	14	14		34	1	30		22	4	11	11	6	8	14					19	15
Region																								
number reporting	356 482	355 345	461 572	462 193	541 001	615 179	651 853	655 019	716 450	741 916	893 992	760 870	754 466	718 799	724 345	818 740	874 721	870 313	834 604	822 454	789 457	808 817	805 578	987 927
percent reporting	36	33	36	36	36	36	36	36	36	35	33	31	35	33	33	28	31	31	31	33	35	35	35	36
	100	92	100	100	100	100	100	100	100	97	92	86	97	92	92	78	86	86	86	92	97	97	97	100

Country data for the Western Pacific: case notification rates (per 100 000 population), 1980–2003

	1980	1981	1982	1983	1984	1985	1986	1987	1988	1989	1990	1991	1992	1993	1994	1995	1996	1997	1998	1999	2000	2001	2002	2003
American Samoa	6	18	17	22	32	13	20	21	29	11	19	6	2	8	8	6	0	11	5	7	5	5	3	5
Australia	10	9	8	8	8	7	6	6	6	6	6	6	6	6	6	6		6	5	6	5	5	5	5
Brunei Darussalam	102	143	120	131	118	107	92	80	52	51	56		66	57				51		83	92	63	66	58
Cambodia	39	29	116	103	132	125	122	104	118	84	67	108	155	123	136	127	126	129	136	150	144	142	178	199
China			10	11	14	21	24	23	27	27	33	29	27	29	30	42	41	38	36	36	36	37	36	47
China, Hong Kong SAR	160	150	144	137	145	138	135	131	125	119	114	109	112	110	104	0	103	110	117	112	111	105	89	80
China, Macao SAR	437	226	87	163	229	186	131	117	92	76	92	86	75	72		98	136	134	107		100	102	84	80
Cook Islands	207	56	108	165	114	204	96	90	111	6	5	43	64	32	21		0	0	5	16	11	11	5	0
Fiji	33	28	24	27	24	32	28	24	23	30	31	34	33	24	37	26	26	22	21	24	18	22	18	21
French Polynesia	50	42	41	47	47	45	48	44	34	38	30	25	41	38	42		39	41	46	41	27	26	27	20
Guam	52	38	44	42	46	31	40	27	32	57			43	50	66						35	40	32	14
Japan	61	56	54	52	51	48	47	46	44	43	42	41	39	39	36	34	33	33	35	32	31	28	26	25
Kiribati	252	317	321	207	177	161	197	164	303	172	95	125	135	131	330		414	578	339	308	300	222	227	324
Lao PDR	238	78	141	137	185	118	41	91	186	73	44	46	23	47	25	18	30	39	43	47	42	45	47	49
Malaysia	82	82	82	78	69	67	67	67	65	61	66	60	61	64	59	58	61	63	64	66	65	63	60	64
Marshall Islands	20	22	36	43	33	40	94	79	26	16		57	113	131			122		98	81	67	108	97	113
Micronesia			86	90	90	77	68	109	84	72	381	354	110	146	164	161	117	99	115		85	97	117	91
Mongolia	70	64	76	84	89	157	143	120	121	103	7	71	65	61	73	116	143	123	119	135	124	139	150	151
Nauru	0	26	104	0	0	0	96	70	90	0	74			38				17			33	24	39	23
New Caledonia	76	88	81	114	94	67	62	46	68	76	84	80	78	57	51	45	53	44	44	37	44	28	29	16
New Zealand	15	14	14	13	13	11	10	9	9	9	10	10	9	8	10	11	10	9	10	12	9	10	9	10
Niue	29	0	64	101	35	0	192	0	123	0	0		90	46	92	0	95	0		49	0	0	203	0
Northern Mariana Is		140	370	331	233	232	52	164	72	69	64		137		87	87	88	153	152	99	107	79	70	57
Palau	140	81	135	108	151	191	93	266	117	20		39	25	153	245	111	28	83		170			55	44
Papua New Guinea	78	76	81	85	98	94	77	59	109	85	61	81	59	167	117	171	106	161	222	251	227	291	95	322
Philippines	234	237	207	205	287	278	276	288	314	364	519	332	369	272	269	174	237	274	223	196	158	139	151	168
Rep. Korea	236	255	257	230	212	214	215	210	177	165	149	134	110	106	86	94	87	72	75	69	47	79	74	71
Samoa	38	32	28	26	24	27	41	18	18	23	27	27	16	30	27	27	19	19	13	18	25	13	18	15
Singapore	112	98	86	80	81	72	64	57	58	55	53	59	56	56	50	54	54	53	56	46	43	37	36	38
Solomon Islands	116	132	132	119	128	139	104	115	124	158	120	94	107	105	92	94	77	80	72	68	69	65	55	61
Tokelau	0	64	0	0	0	121	0	546	61	0		63	64		0	131	0		30	0	0	0		
Tonga	66	50	46	51	56	50	36	25	14	36	23	20	29	33	23	20	22	21		22	24	12	28	15
Tuvalu	441	235	154	291	112	393	327	262	281	299	260	334	329	303	202	378			181	136	157	155	124	283
Vanuatu	152	77	141	156	146	94	97	65	83	99	94	150	122	70	91	46	71	101	95	63	77	87	49	49
Viet Nam	81	80	93	76	76	79	79	90	83	81	76	89	82	75	72	77	101	104	115	115	115	115	118	114
Wallis & Futuna Is	208	209	42	139	112	109		256	7	220		159	29	79	78	43	57	98					130	102
Region	**27**	**27**	**34**	**34**	**39**	**44**	**46**	**45**	**49**	**50**	**59**	**49**	**48**	**46**	**45**	**51**	**54**	**53**	**50**	**49**	**47**	**47**	**47**	**57**

WPR

Country data for the Western Pacific: new smear-positive cases, 1993–2003

	Number of cases											Rate (per 100 000 population)										
	1993	1994	1995	1996	1997	1998	1999	2000	2001	2002	2003	1993	1994	1995	1996	1997	1998	1999	2000	2001	2002	2003
American Samoa	1							2	2	1	2	2	8		0				3	3	2	3
Australia	557			0	226	203	285	251	228	210	113	3	4		0	1	1	5	2	1	1	1
Brunei Darussalam	68				0		102	84	95	112	121	24				0		31	25	28	32	34
Cambodia		11 058	11 101	12 065	12 686	13 865	15 744	14 822	14 361	17 258	18 923		99	97	102	104	111	123	113	107	125	134
China	84 898	104 729	134 488	203 670	236 021	202 817	201 775	204 765	204 591	194 972	267 414	7	9	11	17	19	16	16	16	16	15	21
China, Hong Kong SAR	2 429		1 677	1 774	1 943	2 091	2 020	1 940	1 857	1 890	1 779	41		27	28	30	32	30	28	27	27	25
China, Macao SAR	108		141	258	325	276		160	157	147	138	27		34	61	76	63		36	34	32	30
Cook Islands	4	1					1		2			21	5				5			11	5	0
Fiji	58	60	68	69	66	74	65	62	73	75	70	8	8	9	9	8	9	8	8	9	9	8
French Polynesia		38		37	41	34	33	29		28	21		18		17	18	15	14	12		12	9
Guam		40						43	47	31	21		28						28	30	19	
Japan	17 890	16 770	14 367	12 867	13 571	11 935	12 909	11 853	11 408	10 807	10 843	14	13	11	10	11	9	10	9	9	8	8
Kiribati	99	184		144	50	52	59	54	64	82	99	131	240		182	62	64	71	64	75	95	113
Lao PDR			478	886	1 234	1 494	1 719	1 526	1 563	1 829	1 882			10	18	25	30	33	29	29	33	33
Malaysia	6 954	6 861	6 688	7 271	7 496	7 802	8 207	8 156	8 309	7 958	7 989	36	35	33	35	35	36	36	35	35	33	33
Marshall Islands	12		15	12	14	11	17	11	15	18	20	26			25		22		22	29	34	38
Micronesia			9	14	9	14		15	8	22	27			8	13	8	13		14	7	20	25
Mongolia	86	145	455	769	1 171	1 356	1 513	1 389	1 631	1 670	1 541	4	6	19	32	48	55	61	56	65	65	59
Nauru		2					2	4	2	2	1											
New Caledonia	16	28	21	26	24	26	22	20	19	21	14	9	15	11	13	12	13	10	9	9	9	6
New Zealand	91	61	78	90	83	106	94	74	68	88	106	3	2	2	2	2	3	3	2	2	2	3
Niue	0	0	0	1	0	0	1	0	0	1	0	0	0	0	47	0	0	49	0	0	51	0
Northern Mariana Is			14	26	21	26	15	27	19	21	16			25	45	34	41	22	39	26	28	20
Palau	8	11	9	4	7		20			9	5	49	66	52	23	39		106	39		45	24
Papua New Guinea			1 652	652	1 195	2 107	1 914	2 267	1 122	926	3 231			35	14	24	41	37	43	21	17	57
Philippines	92 279	87 401	94 768	86 695	80 163	69 476	73 373	67 056	59 341	65 148	72 670	141	131	139	124	112	95	99	89	77	83	91
Rep. Korea	16 630	13 266	11 754	11 420	9 957	10 359	9 559	8 216	11 805	11 345	10 976	38	30	26	25	22	22	21	18	25	24	23
Samoa	21	18	15	9	14	7	17	13	11	19	12	13	11	9	5	8	4	10	8	6	11	7
Singapore	513	861	455	519	436	482	465	248	357	549	586	16	26	13	14	12	13	12	6	9	13	14
Solomon Islands	155	114	109	90	113	140	93	109	118	108	138	44	31	29	23	28	34	22	25	26	23	29
Tokelau		0	1	0	0		0	0	0		0		0	66	0	0		0	0	0		0
Tonga	16	17	9	14	11	16	10	15	8	23	11	16	17	9	14	11	16	10	15	8	22	11
Tuvalu	2	1	6					0	0	0	0	22	11	63				0	0	0	0	0
Vanuatu		62	30	50	66	38	43	63	57	38	40		37	17	28	36	20	22	32	28	18	19
Viet Nam			37 550	48 911	50 016	54 889	53 805	53 169	54 238	56 811	55 937			52	66	67	72	70	68	68	71	69
Wallis & Futuna Is			3	3	1				1	7	7			21	21	7					7	48
Region	**222 895**	**241 732**	**315 946**	**388 346**	**416 952**	**379 699**	**383 884**	**376 443**	**371 577**	**372 221**	**454 732**	**14**	**15**	**20**	**24**	**25**	**23**	**23**	**22**	**22**	**22**	**26**

Notes

Brunei Darussalam
Treatment outcomes are for laboratory-confirmed cases, and for nationals only. Non-nationals are deported to their country of origin after two weeks of treatment or conversion to smear-negative status.

Cambodia
The latest estimate of the incidence of TB does not take into account the results from a recent disease prevalence survey.

China
The NTP notes that age and sex data are incomplete. Relapse notifications include both smear-positive cases and smear-negative/-unknown cases.

China, Hong Kong SAR
Patients' outcomes are assessed at 12 months after diagnosis.

Guam
Of 9 smear-negative, culture-negative cases, and 3 cases with smear and culture not done, all 12 completed treatment.

Malaysia
Age and sex data are for all new cases.

Palau
DOTS coverage was not reported, but assumed to be same as in the previous report.

Singapore
All data refer to TB cases notified among resident population.

Tokelau
DOTS coverage was not reported, but assumed to be same as in the previous report.